ID0996757

PANDEMIC DIARIES

MATT HANCOCK

PANDEMIC DIARIES

THE INSIDE STORY OF BRITAIN'S BATTLE AGAINST COVID
WITH ISABEL OAKESHOTT

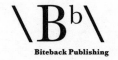

Biteback Publishing

First published in Great Britain in 2022 by
Biteback Publishing Ltd, London
Copyright © Matt Hancock and Isabel Oakeshott 2022

ISBN 978-1-78590-774-6

10 9 8 7 6 5 4 3 2

A CIP catalogue record for this book is available from the British Library.

Set in Minion Pro and Proxima Novo

Printed and bound in Great Britain by
CPI Group (UK) Ltd, Croydon CR0 4YY

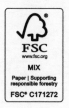

FSC
www.fsc.org
MIX
Paper | Supporting
responsible forestry
FSC® C171272

This book is dedicated to all those who worked so hard to save lives and help our country get through the Covid-19 pandemic, and to my wonderful children, who sustain me.

CONTENTS

PROLOGUE

In human history, there has never been anything like the speed and intensity of the pandemic which swept the world in 2020. Governments did their best, but most struggled to respond to the remorseless virus and our fast-changing understanding of how it should be fought. The cost in lives, livelihoods and lost health and opportunities was incalculable.

I was in the hot-seat. From the first warning signs in Wuhan through to the massive national response, I was at the centre of events. It was the most important thing I have done in my life and I gave it my all. I am proud of what we achieved, especially on the vaccine, but there is much to learn for the next public health crisis of this kind, which I am sure will happen in my lifetime. That's why I have written this book: to tell the story of what actually happened, as I experienced it. What follows is the first and most detailed account of the pandemic from inside government. Written as a diary, sometimes hour by hour but mostly day by day, it charts the key events and how I felt about them at the time.

Of course, I didn't have time to keep a detailed diary in the midst of the maelstrom, nor would it have been right to do so. For the best part of eighteen months, I spent almost every waking hour managing our response, alongside the many amazing healthcare professionals, carers, public servants and other key workers who did so much to save lives and keep the country going.

My typical day started at 6 a.m., checking overnight messages and the news. Typically I would be responsible for over half of the stories on the BBC each morning when I woke. I would see my family for half an hour over breakfast and leave for the department at around 7.30 a.m. I would generally have twelve to fifteen meetings per day, mostly in my cavernous office on the ninth floor of the Department of Health on Victoria Street, overlooking Parliament and half of London, or in the Cabinet Room in 10 Downing Street. My diary would be constantly moving. On particularly busy days my private office, which operated on a shift system to keep up with the workload, would schedule me five-minute breaks to go to the loo. Every day, I would respond to literally hundreds of emails and messages and dozens of phone calls. At night I would typically read and comment on around twenty extensive papers in my red box. All this was in addition to the press conferences, parliamentary statements, social media posts and videos and TV and radio interviews, of which I naturally did more than any other member of the government. I always tried to get to bed by midnight, because I always needed to be functioning the next day.

I say none of this for sympathy and deserve none. I chose to accept the role of Health Secretary and a pandemic is an occupational hazard, as war is to a soldier. To serve in this way was an honour. All I can say is that I did everything I could.

The account that follows has been meticulously pieced together from my formal papers held by the department; contemporaneous notes and voice memos; my communications with ministerial colleagues; interviews with many of the participants and myriad other emails and messages that record what happened and why particular decisions were taken. Anything directly quoted is from a recorded source. It is not a memoir – though I have included a chapter of reflections with hindsight as an epilogue.

I have not been exhaustive. To do so would make the book unreadable. The task of a comprehensive assessment rightly falls to the public inquiry, which I enthusiastically welcome, and to which I have made available all my materials. Instead I have tried to focus on events in which I was directly involved. I have included some of the lighter moments to try to give a sense of what it was really like. Amid the enormous hard work and heavy sense of responsibility, there were of course chinks of light, though I was always mindful of the very serious situation and the fact that many families tragically lost loved ones – including my own.

I have tried to be fair to those with whom I worked. So many people worked so hard in the national interest. I was supported by an amazing team of ministers, advisers of all kinds and an extremely talented civil service and wider team. I have included the names of the most senior figures and those with whom I worked most closely. I am incredibly grateful to them all.

I was supported throughout the worst times by my family and by Martha, none of whom I saw enough of, and I am grateful for their support. In writing this book I have also had the help of another incredible team: my researcher, Asher Glynn, who pulled together a vast quantity of material and turned it into a coherent mass; Jack Grimston, who put it into rough diary form and interviewed me to improve my recall of events; my fiercely loyal and effective communications adviser, James Davies; the diligent Josh Dolder; and above all Isabel Oakeshott, whose tenacity at getting me to remember the most telling detail and gift in improving my drafting to create a compelling account are second to none. Without all these people the book would not have been possible. I am also enormously grateful to Elizabeth Hitchcock, Bobby Bennett, Harry Pearce Gould and Chloe Osborne in my constituency team for helping me do my job as MP, and to Rachel Hood and the West Suffolk team for their support throughout it all.

Throughout the project, Gina's love and advice in helping me articulate how I felt about what happened – as she did throughout the pandemic – were invaluable. Most of all I am grateful for the love of my children, who have given me plenty of advice about this book, and to whom it is dedicated.

JANUARY 2020

I woke up in Suffolk after a quiet New Year's Eve. Last time I pulled an all-nighter was a couple of weeks ago after the general election. As I was waiting for my result in my constituency in Newmarket, Conservative HQ called asking me to go to a victory rally in Westminster at 6 a.m. High on adrenaline, I hammered down the motorway to London, rolled into the QEII Centre and found myself standing in a massive placard-laden crowd next to an exuberant Boris, who was waxing lyrical about delivering on our manifesto commitments to the NHS. Turning to me, he declared that I would make sure that we honoured our election promises on the NHS. I knew my job was safe.

As I then made my way out of the room, I saw my three brilliant special advisers – Jamie Njoku-Goodwin, Emma Dean and Allan Nixon – somewhat the worse for wear from the election night party. Looking at the state of them – Jamie still in his shades – it must have been quite a celebration.

At 7 a.m., we trooped bleary-eyed back to my office on the ninth floor of the Department of Health and Social Care (DHSC), only to discover that it had been completely emptied of my personal effects. My bookshelves, normally packed with biographies, policy tomes and the various Acts of Parliament I've proudly steered onto the statute book, had been stripped bare. My stuff was all in boxes. They had clearly been preparing for a changing of the guard: British politics is brutal. We cheerfully put it all back in place and got to work.

So a new political year begins, with an eighty-seat majority. Politically, things look good. Five years in office and a civil service team super-responsive to the clear mandate – something they have been missing for some time. Boris says he's going to 'get Brexit done', and he means it.

As for me? I'm in reasonable shape. I could be fitter, but it's not terminal decline. Plus, I love my job and am fired up about delivering our manifesto promises and seizing on the massive improvements to healthcare that are just around the corner: in cancer, dementia and preventative healthcare we are on the cusp of a revolution every bit as big as the digital revolution in every other part of life.

As much as I'm savouring the idea that we might just have achieved a two-term victory, the past five years have been a long and painful lesson in just how unpredictable this business is. Standing in my kitchen in Suffolk, I scanned my New Year's Day copy of *The Times* for clues as to what might be lurking around the corner. The only thing on my patch was a news-in-brief story about a mystery pneumonia outbreak in China. There were enough people in hospital for Beijing to have put out an alert. It reminded me a bit of SARS (severe acute respiratory syndrome) back in 2003, which killed hundreds of people, mainly in China and Hong Kong. I asked private office to put together a briefing and made a mental note to raise it when I got back.

THURSDAY 2 JANUARY

I have two or three mega things to sort this year; a series of other worthwhile challenges (e.g. cutting the eyewatering cost of clinical negligence); and endless minor irritations. In the mega category are the forty new hospitals and 50,000 more nurses we promised during the election campaign. I backed these pledges and truly believe they're achievable, but they just won't happen unless I apply relentless pressure to all the parts of the machine that need to crank into action.

Likewise, the NHS is crying out for a more modern, tech-enabled approach. It's the only way to make it sustainable in the long term, and if like me you really believe in the NHS, you've got to reform it to bring it into the modern age.

Among multiple items in the minor irritation category is a somewhat random proposal that's come up to ban menthol cigarettes. 'Remind me why we're doing that?' I asked my team. Cue blank faces all round. The only reason anyone could come up with is that Brussels told us to. So we are bringing in an EU law after we leave the EU with no justification except that it's an EU law?

Bonkers.

FRIDAY 3 JANUARY

Every Health Secretary spends winter worrying. Last autumn I took a deep dive into why we always seem to have a crisis. There's a general assumption that it comes down to extra demand. I've done the analysis and found that this is only half true. In fact, the busiest month for patients turning up at A&E is not actually winter at all; it's July. But staffing doesn't get matched to demand. Add to that the entirely preventable action that should keep people out of hospital but doesn't happen. Both of these are entirely fixable and I intend to sort them.

Another thing that would make a huge difference is if all frontline staff were vaccinated for flu. I've long thought it should be mandatory. A bad flu season is the difference between just about coping and complete meltdown for the NHS. Surely if you give your life to caring for people, protecting them from disease is a must?

Perhaps surprisingly – given his strong libertarian leanings – Boris agrees. When I raised it with him straight after the election, his response was: 'Just get on with it.' Unfortunately, the doctors' and nurses' trade unions – the British Medical Association (BMA) and the Royal College of Nursing (RCN) – are dead against the idea, so it's not easy.

Sky News called this evening, wanting me to do a short clip tomorrow morning about embracing technology in the NHS. Sadly they don't have a truck with a camera within reach of our farmhouse in

3

Suffolk, so it was a non-starter. I've learned the hard way that when I'm giving interviews here, Skype is not an option – especially not when talking about technology. Last time I tried, I was mid-flow, waxing lyrical about digital transformation, when the connection died. Not the best look for a champion of innovation.

SUNDAY 5 JANUARY

More in the papers on the new disease in China. There are now fifty-nine cases; seven of these patients are seriously ill with breathing problems. The WHO (World Health Organization) has got involved via its east Asia head office in Manila.

There are jitters in Hong Kong and Singapore, including a suspected case in a three-year-old Chinese girl who'd recently been to a city called Wuhan. Almost nobody here has heard of it, but it's vast: almost 10 million people, about 700 miles south of Beijing; the capital of Hubei province. Looking at it on the map reminded me of one of my first trips to China. It was back in 2007 and I was accompanying David Cameron soon after he became Tory Party leader. He went to another of these vast unknown cities – Chongqing – to give a speech. I remember our Foreign Office man there complaining bitterly that he hadn't seen the sun for six months because the smog was so bad. The Chinese, of course, have no way to describe the Leader of the Opposition. Literally lost for words, they strung up a huge banner saying, 'Chongqing University welcomes David Cameron: Next Prime Minister of United Kingdom'. Obviously David was delighted, but it hammered home the absurdity of autocratic regimes. They simply had no concept of official political opposition.

Re. the virus, I asked my private office for a full briefing tomorrow morning. I don't like it when the best information I'm getting is from the newspapers.

MONDAY 6 JANUARY

First day back in the office. There's a tangible sense of optimism. Big focus on delivering our manifesto commitments and living up to the faith people put in us, many for the first time.

I had a meeting with our new CMO (chief medical officer), Professor Chris Whitty, and his team to talk about mandatory flu jabs. He gave the cases for and against. Doctors are already obliged to be vaccinated against hepatitis, but that's a one-off. This would be a major expansion. Chris sees both sides of the argument, but senior NHS figures have put it in the 'too-difficult' box because of trade union opposition. I think that's an abdication of leadership. It would save thousands of lives.

While I had so many experts in the room, I took the chance to ask what we know about the new disease in China. Chris and his team told me they're across it, though there's not much to go on. They're trying to get whatever information they can out of the Chinese and the WHO. There's a suggestion of a link with a so-called wet market – one of those medieval-style places with caged live animals which are slaughtered right in front of you. This one is said to sell pangolins and various other exotic wildlife. Apparently many of the patients are connected to the market in some way. I've seen these places in Vietnam and they are repulsive – shutting them seems a good idea whether or not there's any link with the disease.

We talked about the chances of the virus coming here. Nobody knows, but Chris's view is that we need to be vigilant. I asked to see the emergency plans that were put together after a Whitehall pandemic preparation exercise a few years ago under my predecessor Jeremy Hunt, known as Exercise Cygnus. I also asked about the likely need for a vaccine. It's too early to know whether the vaccines we have stockpiled will work against this, I was told, but creating a new one normally takes many years.

TUESDAY 7 JANUARY

I asked Chris Whitty to pop up and see me again about the new disease. We found out overnight it's not a flu but a novel coronavirus. This is not good news. We've millions of stockpiled flu vaccines – I signed off updating the supply last year – but nobody has ever invented a vaccine against a coronavirus.

I appointed Chris as chief medical officer last year after Dame Sally Davies retired. He'd been the chief scientist in the department for several years and had a hugely respected and broad career; very varied and mostly international. I'd first come across him when he played a key role in stopping the spread of Ebola as it threatened to escape from west Africa in 2015. His careful, diligent approach and fierce intelligence made him the obvious choice. Inside the department there are lots of Chrises, so he is known formally as CMO and informally as the Prof.

He told me that Singapore and Hong Kong have started screening all arrivals from Wuhan for symptoms – mainly fever and coughing. Breathing problems seem to come later. There's no evidence yet of human-to-human transmission, which is the critical tell-tale sign of a potential pandemic, but it's too early to tell.

At 7 p.m. we had the first vote of the year in the Commons. I found the PM in the voting lobby looking like he'd had a good Christmas and revelling in all the congratulatory back slaps from colleagues. We walked through the lobby together, and I told him about the new disease.

'You keep an eye on it,' he said breezily. 'It will probably go away like all the others.'

Hmm. I can see why he thinks so: SARS and MERS were big false alarms for the UK. We are both optimists – and I hope he is right – but it's my job to keep a watching brief.

In more trivial news, a picture of my Union Jack socks has somehow gone viral after I was pictured on my way into Cabinet yesterday. My old university friend and communications specialist Gina Coladangelo was not particularly impressed and messaged saying I shouldn't wear them too often. I thought I was being patriotic, but she thinks they're a bit UKIP.

THURSDAY 9 JANUARY
A bad start to the day: getting a kicking over GP numbers on Radio 4's *Today* programme and not being able to kick back. Ministers are

banned from going on the show by No. 10, so our defence was limited to a lame official statement tagged onto the end of what was a long and emotive report. Dominic Cummings, Boris's chief adviser, sees the *Today* programme as an anti-Tory resistance bunker packed with Islington Remoaners and doesn't think we should dignify it with our presence. I think that is very pig-headed. It's a major national media outlet with 6 million listeners. We are cutting off our noses to spite our faces.

Later I got my first written briefing about the virus from the department. They still don't know a lot, but it looks like our carefully laid plans for a flu pandemic aren't going to be much use. This virus appears to have a much longer incubation period, though I am reassuringly told that the six known coronaviruses aren't transmitted by people without symptoms. Encouragingly, it doesn't appear to affect children. However, there is a possibility that domestic animals may be what scientists call a 'reservoir' of the disease. Apparently felines are a particular worry. Here's hoping that particular concern proves unsubstantiated. The Great British public put up with mass culling of cows, pigs and sheep during BSE and foot-and-mouth disease, but God help any politician who comes for their pet cats.

The body responsible for tracking and protecting us from pandemics, Public Health England (PHE), wants to publish some generic infection control advice tomorrow. It's a rehash of existing advice, so no big deal. Since they're the experts, I say fine. The more information out there the better.

What is a big deal is that PHE is now categorising the virus as a 'high-consequence infectious disease'. It means that anyone treating patients who might have it will need to wear hazmat suits. Luckily we stockpiled huge amounts for a potential flu pandemic. Meanwhile work is under way within PHE to develop a test for the virus. They can do this once the Chinese publish the genome, which could be any day. It's amazing that we can develop a test for a microscopic organism so quickly.

FRIDAY 10 JANUARY

I went up to Doncaster to visit the Royal Infirmary. The building is knackered. I dropped heavy hints that it could become one of our promised forty new hospitals. I told the local paper that the new MP, Nick Fletcher, has been on my case non-stop about it, which is true. A Tory MP in Doncaster? I still find it hard to believe. If we're going to keep the red wall painted blue, decent hospitals are essential, but they will not materialise unless Rishi Sunak, the Chief Secretary to the Treasury, is onside.

SATURDAY 11 JANUARY

First death from the virus in China – at least, the first one they've told us about.

The victim died two days ago and was a regular customer at the wet market. He's said to have had various pre-existing health conditions. We still have no idea how infectious or serious this thing is. The hope is that it might just fade away like SARS.

More positively, the Chinese have published the genetic code. It turns out they actually completed the work two days before sharing the results, which is annoying, but at least the ball's now rolling and they're being surprisingly open. We can get going on tests and even start the process of developing a vaccine. Normally, the Chinese make a lot of noise about wanting to work together and having 'high-level dialogue' etc. while giving nothing away.

Sir Keir Starmer, who looks like the frontrunner in the Labour leadership contest, has launched his campaign in Manchester. The hard left seem to think he might be the new Tony Blair. Not likely: he may be clever, but he seems a bit dreary. Anyway, anyone's better than Jeremy Corbyn.

SUNDAY 12 JANUARY

The WHO has published its first analysis of the disease. Initial data shows that it has a lower mortality rate than SARS but is much more infectious. Counter-intuitively, that means if it spreads, the total number of deaths will be higher – a lower mortality multiplied by a very large number of cases. I've got a bad feeling about this. Other than it apparently not affecting children, each new fact we discover is bad. The advice from my scientists is excellent, but I'm not getting much of a response from the rest of the system.

If it's a 'low mortality but high infectiousness' disease, it's going to be difficult to explain to people. Discussing risk is one of the hardest things to do in politics. Get one word or phrase wrong, and the consequences can be dire: either increasing the very risk you're trying to avoid or changing people's behaviour in some way that is not helpful. Tricky.

I took a call from Gordon Sanghera, chief executive of Oxford Nanopore, which designs tests based on genetic sequencing. He reckons they can come up with something in a matter of days. I've seen their DNA testing devices – they're amazing – so I believe him. If this could be infectious enough to spread worldwide, we'll need all the technology we can get.

MONDAY 13 JANUARY

NERVTAG (the New and Emerging Respiratory Virus Threats Advisory Group) held a teleconference on the virus this morning. It's a high-powered group of scientists specialising in novel respiratory illnesses, chaired by Peter Horby, the Oxford specialist. Professor Neil Ferguson, of Imperial College, London, is a member. Jonathan Van-Tam, one of Chris Whitty's three deputies, attends as an observer.

I wanted to know whether we need to start screening people at airports. Definitely not, according to NERVTAG. They think screening at airports will only slow the virus getting to the UK down a bit. Knowing his love of flying, Grant Shapps, the Transport Secretary, would go ballistic if we even suggested it. What would make a massive difference is if the Chinese stopped people leaving Wuhan. I'm struggling to see how they justify letting people flood out of the city when they know there's such a big potential problem.

One thing that is reassuring the scientists is that there has never been a coronavirus known to transmit without symptoms. But there's always a first time and if this advice is wrong, and there's a chance the disease is being transmitted asymptomatically, it will probably have spread quite widely outside Wuhan already.

My attitude is it's vital we base our decisions on science, not my hunches. I'm lucky to be surrounded by some of the best scientists in the world. Then again, it's also my job to challenge the experts from a lay perspective. I asked Sir Chris Wormald, my Permanent Secretary at the DHSC, to come into my office this morning with the top team to think through how we should handle what is clearly going to be a very science-driven response with wider issues to consider. He advised me to think about it this way: 'We should be *guided* by the science.' That doesn't mean blindly following it; it means taking the science as the starting point.

All this goes to the core of decision making. As a minister, you constantly have to take decisions. Civil servants typically give you options, whether in a paper or in a meeting, usually highlighting their preferred choice. Special advisers give you a rounded view on the advice, taking in the political and wider considerations. Sometimes what's recommended is the best course of action, but not always. The best decisions often come when the team argues it out in front of you. I hate it when they stitch it up in advance, agree a preferred approach and present it as a single, unanimous recommendation. Sometimes you find out afterwards that there was a huge row about how to present a unified front when you actually wanted to see the argument. Civil servants are generally very bright, committed people but too often hate any confrontation in front of the minister. I want to know what they really think.

We agreed that PHE should put out more guidance saying the risk to people in the UK is still 'very low' and advising anyone visiting Wuhan to wash their hands and 'minimise contact' with live birds and animals in markets there. (You'd think people would wash their hands anyway if they go round touching live bats at market stalls...) We've also been poring over contingency plans in case this gets really bad. Officials earnestly inform me that every local authority and every NHS organisation in the country has a pandemic preparedness plan 'on the shelf' ready and waiting. The question is whether these documents are worth the paper they're written on. I've asked to see a random selection.

The good news is we've got a billion items of disposable personal protective equipment (PPE) stockpiled and ready to dispatch to hospitals if required. It's stashed away at a secret location in the north-west, where it's been gathering dust – hopefully not literally – since it was put together in 2009.

At the moment the response is still very much within our remit in the Department of Health – hospital capacity, nursing numbers, any legislative changes we might need, testing and the very early work on a vaccine – but the rest of government will need to crank up in case this goes global. So far I am not getting much back – the system is preoccupied with delivering Brexit at the end of the month.

TUESDAY 14 JANUARY

Andrew Wakefield, the 'doctor' who got struck off for his outrageous scaremongering over the MMR jab, has reared his ugly head again. Just when we may need a vaccine for a deadly new disease, he's plugging some new film called *Vaxxed II: The People's Truth*. Apparently it's being marketed on secret Facebook groups. I cannot believe that he's still in circulation, spreading his misinformation. Or that he used to date the supermodel Elle Macpherson. How did that happen?

I don't want any of his latest nonsense getting any traction, so I issued a statement about the wonders of modern vaccines and the dangers of listening to misleading tripe.

Meanwhile PHE has come up with a diagnostic test. You've got to hand it to them: China only published the genetic code three days ago, and they've already figured out how to spot it in a drop of saliva. I had a spare hour this afternoon, so I popped into Chris Whitty's office to discuss the latest developments. I noticed that he has a Union Jack flying from his balcony, which I hadn't clocked before. The Prof is a committed internationalist who has spent most of his life in developing countries where he thinks he can do the greatest good to the greatest number. Clearly he's also a patriot.

We discussed what we know about the virus and he stressed the importance of the R number: the average number of secondary infections produced by a single infected person. This determines how fast the disease spreads. One of the joys of being a minister is getting the best advice the British government has to offer. It felt like a tutorial from a world expert, which, in a way, it was.

I was struck by the similarity of Chris's epidemiology to my economics experience at the Bank of England. Both are about the interaction of science and human behaviour. The statistical techniques are almost identical – all about the interaction of linear and exponential growth.

I asked about a vaccine. He says there are effectively two types: one that's 'pandemic-ending' and prevents people getting ill and passing on the virus; the other that's 'pandemic-modifying', meaning it helps prevent illness but doesn't stop the disease in its tracks. The experts seem to agree that with something spreading as fast as it is in China, it's best not to count on eradication.

Rosie Winterton, the Labour MP in Doncaster Central, is furious that I didn't tell her I was going up to her patch the other day. My bad. It's a rule with ministerial visits that you should tell the local MPs. Rosie got very huffy and demanded to speak to Chris Wormald, which would have been a complete waste of his time. Allan Nixon, whose job is to manage my links with MPs, generously offered to take the blame, but I decided to call her personally and grovel, and she couldn't have been more gracious.

WEDNESDAY 15 JANUARY
Parliamentary business carries on as normal. Today was the second reading of the NHS Funding Bill, which I'm piloting through the Commons. Under the circumstances, it feels like a sideshow. However, I can't scrap it or delegate it to someone else as it's a direct instruction from Dom Cummings, who essentially controls the No. 10 machine.

He is aggressively unpredictable. Last year he destroyed many careers as he drove Brexit through, so I pick my battles.

In essence, the Bill is a PR exercise designed to show voters that we're committed to funding the NHS properly, which we always have been anyway. I wanted to include in it the important, substantive reforms that I've been working on for over a year now, but Cummings said no. By conceding, I secured No. 10's commitment to a future Bill later in the parliament. The irony is, this Bill is so worthy and dull that nobody's noticed we're doing it, meaning it's not even working as a piece of spin.

Nobody in Westminster's talking about the coronavirus either, and Downing Street isn't keen on me making a statement to Parliament, as they want to keep the media focus on Brexit. A pandemic isn't part of their gameplan. Chinese New Year on 25 January could be critical. Millions of people will be moving around within China and flying in and out for the celebrations. If the authorities don't get their act together, the virus will go haywire.

FRIDAY 17 JANUARY

A second coronavirus death in Wuhan: a 69-year-old man. It happened two days ago, but we've only just been told. That openness I was talking about? Pretty fleeting. The Chinese are reverting to type.

The US has introduced health screening for arrivals from Wuhan at airports including San Francisco, New York and Los Angeles. I'm uncomfortable about how little we're doing here and raised it again with the PHE team, but the clinical advice is very clear that action at the border won't make any significant difference. The clear consensus, as articulated by the Prof, is that if it's coming, it's coming. So far, it's all about handing out leaflets to people coming off flights from Wuhan. Instinctively, my team and I feel this can't be enough, but whenever I push on it with officials, they are dismissive.

I was slightly surprised to find myself on the front of today's *Independent*. Apparently I've lost a court case over suspending NHS pension payments to staff convicted of crimes. This was literally the first I or anyone on my immediate team had heard of either the policy or the court case. The Department of Health is an enormous beast and legally all the work is done in my name. So if we're sued, technically it's the Secretary of State who is sued, whether or not he or she had anything to do with the decision. It's an antiquated quirk of the legal system and a gift to journalists. But the Department of Health is tiny compared to all the quangos. Over decades of piecemeal reform, a slew of quangos has grown up, all with different accountability. Cummings and I share an agenda to streamline the whole set-up and rescind the formal independence of NHS England, which I have never supported. After all, we're talking about £130 billion of taxpayers' money and millions of lives. Ultimately the Secretary of State – not an unelected appointee – should be responsible for the budget and performance. Privately, Cummings has made it clear he wants to go further and replace Sir Simon Stevens, chief executive of NHS England. A few days before the 2019 election he sent me an excitable text on the matter, saying we needed to 'talk serious turkey on the fundamentals'.

'2020 must be the year we make mega breakthroughs. We need to replace Stevens and change your powers!' he said. I told him I'd think about possible candidates but parked it. Simon is widely respected, was brilliant to us Conservatives during the election campaign and is set to go next year anyway. Any earlier departure needs to be handled with care.

Speaking of Stevens, on his recommendation, last night I watched *Contagion* in bed on my laptop. It's got an all-star line-up: Kate Winslet, Matt Damon, Jude Law, Gwyneth Paltrow and a load of other big names. It's a fast-moving thriller about a new virus in China that jumps from bats to humans, spreads round the world like wildfire and kills millions while scientists race to find a vaccine. Whole cities are put into quarantine and social order cracks. Simon told me it's based on excellent epidemiological research and the medics really rate it. The potential parallels are unsettling. In the movie, a vaccine is the only way out – though the real tensions only build after the jab is developed, as everyone starts fighting over who gets it.

When I woke up today I was briefly unable to distinguish fiction from reality. Were millions dying on my watch? Had the pandemic gone global? Thank God, no. Later at the department, the Prof asked for a word. He entered my office with some trepidation, accompanied only by Natasha Price, my principal private secretary, which is normally bad news. Calmly, in his ultra-reasonable way, he explained that he thinks the virus has a 50:50 chance of escaping China. If it gets out of China in a big way, he says it will 'go global'. Quite what this would mean, nobody knows, but even with the low risk to any one person, a very large number of people will die. Instantly, I thought of *Contagion* and of the role of a vaccine.

TUESDAY 21 JANUARY
On the way into the office I called the PM and told him about the 50:50 chance. He was very matter-of-fact. He says he knows it's bad news when I call him at seven in the morning.

There's now a case in Guangdong, almost 1,000 kilometres from where it all started, and the Chinese authorities are formally saying it can be transmitted from human to human. Lab tests have also confirmed the first case in the US: a 31-year-old man in Washington state who flew in from Wuhan on 15 January. He didn't have any symptoms when he arrived so wasn't picked up by airport screening. He went to the doctor when he felt ill a few days later. The early evidence is that it takes up to fourteen days from infection to first symptoms appearing. That is one hell of an incubation period. You can see why the scientists think airport screening is a waste of time.

In the US they also started researching vaccines straight after the virus genome was published. Anthony Fauci, director of the National Institute of Allergy and Infectious Diseases, who's heading the US government's response, says he reckons clinical trials are a few months away and that a vaccine could be approved some time next year. Our scientists are also already on it. Amid all the uncertainties, one thing's clear: if this thing is a killer, and it 'goes global', as the Prof put it, we will be in a terrifying, hurtling, global race for a vaccine – or a cure.

The speed and determination with which we enter that race, and keep running until it is won, will change the fate of millions of lives. I am determined the United Kingdom will play its part.

Tomorrow, we are going to raise the risk level from very low to low. PHE has also agreed to contact travellers who've come back from Wuhan in the past fourteen days to check they have had the latest public health advice – in other words, to go into isolation if they have any symptoms. I'm uneasy that we're not doing more at the borders, but the experts are still adamant it's not worth the cost – but at least we got some movement.

As for the Chinese, they're in a parallel universe. President Xi Jinping has made a great play of declaring that stopping the spread is a top priority – yet people are flooding in and out of Wuhan for Chinese New Year. Meanwhile local authorities held public banquets for 40,000 folk at the weekend. Seems completely mad.

I asked the Foreign Office whether we could exert a bit of diplomatic pressure to make them see sense. 'Don't even bother trying' was the gist of the response.

Cummings is beginning to up the pressure on removing Simon Stevens. He messaged me before 7 a.m. today asking where we're at. I am trying to find out how Simon himself really feels via a mutual friend, Lord Ara Darzi, since No. 10 seems so set on it.

WEDNESDAY 22 JANUARY

The Whitehall machine is slowly waking up to the fact that we might have a problem. The Scientific Advisory Group for Emergencies (SAGE), chaired by the Prof alongside Sir Patrick Vallance, the government's chief scientific adviser, has met to discuss the virus.

Patrick's background is both as an academic and with the pharmaceutical company GSK, so he has a lot of relevant experience on vaccines. He's brisk, business-like and very straightforward: my kind of scientist.

SAGE backs NERVTAG on screening at airports – or rather not screening at airports. They think there would be so many false positives and false negatives that the whole exercise would be meaningless. They say leaflets, posters and announcements over the tannoy are enough for now. Anyone who's been to Wuhan and feels ill within fourteen days should get tested. We're also putting plans in place to isolate anyone suspected of having the virus and to track down anyone they've been around so we can see how they're feeling. This sort of contact tracing happens all the time for rare outbreaks like legionnaires' disease. Public Health England tell me their contact tracing systems are the best in the world, or at least, top-rated by the World Health Organization.

While the PM is now quite engaged, the Downing Street machine dominated by Cummings is completely uninterested. At least this means he's not interfering. Our relationship is one of wary mutual respect. We've known each other for years, since my first governmental job as Skills Minister at Education, where he was Michael Gove's senior adviser. When he's in a good mood, he calls me 'Comrade', but that's as far as his banter goes.

Moreover, he can be extraordinarily high-handed.

Last summer he sent me a foul-mouthed rant accusing one of my SpAds of 'slagging off Boris'.

'Speak to him and tell him – shut your fucking mouth about Boris, if Dom hears one more whisper he will just fire you instantly and he doesn't make idle threats, OK?'

He claimed other people were telling him he should just fire my SpAd on the spot but that he wanted to give me a chance to sort it out.

'If you actually don't want him any more tell me and I'll bin him Monday. I've got zero time to spend on this sort of crap...' he ranted.

I think he grudgingly accepts me as politically useful and I share his reforming zeal, but I keep my distance. I've never forgotten the shameless untruth he told me the day before Boris prorogued Parliament to get Brexit through. Remainers were going nuts, saying it was undemocratic, a constitutional outrage etc. He and I had lunch together that day and he told me point-blank that they weren't going to do it. The following day, they went ahead. That level of deception from Cummings was shocking.

The Prof came into my office in between meetings to take me through SAGE's conclusions. The R number, which is critical, is currently above 1, meaning the disease is spreading exponentially.

There are three flights a week from Wuhan to the UK. Today PHE announced there would be health officials at airports asking people coming off these flights if they are feeling OK, handing out advice leaflets etc. I think this is far too little and I'm increasingly worried, but the expert advice is adamant. Anyway, it's already been overtaken by events. Beijing has finally swung into action and the entire city of Wuhan goes into quarantine from tomorrow morning. There will be no more transport in or out, including planes, trains and buses. Warning lights are also flashing further afield. Most cases are still in Wuhan, but there are others in Beijing, Shanghai, Hong Kong and Macau, Thailand, Korea, Singapore and Japan – as well as the case in America.

I called the WHO director general, Tedros Adhanom Ghebreyesus, to try to encourage him to declare a public health emergency of international concern (PHEIC), which is a way of ratcheting up the global response. I got to know Tedros through Sally Davies, the former CMO. He and I would talk on the phone. As a former Foreign Minister of Ethiopia, he's very good at the personal relationships and amazingly informal for someone in such a global role.

If we're going to get ahead of this, there needs to be a really high level of international cooperation. The Americans aren't leading because Trump wants to pull out of the WHO. It's a manifest example of the damage his presidency is doing. The Chinese aren't keen – presumably because they're seriously embarrassed to have started this pandemic and are desperately hoping it somehow all goes away. In the end, I was told it can't be done this week anyway, because one of the people who needs to sign off a decision like that is stuck on a long-haul flight. Seriously?

As for us, we *have* to call a COBRA emergency committee meeting. That's the way to inject some urgency into the Whitehall system. I've asked for one off the back of the SAGE meeting – but I need Cabinet Office sign-off to set up the machinery. COBRA meetings are important because their conclusions are automatically taken as agreed government policy, and so their writ runs across Whitehall. That means the chair is in a powerful position to get other departments to act. Cabinet Office officials are fretting that if we call a COBRA and this thing doesn't turn out to be that big a deal, we'll have egg on our faces. Not ideal, but better that than sleepwalking into a much bigger problem. I don't want a COBRA just so it looks like we're doing something: I want to wake Whitehall up to this threat.

Chris Wormald told me he's now working 100 per cent on coronavirus and has delegated everything else to his deputy, David Williams. Thank God Wormald gets it. He's very good in a crisis. He was also at Education in the Gove days, and we've always got on well. I watched him deal with teachers' strikes and endless coalition rows over budget allocations. As for Williams, he's normally the one who looks after the money. He made his name sorting out the great black hole in defence spending in the 2010s and is now responsible for the £130 billion departmental budget. If I want to do anything that needs cash, he's the one I call. A quick shrug or nod is enough to signal he can find the budget.

I found out tonight that Sir Mark Sedwill, Cabinet Secretary and head of the civil service, is blocking my push for a meeting of COBRA. Infuriating! I will have to talk to him.

In the evening, I went to *The Spectator*'s Parliamentarian of the Year dinner. It's always good fun – a raucous and boozy evening for the Westminster village involving awards for various politicians, sometimes for fairly dubious 'achievements'. I came away empty-handed as usual, and really shocked that no one else seemed bothered by the virus at all. I saw the indomitable Andrew Neil, but when I started talking to him about it, he seemed desperate to get away.

THURSDAY 23 JANUARY

No. 10 has grudgingly agreed to let me make a statement to the Commons about the virus. The Prof joined me in my office for ten minutes as I was drafting the script to go over it and help prep me for questions. His air of calm authority comes from a long career fighting infectious diseases in the developing world. A few years ago, he ran a UK programme to help Sierra Leone manage an Ebola epidemic. He said the most important lesson he has learned is what he called 'shoe leather epidemiology', which basically means gathering as much information as you can from the ground. Not massively useful in this case, unless I hotfoot it to Wuhan. He left me sobered. He repeated his dictum that there's a 50:50 chance the Wuhan quarantine won't work and we'll face a global outbreak. The only way to keep it contained is to stop all travel out of China, but obviously that's not our call.

Anyway, it may already be too late. Apparently about 300,000 people poured out of Wuhan by train just before the quarantine deadline. Unbelievably, the authorities only started closing roads out of the city today. The city's health system is now swamped and they've started building an emergency hospital. This being China, we're not talking about months or years of construction – we're talking days. When all this is over, perhaps I should get them to come and put up our forty new hospitals. That way we'd definitely have a full set of gleaming new buildings well before the 2030 deadline.

The Prof's warnings were weighing on my mind when I stood up in the Commons. I wanted to set out the facts and show we've got a grip without causing unnecessary alarm. Putting it diplomatically, the official case numbers coming out of China – 571 confirmed by this morning, including seventeen deaths – are somewhat low-balled, but I didn't get into any of that. Instead I focused on the 'proportionate, precautionary' measures we've been taking, emphasising the 50:50 chance it will still come here. Hopefully this will concentrate minds in No. 10.

Allan is feeling awful and thinks he has flu. I texted to ask if he's been to Wuhan lately.

He didn't reply.

No. 10 are still saying calling COBRA would be 'alarmist'. What utter rubbish. It's not alarmist when there's a 50:50 chance of a pandemic hitting Britain. I told my team to push back hard. They are being fobbed off by Cummings's sidekicks.

FRIDAY 24 JANUARY

The first British people directly affected by the new virus are on a cruise in south-east Asia. There's been an outbreak on board a ship called the *Diamond Princess*, and the passengers are corralled in their cabins while the crew run around trying to work out what to do. Poor people. They've spent a fortune on what they thought would be the holiday of a lifetime and are now imprisoned on a giant floating petri dish. Instead of sipping pina coladas on the sundeck and stuffing themselves at the buffet, they are stuck in rooms the size of a bathmat, waiting for morsels of food to be shoved under the door and praying the Wi-Fi doesn't pack up. This is one for the FCO (Foreign & Commonwealth Office), though I'm not sensing a great deal of urgency over there. For now I've put Emma Dean, my policy SpAd, and Emma Reed, the department's director of emergency response, onto it.

While I was seeing what we could do to galvanise Foreign Secretary Dominic Raab's team, I received a breezy message from David Cameron saying he'd just got back from the World Economic Forum in Davos. He said he was disappointed I wasn't there batting for Global Britain. It was a sly dig as he knows perfectly well that Cummings thinks Davos is part of the Axis of Evil and would never let any of us go.

Minor triumph: I have finally been allowed to convene COBRA. Since Downing Street still isn't interested, I'll probably be chairing. Right now Cummings thinks Covid is a distraction from our official withdrawal from the EU next week. That's all he wants Boris talking about.

There are times when ruthless focus is needed. Unfortunately, Cummings is ruthlessly focusing on the wrong thing.

So far, we've done fourteen tests in the UK, all negative. How long till our first case?

SATURDAY 25 JANUARY

Signs of life from Cummings, who messaged asking if we're on top of things. 'To what extent have you investigated preparations for something terrible like Ebola or a flu pandemic? Are we ready for Ebola or a flu pandemic?' he enquired. Welcome to the party, 'Comrade'. What does he think I've been doing for the past three weeks?

I patiently reply, explaining where we are up to. 'Great,' he says. This is progress.

The FCO have now advised against all travel to Hubei province. I think we need to go further, and cover far more of China, and that we'll need to withdraw Brits from Wuhan. I try to raise these points with the FCO, but I'm told in no uncertain terms that travel advice is a Foreign Office matter, and that because of the time difference their team in Wuhan are all asleep. So I called Dom Raab. He is happy to order the evacuation and will look again at the travel advice. Right now, testing is focused on travellers coming back from Wuhan. Having developed one of the first tests, there seems no urgency to expand capacity. I am constantly pushing PHE to go faster, and to use the private sector – people like Gordon Sanghera, who has been on this since Day 1.

I want everyone returning from Wuhan to be tested, but PHE says the tests are worse than useless if you don't have symptoms. This is a critical issue. If the tests we have don't work on people without symptoms, we need ones that do.

An update on the vaccine: Professor Robin Shattock from Imperial College London says he's already got two candidates that will be ready to test on animals next month. Chris Whitty is still saying it could take years. I think we can do better. I've called a meeting on Monday to go through everything. Vaccines are obviously the way out – whether just for China or for us all. A ponderous 'business as usual' approach is not an option.

SUNDAY 26 JANUARY

The papers are full of the Wuhan evacuation, with editorials screeching for testing of everyone who arrives. PHE is still opposed. I instinctively disagree but want to respect the scientists. Meanwhile the FCO machine is struggling to grind into second gear. This morning I discovered that officials are still working up advice on 'whether' to evacuate, not 'how' – when Raab has already made the decision!

The *Telegraph* has a story about a Chinese report of the possibility of asymptomatic transmission. This is really worrying. I asked officials for advice on this for tomorrow's meeting. PHE is adamant that a coronavirus can't be passed on, and that tests don't work on people without symptoms. These are two killer facts, so I want to push them, and leave them in no doubt that we need to expand testing.

Fellow MP Owen Paterson messaged. I shared an office with his wife Rose when I first worked in Westminster, and he always looked out for me. He put me in touch with Peter FitzGerald, boss of Randox, the biggest UK testing company, based in Northern Ireland. They reckon they can create a test in three weeks max that could produce a result in two to three hours. To develop it, they need samples of sputum containing the virus. I know PHE has some through its international work, and they should share it. I emailed FitzGerald straight away asking for more detail. The best work in medicine tends to happen through collaboration and we need to get cracking.

MONDAY 27 JANUARY

As I was driven to the office early this morning, the *Today* programme was on the radio. I had my head down finishing off the papers in my weekend box so was only half listening. My ears pricked up as PHE came on to talk about the pandemic. Their spokesman sounded dangerously complacent, saying everything was under control, nothing much to see here, we have this covered etc. I jerked my head up out of my paperwork and gazed out over Hyde Park as I heard reassurance after reassurance. Yet I keep hearing that arrivals from China are breezing through Heathrow without even being screened. They haven't got the testing industry up and running, and there's a 50:50 chance of a major pandemic hitting Britain. What on earth are they doing?

Screening is the absolute least we should be doing. I want people arriving back from Wuhan to be quarantined, not just screened.

So by the time the meeting started at 9.45 I was in full 'action this day' mode. The Prof opened by saying that the measures by China appear to be having some effect and that the R number is likely to fall. I pushed him on my worries about asymptomatic transmission. He said that the global scientific consensus is still that this is unlikely. But is 'unlikely' unlikely enough? If you can get it, pass it on and show no symptoms, it will be impossible to manage. I really, really want answers on this one.

We discussed the vaccine briefly, but the right officials weren't in the room. So I called another meeting, tomorrow, to go through the vaccine specifically and what we can do to accelerate it. At Chris Wormald's suggestion, I also asked for the 'reasonable worst-case scenario' for this disease in the UK so we can interrogate the numbers. Only then can we figure out whether our contingency plans are up to it.

I also pushed on a travel ban from China. Sounds extreme, but other countries are now doing it. Again, I met resistance. The response was that this is an FCO responsibility. But surely the FCO need to be driven by the health advice? I asked the Prof to talk to them. He is the CMO for the whole government, so the FCO machine should listen to him.

I got an update too on getting Brits out of Wuhan. We think there are 200–300 UK citizens out there. I made clear my view is that anyone we bring back to the UK should go into quarantine – no ifs or buts. The lawyers insisted it should be voluntary. I think that's utter rubbish. If we're offering people a free flight out of Wuhan, why on earth should it be up to them? If you don't want to quarantine, don't get on the plane! I asked for further advice into how to make this happen – not whether to.

Peter FitzGerald from Randox got back to me with the technical details of what he needs to develop a test. I've told PHE to be helpful. More importantly, they need to track down everyone in the UK who has come back from Wuhan in the past fourteen days. They'll be asked to stay at home and contact the NHS if they have any symptoms. PHE thinks there are 1,460 individuals in this category. They've set up a hub at Heathrow already, but for some reason are waiting until Wednesday to do the same at Gatwick and Manchester. Why so slow?!

Meanwhile the virus continues its relentless spread. Germany has confirmed its first case. The patient reported feeling ill on 23 January and seems to have caught it from her parents, who'd been to Wuhan and tested positive, even though they showed no symptoms. I got straight on to Jens Spahn, my opposite number in Germany. He told me the evidence on asymptomatic transmission was 'tentative' but they are worried and keeping a close eye on it.

I trust what Jens says. We're a similar age, both natural optimists and on the same part of the political spectrum – cheerful centre right. I've known him since we went out for beers to celebrate his birthday during a particularly tedious G7 meeting in Paris. Normally the host government puts these meetings on in spectacular places, showing off the best of what their country has to offer. For reasons best known to themselves, the French decided not to hold it in some splendid chateau or five-star hotel, electing to host the whole thing in their dreary Department of Health. After listening to one too many dull speeches, Jens and I did a runner and went to a little cafe round the corner. Feeling somewhat rebellious, we ordered some beers and sat in the sunshine, hiding in plain sight. He's entertaining, irreverent and we can be pretty open with each other. I'm glad he's there.

Amid all this my team is still getting calls from No. 10 and being dragged into meetings on how we're going to deliver manifesto commitments. I'm going to have to delegate. I want these commitments to happen but have to prioritise. Coronavirus is the first thing I think about when I wake up and the last thing I think about when I go to bed.

TUESDAY 28 JANUARY

A proper 'oh shit' meeting today. In the early afternoon, with the pale winter sun streaming in through the floor-to-ceiling windows, the whole team gathered in my office to go through the reasonable worst-case scenario I requested. There were about thirty people perching on every flat surface in my office overlooking what I think is the best, most spectacular 270-degree view of central London. The office is dominated by a massive circular Damien Hirst portrait of the Queen, which I brought with me from my days in the Culture Department, when I got the pick of the government art collection. When I was promoted to Health Secretary I made sure it was whisked off to my new office before my successor could get his hands on it.

The room was full of clinicians, junior ministers, special advisers, policy experts, PHE and NHS colleagues and experts like David Halpern, who is highly skilled at changing public behaviour without being too heavy-handed. He used to run Cameron's 'Nudge Unit', which tried to do things like get people to pay their taxes on time by telling them that all the neighbours do it. The PHE leadership were there and sat near the table.

In his characteristically understated way, sitting at the back peeling a tangerine, Chris Whitty quietly informed everyone that although there is currently no sustained transmission outside China, in the reasonable worst-case scenario as many as 820,000 people in the UK may die. Although the risk of death to each individual is low, the transmission is so high that almost everyone would catch it, in up to three waves, each lasting about fifteen weeks. The whole room froze. We are looking at a human catastrophe on a scale not seen here for a century.

I asked what we needed to do to accelerate a vaccine. The problem is no one has ever created a vaccine for a coronavirus before. I noticed that Professor Van-Tam, who was sitting on my left, kept putting his hand up asking to speak, in an impeccably formal manner. This was pretty unusual: when I chair meetings, I try to keep it fairly informal and encourage everyone to contribute. Before I make a decision, I like to be challenged. When called, JVT – as he signs off his emails – spoke with a natural authority. He said developing a vaccine normally takes five or ten years, but there's a team in Oxford working on an Ebola project that can easily be switched to the new disease. If everything's fast-tracked, we could do it in a year to eighteen months.

'I want it by Christmas,' I said.

JVT set out how we can get on with fast-tracking and funding vaccine trials. This phase normally takes years. To speed things up, we will need to change the law. Thankfully we can do this by secondary legislation, not a full-blown Bill. No problem, I said. I have the legal power to make a change and this is an urgent national requirement. The relevant regulations and approvals come from the Medicines and Healthcare Products Regulatory Agency (MHRA) – and having voted to leave the EU, we no longer have the complication of getting European Medicines Agency agreement.

The mood in the vaccines meeting was grimly determined, with an overriding sense that this could well be the biggest challenge of our professional lives.

We went through the other problems we had to deal with: testing (I pushed PHE again on expansion and harnessing the private sector); asymptomatic transmission (apparently I'm getting a paper tonight); and how people will respond if we have to ask them to change their behaviour (unclear).

We are starting to think about how the social media companies can help. Jamie has spoken to Twitter and they're going to tweak their algorithms so when people search for 'coronavirus' and various other key terms, they'll go to our official guidance page.

Meanwhile Raab relayed a request from the Chinese Foreign Minister for us to put goggles, masks and other equipment on the flight out to Wuhan. We should definitely do this as we want to set a high standard for international cooperation. We're bound to need help from others further down the line. In the same spirit, we're going to offer any spare seats on the flight back to non-British nationals who need to get out. They'll have to get straight home from wherever we land them in the UK without transferring to other airports. Otherwise they'll be carted off to quarantine.

Jim Bethell, a friend who's the whip in the House of Lords covering DHSC business, passed on the latest from his mates in Hong Kong, who say everyone's terrified, restaurants and public transport are deserted and expats are fleeing. Sobering.

WEDNESDAY 29 JANUARY

There's brass neck and then there's former Tory MP Sarah Wollaston. This pro-EU hardliner went off the reservation over Brexit, defected to the Lib Dems via the embarrassing Change UK and then spent weeks trying to portray Boris as some kind of tinpot dictator. Only last month she stood against us in the election as a Lib Dem. Now she's written to me all, 'Hi Matt, hope all is well?' as if nothing'd happened, lobbying for us to make her chair of NICE (the National Institute for Health and Care Excellence), presumably on the grounds that she's a GP and chaired the health select committee. I could not believe the cheek of it. I bounced her request off Dom, who was suitably disgusted.

'No way! PM would hit roof! She's called for most of us in No. 10 to be arrested!' he exclaimed.

'Quite. I thought extraordinary that she asked,' I replied.

PMQs today was surreal: not a single question on the virus. I stood by the Speaker's chair thinking, 'Every single question you lot are asking will be rendered completely irrelevant in a few weeks.'

After yesterday's shocking meeting, today we had a more pragmatic discussion. The Prof has helped crystallise my thinking on how we phase our response to the virus, at least in the early stages. He popped upstairs to propose four elements. First, we try to contain isolated outbreaks. Then we try to delay the spread. If containment doesn't work and the virus spreads to the general population, we move on to mitigating and slowing its effects, and throughout we research for treatments and a vaccine.

Feeling like a broken record, I pushed PHE again about asymptomatic transmission. Their latest paper says almost nothing – not even a provisional finding. I don't get why it's taking so long to get an answer on this – not just here but around the world. I called Tedros again to have another go at persuading him to declare a public health international emergency. My sense is he's terrified of upsetting Beijing. I asked him about unofficial reports from China that there was asymptomatic transmission and he played it down, blaming 'translation issues' as if the glaring lack of information coming out of China is all some kind of perfectly innocent communication problem. Sensing I was a bit sceptical, he doubled down, claiming to be 'impressed by their transparency'. What?! The Chinese made their comments about asymptomatic transmission three days ago and the WHO still hasn't checked if they were reported correctly. Unbelievable! Doesn't anyone there speak Mandarin?

My view is that Tedros is trapped by the politics. While the US and UK are the WHO's biggest funders, we play with a straight bat. China runs various projects in his private office, so he is scared stiff of upsetting them. You can't fault the WHO's science, but the politics is awful. It's going to be a serious issue if we have a global disease and the main global health body adopts the Chinese approach to information flow. If asymptomatic transmission is happening, then the odds are that the disease is already out of control.

Confirmed cases in China are now up to nearly 10,000, plus more than 100 others in twenty-two other countries. We're testing a trickle of people here and 50:50 is looking increasingly optimistic. British Airways has suspended all flights to and from mainland China, but more than a month since this thing started, international travel is still pretty much business as usual. I am haunted by *Contagion*…

We finally held our first COBRA. The underground bunker room was packed. Ben Wallace at Defence, Dom Raab and Simon Stevens sat at the top of the table as officials typed action points and conclusions real-time onto the screens above our heads. We went through the reasonable worst-case scenario and ministers were sent away to work out what they'd have to do if that happened. We discussed the evacuation plans. The FCO is getting a kicking over the evacuation from Wuhan because British citizens aren't allowed to bring their other halves. Actually, it's the Chinese authorities who are banning their citizens from leaving, even if they're dual nationals. We want to be compassionate, but the Chinese Communist Party doesn't really do touchy-feely. The French and the Americans have hit exactly the same problem.

THURSDAY 30 JANUARY

The Wuhan Brits are on their way back to Britain courtesy of the RAF. We filled the outward flight with PPE for the Chinese. Given the scale of the crisis they're facing, it's only a gesture, but it's better than nothing. Obviously we can't afford to run down our own stocks in case things get really bad here. I've asked for an audit of exactly what we've got.

Before the evacuees left China I had a showdown with officials and lawyers over what to do with the evacuees when they land at RAF Brize Norton. PHE thinks they should be greeted with a smile and a leaflet and asked nicely to go home and stay there for a couple of weeks. I think that's incredibly naive and said they should go straight into quarantine. PHE hit back with a whole series of reasons why this would be too difficult and started hand-wringing about human rights. They're worried we could be hit with a judicial review.

'OK,' I said, 'let's get them to sign a contract before they board. In return for the flight, they agree to go into quarantine. No contract, no flight.'

I was told the contract wouldn't be legally enforceable and was too draconian. 'Do it anyway,' I instructed. It's what the public will expect. Amazingly, they fell into line. Bit edgy, and maybe some judge somewhere down the line will raise an eyebrow, but at least we'll have a written commitment from them agreeing to go into quarantine. This flight isn't a freebie – it's their last chance to get out, thanks to the British taxpayer, and it's a quid pro quo.

I was on a visit to Porton Down, to see the high-security testing and vaccine production capabilities, so I asked Jo Churchill, my constituency neighbour and junior minister responsible for public health, to go up to the former nurses' quarters at Arrowe Park Hospital, where the evacuees will be accommodated, to make sure it's comfortable. She's insisted on packs of toiletries and more towels. Alarmingly, she also messaged me to say the passenger numbers on the plane manifest don't tally with the numbers the FCO gave us, so we're not exactly sure how many people are arriving. Nothing could exemplify the woeful lack of information about this crisis better than the fact that we don't even know how many people are on the evacuation plane.

Later, once back in the office, I talked to Chris Wormald and Allan about our general approach and the risk of judicial reviews in coming months. I'm adamant we have to prioritise the concrete here and now, not what some vexatious litigant might hit us with later. This is about saving lives. My view is that we deal with legal headaches later, when people aren't actually dying. I have instructed the team to ignore the noise and do what is best to keep people safe. After all, while liberal individualism may be the best way to organise a society in normal times, in a pandemic, the harm principle applies to anyone who might be spreading the disease. Even liberals should support fairly draconian action to protect others. You've got to be a hardcore libertarian to disagree. This is at least something the pandemic preparedness plan has furnished us with. There's a whole draft Bill ready to go that was written as a result of the Cygnus exercise. I've asked Wormald to work on the legislation so it reflects the pandemic we're facing, not the flu pandemic anticipated by the exercise. We need to remove any ambiguity. There will be times when some people will need to quarantine to protect others. It will need rock-solid legal underpinning.

The WHO has finally got its act together and declared the virus a PHEIC. This is a wake-up call for everyone around the world and it means we can all work to roughly the same principles. The WHO has advised every country to bring in proper surveillance, isolation, contact tracing and prevention to try to slow the spread. Countries must also share full data with WHO. No exemption for China. (Good luck with that one.)

Following that announcement, the four UK CMOs (the Prof and his opposite numbers in Scotland, Wales and Northern Ireland) have raised the risk level from low to moderate. It's vital that all parts of the UK move in lockstep. We can't have our response undermined by petty devolution politics.

Yesterday I got a slightly frosty message from Ben Wallace reminding me that the Department of Health should not talk about how the armed forces will help in this crisis unless and until he has signed it off. He's right. The military are his assets, not mine, as I reminded my team. I think he felt a bit guilty about his huffy tone because he imme-diately followed up with an emollient message assuring me that they will do whatever is required to help. I don't doubt it.

Endless rumours flying round about cases in this or that part of the country. We're being contacted by jumpy new MPs every time they hear something. We're not going to investigate each time we're asked, so we just keep repeating the facts: namely, that there are no confirmed cases here.

PHE's audit of PPE came back and did not lighten my mood. The paperwork is all over the place. There's no clear record of what's in the stockpile, and some kit is past its 'best before' date. I've instructed officials to work out what we need fast, and buy in huge quantities.

FRIDAY 31 JANUARY

Brexit Day – and the virus is here. Nearly four years after the referen-dum (feels more like twenty) we are officially out of the EU. According to the Downing Street grid, today was meant to be about celebrating this historic moment, our new horizons etc. Instead it kicked off with Chris Whitty announcing the arrival of the disease. Downing Street are furious. I am daunted.

I got a call from my private secretary at half past midnight last night to tell me we had two confirmed positive cases: a Chinese student and his father, who'd flown in from Wuhan to visit him. After they report-ed ill on Wednesday night and then tested positive, health officials in full hazmat suits turned up on the doorstep of the flat where they were staying in York and carted them off to hospital. Our protocols worked seamlessly, and to give the patients their due, they behaved impecca-bly, isolating in their apartment from the moment they fell ill, along with the student's mother. Curiously, she's tested negative, showing what a lottery this virus may be.

To the dismay of some colleagues, the PM pressed ahead with a long-planned Brexit-themed Cabinet meeting in Sunderland. These symbolic displays of our (very real) commitment to voters beyond the M25 are not universally popular among colleagues. Theresa May's Chancellor Philip Hammond was always particularly unenthusiastic, adopting an even more lugubrious expression than usual whenever he was forced to traipse around the country.

The north-east is Leave country and Sunderland was the first place to declare its results on referendum night. At the Cabinet meeting, held at the National Glass Centre, Boris laid out his buccaneering vision of Britain's future, while I brought everyone down to earth with a coronavirus update. I mentioned the potential 820,000 deaths figure and the reaction was somewhat 'shrug shrug' – essentially because they didn't really believe it. I am constantly feeling that others, who aren't focused on this every day, are weeks behind what's going on.

While we were all trooping back to London, the Wuhan flight touched down at Brize Norton. In front of cameras, the evacuees were instantly whisked off for a two-week staycation courtesy of Her Majesty's government. In another example of the complacency of PHE, the elaborate measures we'd taken to ensure the whole thing didn't become a super-spreader event were somewhat undermined by an embarrassing oversight. The RAF crew and all our officials were in full hazmat suits, but the poor coach drivers taking them to Arrowe Park were in their normal work clothes. I had personally insisted that everyone on the flight – crew included – be protected in PPE. I hadn't thought I'd need to be so precise as to say the same precaution obviously had to apply to the bus drivers. So I couldn't believe it when I watched the buses trundling out of Brize driven by blokes with no protection at all. Who on earth would give protection to air crew but not bus crew?

Jamie Njoku-Goodwin, my media adviser and the best person in Westminster at looking round political corners, pointed out another potential problem: the four coaches PHE had hired belong to a company called Horseman. Their logo was emblazoned in large letters on each coach. Cue potential headlines about the 'four horsemen of the apocalypse'. Not exactly ideal optics.

Once the evacuees were safely in situ, I spoke to all the Merseyside

MPs in an effort to keep them onside. One Labour MP made a moronic comment about the Tories hating Liverpool and 'now we're sending the plague there', but the rest were very reasonable.

This evening I went to Downing Street to the Brexit celebration party. I stood next to the Chancellor of the Exchequer, Sajid Javid, as Cummings stood on the podium and literally burst into tears. He couldn't manage more than a sentence. Here was his life's work complete! The PM made a strong speech in praise of his right-hand man and, after everyone counted down to midnight, banged a little gong on the table to mark the moment of exit. Sajid just stood there looking perplexed throughout. It was a strange feeling being at a celebration for an event I'd voted against, but wanted to be delivered, yet fundamentally thought would soon feel small compared to what was coming down the tracks.

Perhaps Sajid was so quiet because he's worrying about coronavirus. Earlier today he messaged asking why we're still allowing flights from the UK to China. I told him PHE doesn't think it's worth closing them down unless it's done with other countries, though, given the scale of the reasonable worst-case scenario, personally I'd rather go belt and braces.

Apparently one of Sajid's contacts is a highly respected global expert on disease and told him privately that he thinks there is a 30 per cent chance this will be massive and that 'millions' will die. Saj was at pains to point out that he doesn't necessarily believe these apocalyptic figures, but he's clearly troubled. I asked if he wanted a personal briefing from the CMO, and he accepted, adding that he's 'v concerned'.

Meanwhile endless glitches to sort out. Merseyside Police complaining about having to provide security at short notice; Simon Stevens's office asking how many double rooms and how many single, as if we're some kind of travel agency; and Jenny Harries – another of the Prof's deputies – is going to liaise with the FCO about the situation with international flights, hopefully ahead of Raab advising against all travel to China.

Amid the torrent, I've told the team it's absolutely vital that we don't let up the pace on manifesto commitments. We're ensuring that the teams working on them are totally free of coronavirus work. Wormald is putting undistracted senior officials in charge of these programmes.

Jim Bethell warned me this evening he would be late for the Monday morning meeting because 'blush, blush' (his words, not mine) he's been assigned to welcome the Sultan of Brunei to Britain on behalf of Her Majesty.

'If I'm wearing a bling new watch, it was a present from my wife, promise,' he quipped.

As a government whip in the Upper House, Jim is also a Lord in Waiting to the Queen so gets called on to do stuff like this. Nice to see our whip getting all the glamour.

FEBRUARY 2020

SATURDAY 1 FEBRUARY

The Chinese authorities have gone full totalitarian, locking people indoors and only letting them out to get what they need to survive. In Hubei, only one person per household is allowed out every two days for food and other essentials. Funerals have been banned and bodies just have to be dealt with at the nearest crematorium straight away. Terrifying.

I was brooding over all this at home when I thought, 'Thank goodness for Chris Whitty.' I sent him a WhatsApp saying how brilliant he's been this past week, which is true. So many people are commenting about how reassuring he is when he makes public statements. I told him I hoped he'd get some rest this weekend, though I doubt it.

There are now nearly 12,000 confirmed cases of the virus worldwide. Of those, 259 have died, all in China. Spain has had its first case, the US is up to eight and numbers are growing in Australia, Japan, Singapore and across east Asia.

PHE wants to do a national anti-obesity TV advertising campaign, but the Cabinet Office took one look at the proposal and threw it out. I asked the Prof what he thought and he replied that PHE comms can sometimes be 'a curate's egg'. He's so diplomatic. That's the end of that then.

SUNDAY 2 FEBRUARY

Chaos at Arrowe Park after an attempted jailbreak by one of the evacuees last night. Natasha rang to say the guy is very upset and is demanding to be tested and released if it comes back negative. Our advice is that if people are asymptomatic, they probably won't test positive even if they have it, so security are under strict orders not to let him leave. The details are murky, but apparently he has packed his bags and is standing by the doorway, getting increasingly irate. The security are not sure how long they can stop him from doing a runner.

With the lawyers' advice ringing in my ears, I was feeling a teensy bit nervous about the whole scenario, so we decided to see if we could find a magistrate willing to apply the emergency section of the 1984 Public Health (Control of Disease) Act to enforce the contract the guy signed when he got on the flight. The Act is very outdated in many ways, including needing a magistrate to sign off on the detention of someone for public health reasons. After something of a scramble, the department identified a local Liverpool magistrate – who coolly informed us she would not play ball. Apparently she considered the measure disproportionate. Rapidly running out of options, I came up with the idea to tell our potential absconder that if he disappears, he will have to reimburse the Great British taxpayer for his share of the cost of the very expensive evacuation flight. The lawyers were happy with that, so we went ahead. Taking everything into account, including all the time spent by FCO officials, lawyers, doctors etc., his bill would have been gargantuan. Thankfully it did the trick and he's staying put.

Taking a breather this evening, I was exchanging messages with Ed Argar on the NHS Bill as we both watched England lose to France in the Six Nations. Ed is my absolutely rock-solid number two in the department, undemonstrative, efficient and shrewd. As I spend more time on Covid, he's going to have to spend more and more time on everything else. I told him it's important the forty hospitals we are building per our manifesto commitment are not only new but beautiful. Too many of these buildings are just utterly depressing. I asked Ed to draft in Nick Boys Smith of Create Streets, who is the big advocate and guru of aesthetic development, and he enthusiastically agreed.

Tomorrow's *FT* has a great story about Nissan doubling down on its investment in the UK. Their Sunderland plant is such an icon of the Thatcherite revival of the car industry. It's a huge vote of confidence in post-Brexit Britain, especially from such a previously ardently pro-Remain firm. Nice to see the story reported by the most fanatically pro-Remain newspaper.

First coronavirus death reported outside China: a 44-year-old man in the Philippines. That emergency field hospital they started building in Wuhan ten days ago is finished already. Incredible. Everyone says it could never happen here. It pains me to say it, but I fear they're right.

MONDAY 3 FEBRUARY

'When SS off?' Cummings asked. He's not letting go of this mission to get rid of Simon Stevens, despite the fact that we're about to be hit by a pandemic. 'We must get on with it now,' Dom added. 'Announce next week as part of reshuffle frenzy and it will all get lost in that.'

I made a mental note to check with the PM. Does he really want Simon Stevens forced out?

More positively, I was able to tell the PM we've formally allocated £5 million seed funding for a new hospital in his constituency – one of the forty.

'Hooray!' he replied. 'Spades in the ground next year!!'

'Inshallah,' I said, not feeling quite as optimistic.

In the splendour of the old Royal Naval Hospital in Greenwich, he gave what was supposed to be a historic speech on Brexit, setting out a rather excellent free trade vision for the future. He touched on the virus, warning against rushing to close borders as this could be used as an excuse to put up unnecessary trade barriers 'beyond what is medically rational, to the point of doing real and unnecessary economic damage'. I can live with that, although it doesn't give us much wiggle room.

But the speech was completely overshadowed by events. In Wuhan, the army has taken over delivery of medical supplies. The Shanghai Stock Exchange was down 8 per cent for the day when it reopened after the specially extended New Year break.

SAGE reckons the epidemic is still growing exponentially, probably doubling in size every four or five days. It's possible that as few as one in twenty cases in China are being identified, which would mean the real size of the epidemic is 200,000–300,000 cases.

Given the signs the virus is taking hold outside China, SAGE has also looked again at travel bans. Their view is that there still isn't much to be gained and that we won't keep the infection out. The only benefit would be to buy time, but the evidence suggests reducing imported cases by half would only hold the epidemic up by about five days. To gain a month, we'd need to cut international travel by at least 90 per cent, which would require draconian measures, far beyond China. The boss is clear: we've got to follow the science on this one, and the science is clear: it's not worth it. We agreed to recommend against travel to China, but that's as far as it goes.

There's a debate brewing on face masks. We asked NERVTAG to look into whether they do any good. They say there's no evidence either way that the general public wearing masks would make any difference. If they don't really help, I certainly don't want to impose them on people. I for one would hate wearing them. Afterwards, one of the team sidled up to me and told me that there's a furious global debate on this question. Apparently scientists can't agree at all. The way the virus is transmitted isn't yet understood. For now, the best advice is that health and care workers should wear fluid-repellent surgical masks but not the full respirator kit.

I want the UK to be first in the world to develop a vaccine. It's a huge ambition and I've no idea whether we can pull it off, but we should throw everything at it. Today we pledged £20 million for the international research effort. I talked to the team again and made it very clear that we can't go through the usual laborious regulatory processes. Of course we mustn't cut corners on safety, but everything else *has* to be accelerated. I do not want our scientists wasting their time filling out endless agonising grant applications.

I insisted that things are done in parallel, not in series. This is something JVT has been very hot on. Begin lab trials as soon as possible. Then go straight onto Phase 1 clinical trials, to be complete two to four months after that. Start manufacturing before approval. This would all be unprecedented in the field of vaccine development. In my statement to Parliament today, I thought it best to include details of the evacuation plan for next week. I was about to go into the debating chamber when we got a call from FCO officials. We'd given them an advance copy of the speech and they were in a complete flap, insisting I take it all out. It wasn't worth a fight, so I deleted the section concerned, thinking nothing more of it until this evening, when I discovered that the FCO have announced exactly the same thing themselves from Beijing. Talk about joined-up government…

TUESDAY 4 FEBRUARY

The British-registered *Diamond Princess* is still marooned in Yokohama harbour in Japan, with all 4,000 passengers confined to their cabins for two weeks. It must be horrendously claustrophobic: no exercise, no fresh air and God only knows what they're being given to eat. We know some are British and we're keeping an eye, but it's in the hands of the Japanese.

Jens Spahn came over from Germany, a trip he's been planning for a while. It was great to see him. Germany is following our lead in giving more money to vaccine research. He reckons we should do it together to show Germany and the UK cooperating post-Brexit. His English is impeccable and his attitude is quite rare for a European politician: however disappointed he is that we've left the EU, he understands why people voted the way they did, and that we must deliver on the referendum result.

We talked about what sort of social restrictions may be needed if the virus takes off, though SAGE still doesn't want us to do anything.

As a liberal, I've always believed people make the best decisions for themselves. I've driven the government deregulation agenda for years. Part of the reason I got into politics is because my parents' business nearly went under because of a cashflow problem when a major client went bust. I was a teenager at the time and it was deeply affecting. Now we are contemplating actions that could bankrupt millions of businesses and interfere in literally everyone's lives. It is a very, very strange feeling; not me at all.

Officially, SAGE still hasn't confirmed asymptomatic transmission, though they're edging towards it. So far, the data suggests people could be infectious for as long as two weeks after they first get symptoms. They're sick, on average, for between two and three weeks, but some are suffering for far longer.

After seeing Jens I went over to the Commons to give my mum birthday tea. She and Bob, my stepfather, had come down from Cheshire for the day, and with Martha and the kids we had a lovely time.

The episode over the Arrowe Park wannabe escapee has concentrated minds on our legal powers – or lack of them. Seat-of-the-pants improvisation got the Wuhan lot onto the plane and into quarantine, but it could have become messy. After much to-ing and fro-ing with No. 10, I asked Robert Buckland, the Justice Secretary, if we could add stronger powers onto his terrorism Bill. He's going to look into it. For now we'll have to rely on the existing setup, i.e. police persuasion in the first instance, escalating to a magistrate's order under existing legal powers for seventy-two hours' detention for breach of the peace if things go badly wrong. It's worryingly vague and we have to hope nothing serious comes up. In the meantime, I've chased Wormald on the draft clauses we need to put through Parliament so we have the powers of compulsion if we need them.

WEDNESDAY 5 FEBRUARY

PMQs – still no questions about coronavirus. Colleagues were busy congratulating each other over Brexit, and Corbyn was asking about climate change. In the department, we're focused on how to protect the vulnerable from the virus. Jenny Harries is running the process. First we have to define what conditions make you particularly vulnerable. That's a job for clinicians, which Jenny can do fine – though we don't know much yet and will have to adjust as we get better data from abroad. We then need to identify everyone who has those conditions. Doing that is not easy, because NHS GP data is segregated and held by two private businesses, who can be very tricky to deal with. We then need to check the data makes sense, which means GPs looking down the lists the system comes up with. Then we need to actually make contact. But the NHS's data on people's contact details is famously sketchy. And because this is inevitably going to be imperfect (for example, hard as it is to believe, some people still have their medical records on paper) we then need to have a system that allows people to self-declare that they have one of these conditions and get their GP to vet whether they should go on the list or not.

Even two years ago this would have been completely impossible. Thankfully NHS Digital has been making big strides, as a result of which it is at least theoretically doable. It involves getting patient lists from GPs and pushing the NHS technology to its limits. I've spent my time as Health Secretary so far trying to haul the health service out of the IT Stone Age, with mixed success. We're now somewhere around the Bronze Age – and about to be tested, big time.

Ben Wallace is worried that the FCO is 'setting the pace on the Chinese virus' (as he put it) and that our primary focus should be on UK health, not evacuating expats. 'These evacuation flights are all very good, but in the end this is about the health of the homeland. My view is that the MoD and FCO are simply your facilitators, not the lead,' he said.

Very decently, he offered to have a quiet word with Sedwill, stressing that the Department of Health should be calling the shots. I wouldn't be worried about the FCO taking the lead on what happens abroad if they actually stepped up. The problem is the officials don't seem to get the urgency.

I had dinner with the wonderful Ana Botín, chair of Santander, and some of her friends. Covid was all we talked about. PMQs hasn't caught up yet: outside Westminster, people have gone from not caring to caring about nothing else. I was grilled all evening. Socialising now feels like an extension of our public information campaign. I get asked endless questions, most of which we don't yet know the answer to.

Brexit is finally off the top of the polls as the issue the public are most concerned about, pipped by health, according to YouGov. Not exactly in the circumstances I would prefer, but at least that toxic issue may finally be behind us.

THURSDAY 6 FEBRUARY

A sense of foreboding as a third UK case is confirmed. The patient lives in Brighton and got home from a trip to Singapore last week, after which he went skiing in France. If there's asymptomatic transmission, we're really screwed. God only knows how many people he may have passed it onto in his chalet, during his travels and back here.

Super unhelpfully, the PM's spokesman blurted out the news in the lobby briefing today, going way off script before we were in a position to confirm what had happened. Time to sort out government comms on the virus or it will be a complete shambles when things get more serious.

Rumours Boris will conduct his post-election reshuffle tomorrow. Unusually, I'm not bothered. Under the circumstances, I won't be going anywhere.

FRIDAY 7 FEBRUARY

Grim twist. The Chinese medic who first raised the alert has died of the disease. Li Wenliang was an ophthalmologist in Wuhan and warned his colleagues about a new SARS-like virus in December. He was then given one hell of a dressing-down by local police and had to sign a statement denouncing himself for spreading 'false and illegal rumours'. He got the disease on 8 January and is dead a month later. Pretty sobering, and a dreadful reflection on the irresponsible approach of the Chinese authorities. What a hero.

Another meeting on the vaccine with the Prof, JVT, Wormald and Jim, who I want involved in the vaccine mission. We went through everything we need to do to get things moving as fast as possible. Multiple reality checks from Chris Whitty on how long it might take – he thinks it could be years – and the dire consequences of not doing everything by the book. Teams at Oxford and Imperial College are already making great progress and say the first trial doses should be available in a matter of weeks. My view is we should get them manufacturing straight away, so if the trials come good, we can vaccinate as fast as possible. The pressure if and when one is found to work will be immense.

Meanwhile the Home Office is kicking off over quarantine. They now say we may not have the power to enforce detention, even for seventy-two hours. My lawyers do think, though, that we only need regulations under the 1984 Act, not a whole new Act of Parliament. But parliamentary counsel – the hotshot specialists who actually write the law – say they can't draft anything until everyone agrees, and the Cabinet Office is trying to grab control of the whole thing. It's a classic Whitehall turf battle just as we don't need it. So I called a meeting this afternoon to sort it all out. Finally we got the green light to draft the regulations, and to their credit the parliamentary counsel agreed to spend the weekend writing them.

Coronavirus is becoming all-consuming. For various reasons I'm supposed to be going to Center Parcs this weekend. Not sure how much time I'll have for the adventure playground.

SATURDAY 8 FEBRUARY

Desperate measures may be required at Arrowe Park, where we once again have someone threatening to leave. We still don't have our legal ducks in a row, and Jenny Harries is on standby to hotfoot it up there to try to restore calm. One of the evacuees now claims he never signed the contract, so is under no obligation to stay. Cue frantic calls to the British embassy in China in hopes he's calling our bluff and that we can retrieve our paperwork. If not, Jenny will appeal to him face to face to stay put. The stakes are that high. My real fear is that if one goes, they'll all go.

It turns out that the Brighton skier managed to infect all five other Brits with whom he was holidaying. They're still in France. We're working with the French to track them all down. It's an ominous sign.

SUNDAY 9 FEBRUARY

Strangest ever trip to Center Parcs. I have an old university friend called Dom who – shockingly – had a stroke in his twenties and is now in a wheelchair. For the past couple of years, a gang of us have who have been friends since our student days have been going to Center Parcs together for the weekend. Dom can't work, and we all love to see him. To go away he needs special kit and a disability-friendly venue. Center Parcs do that brilliantly. Unfortunately, I had to spend half the weekend on the phone to officials working on quarantine regulations, trying to issue instructions between trips on the zipwire and to the 'subtropical swimming paradise'. We had to use a little-known emergency procedure meaning the powers become law the moment I sign them and are then approved in Parliament retrospectively. The whole experience was surreal: I approved the final measures while we were packing to leave, trying not to miss anything vital from the lawyers while bundling all my stuff into my bags. Unfortunately, that wasn't the end of the process: to become law, the new regulations had to be physically signed. Demonstrating her customary dedication, Natasha came round to the house with the various documents when I got back this evening, and I did the honours at the kitchen table. Hopefully the changes will remove the ambiguity and with it the problems we had with Arrowe Park. We can't spend our time ringing round grumpy magistrates trying to get them to sign things off on a case-by-case basis.

We're adding a second quarantine centre, Kents Hill Park hotel in Milton Keynes, to accommodate more overseas returnees. In her capacity as Public Health Minister and general fixer, Jo Churchill dropped in at the centre. A good job she did, as it turns out Chris

Whitty has been using his personal credit card to pay for all the extras to make their lives comfortable. What an absolute legend. The Prof always goes above and beyond. But what is wrong with the procurement system that he had to do this himself?

MONDAY 10 FEBRUARY

There are now eight positive cases here, all contracted overseas, including two GPs. Half are linked to the man in Brighton, who – as I feared – turned out to be something of a super-spreader. I called the PM to tell him this thing could go either way: maybe we manage to contain it, but more likely we're going down.

'Bash on,' he said – a typical Boris refrain.

I squeezed in a flying visit to his constituency to bang heads together on the proposed new hospital. Afterwards, I texted him to say the meeting had gone well and that first onsite works should begin this summer. Worst case, it's part built by 2024. Best case, it's finished.

'Yipppeeee,' he replied. Now I just have to make it happen, along with the other thirty-nine we've promised. What could possibly go wrong?

So far, no explosions over the new legal powers. We were worried about how they would be received, but all quiet. It helped that I'd squared off the detail with shadow Health Secretary Jonathan Ashworth, who's very definitely one of the good guys. He was as pleased as we were that Corbyn didn't win the last election.

TUESDAY 11 FEBRUARY

The disease has a new official name: 'Covid-19', standing for 'coronavirus disease 2019'. The WHO came up with it – they were keen the name wasn't place-specific (the Chinese would have insisted on that) and that it's easy to pronounce. More than 1,100 people have now died in China, where they've had nearly 45,000 cases, and that's just the confirmed ones.

SAGE has started working on what lockdown options might have the biggest impact if they're needed. They're all being set out on a big

A3 sheet of paper for ministers to consider. It's dry scientific analysis – but shocking nonetheless. They think there's not much point stopping large public gatherings because things like sporting events are one-offs that will only ever comprise a small proportion of contacts people have with others. People gather more closely and frequently in pubs and restaurants. Religious services and family gatherings are the biggest risk of all, as they bring much closer contacts than anything in public and generally involve older people. Then there's schools. Might we have to shut them too? Since this disease barely affects children, it's hard to see how that would benefit them directly, but if children pass it on we might have to. Think of the impact that would have! Another measure we're considering is household isolation: the idea that if one family member gets Covid, the whole household has to isolate. Nothing like that has ever happened in Britain before.

Driving home down the Harrow Road later, I looked at the crowds spilling out of the pub on the corner and tried to imagine what it will be like if we have to shut these places. I felt like I inhabited another world, that no one outside had yet seen into.

Unhelpfully, No. 10 have been briefing far too definitively that there won't be any flight bans. Big mistake. The reality is we may have to close borders.

After this shock, Cabinet. In a mini-success, I've won the battle to ensure the emergency Coronavirus Bill is DHSC legislation, not run out of the Cabinet Office. Normally it takes months to get cross-government approval for a Bill. This time it was formally approved at Cabinet in principle – subject to wrangling over the detail, no doubt. The emergency regulations we've passed for Arrowe Park are OK, but we need a much broader set of changes – everything from rules around court procedures to powers to pay money out and support businesses much more directly than we ever have before. Cabinet nodded it through without dissent, reassured that it would be a temporary measure. I've been trying to get a meeting with Rishi Sunak, Sajid's number two at the Treasury, to talk about cutting the cost of clinical negligence. His office keep saying they can't find a time on Thursday:

reshuffle day. I wonder if Rishi thinks he's about to get promoted and is keeping his diary clear?

'Have you had the wink?' I asked.

Apparently not.

'Ha! No, nothing that exciting,' he replied, saying he's just back-to-back with meetings.

Actually, I have a wider problem with the Treasury, which just isn't engaging with our manifesto commitments for the NHS. I messaged Cummings saying I need them to play ball so that we can visibly deliver on extra nurses and hospitals by 2024. The Budget is only a few weeks away and they're still proposing to cut £1 billion from our capital budget, which we just can't spare. I've written formally to HMT, but it would help if No. 10 gave them a serious push.

'These are not nice-to-have: they are mission critical commitments,' I told Cummings. No reply so far.

WEDNESDAY 12 FEBRUARY

I was back in the COBRA room today for a civil service exercise to rehearse what we'll do if the virus runs out of control. Whitehall is good at putting these exercises together, and if everyone plays their part, they can be very useful. There was one flaw: there's a reshuffle tomorrow, and most departments had sent junior ministers, many of whom are about to be moved. Surely you do the practice exercise after the reshuffle, not before? There were about thirty of us seated in two rows around the big COBRA table. In front of us were various folders containing scenarios that unfolded as the exercise progressed.

We role-played how we would do our jobs in two months' time if the very worst-case scenario has happened and there are hundreds of thousands of people dying. We were asked to imagine that we'd failed to slow or mitigate the virus and we were reduced to reacting to the calamity. Where in Hyde Park would the burial pits be? Who would dig them? Have we got enough body bags? I sat there thinking, there's no way we can let ourselves get into a position where we need half a million body bags. It just can't happen.

Worst of all was agreeing a protocol to instruct doctors which lives to save. Do we treat the young, because they have more years to live, or the old, because they are more vulnerable? Are all lives saved equal, or is each year of expected life equal? Horrific decisions, presented in such a bald, matter-of-fact way.

Going through the administrative requirements for handling death on such a scale was really frightening. I could tell from the looks on my team's faces that the gravity of the situation had hit everyone. And my conclusion wasn't administrative at all. I resolved I never want to make these decisions for real: we must not let this happen. These scenarios and options are inconceivable. Of course, at a policy level the NHS already takes the view that drugs are cost effective if they cost less than £30,000 per year of quality life saved. That's one thing. But asking doctors to choose between who to treat and who to leave? Dreadful. Whatever it takes, we must not let the NHS get overwhelmed.

These exercises only work if you suspend disbelief and throw yourself into it. I looked across the room to George Freeman, probably my oldest friend in Parliament and the Transport Minister, with whom I shared an office for years. He was earnestly engaging in the make-believe, brow furrowed, playing his part as if it were for real.

Later I went to see the PM to update him on the real world. I consciously had to jolt myself out of the 'worst-case scenario' mentality from the exercise, otherwise I might have given him a much more alarming sit-rep than required.

I took the chance to ask him about Dom's insistence on getting rid of Simon Stevens. It turns out the adviser wasn't speaking for his master at all. Standing in his gilded office behind the House of Commons, Boris said, 'On no account must we force him out. He's done a long stint, so he may want to go, but let him go in his own time.' That was my view exactly too, especially with coronavirus getting worse every day. It was a stark reminder of how little Cummings was representing the Prime Minister's agenda – and how important it is to speak to Boris himself. I find it astonishing that Boris gives so much power to someone with such a blatant disregard for his own agenda or instructions. There's no way any previous Prime Minister I've worked with would let it happen. I resolved not to listen to Cummings unless I knew he had the explicit backing of the boss.

I sent a birthday greeting to Sir Nicholas Soames. I share so many political views with the old grandee, who retired at the 2019 election. He used to call me 'Matty Moo Moos', including once on Twitter, where he achieved some unexpected, late-career fame. Parliament is less colourful now he's gone.

I told Cummings I'm getting worried about progress on our key manifesto commitments on the NHS. These pledges were central to our electoral credibility, not to mention his Vote Leave campaign. Annoyingly, I'm not getting any traction from the Treasury. 'I need them to play ball to visibly deliver on nurses and hospitals by 2024. I am pushing through official channels, but I need some drive from you,' I appealed.

His reply was a metaphorical shrug.

THURSDAY 13 FEBRUARY

Reshuffle day. Massive drama – Sajid Javid has resigned as Chancellor. Totally unexpected.

I wasn't really engaging with the various reshuffle comings and goings, knowing I wasn't likely to be moved. I was sitting in my office (on my director's chair with 'Hancock' across the back, a present from Pinewood Studios on a visit as Culture Secretary) with a team of public health officials when I suddenly realised everyone else was looking at their phones and muttering. I asked Emma what was going on.

'Sajid's resigned over his SpAds,' she told me.

'What? Over SpAds?' I replied in astonishment. Not the most diplomatic reaction in front of my own SpAds, who looked crestfallen. Head, desk. Feeling awful, I did some very hasty backpedalling, explaining that now he's resigned, they'll all lose their jobs anyway. 'That's just how it works when you're a SpAd – zero job security. You're only as safe as your principal,' I said, trying not to sound as if I don't care.

I hoped I made it clear how much I value them – which I really do – and they laughed it off, but I'm not sure they bought it. I felt bad – they are so loyal to me.

As for Sajid, there's history there. Last year, Cummings had one of his SpAds escorted out of Downing Street by a copper after accusing her of leaking information to the media – extraordinary chutzpah from someone who leaks at will – over something she vehemently denied. It was appalling behaviour and Sajid was rightly furious. Apparently Cummings tried to use the reshuffle to shore up his own power base by telling Sajid his remaining advisers would have to answer to No. 10 – i.e. him. Sajid told him to shove it – or words to that effect – and walked.

After the news broke, a few friends wished me luck, tipping me for the Treasury, given I started life as an economist at the Bank of England. Good of them, but now is no time to change Health Secretary, even if Boris were that way minded. In the event, he promoted Rishi to No. 11. No wonder he was so coy the other day – he must have known things were getting very strained between Sajid and Cummings.

My own ministerial team has emerged largely intact. Nadine Dorries thought she might be moved but sent a 'Whoop Whoop!' WhatsApp to everyone this afternoon confirming that she's staying put.

Jo Churchill stays too as the Public Health Minister, as does Ed Argar. Caroline Dinenage, who has been a terrific Minister of State for Social Care, is being replaced by Helen Whately. It's such a difficult portfolio, because you get all the scrutiny but, because social care is delivered by local authorities, you've got very few levers.

As the officials left the room at the end of the meeting, my advisers, Chris Wormald and David Williams stayed behind. The general view here is that Rishi will be easier to work with than Sajid, which is good, because I'm going to need Treasury firepower to get the forty hospitals programme moving.

Annoyingly, Cummings is still banning ministers from appearing on the *Today* programme. Now we're in a crisis, this is beyond ridiculous. We can't afford petty vendettas with the media right now. This morning the Prof very capably stood in as the government representative. He has statutory independence, so Cummings couldn't ban him even if he wanted to. He explained our focus on containment and isolation while numbers remain low, though he made clear we're preparing for the next phase. I was fleetingly grateful for Cummings's ban, or I'd have been on the show myself, trying to field a bunch of awkward questions about the reshuffle.

Away from political machinations, my scientific advisers are increasingly pessimistic. SAGE is now of the view that China has failed to contain coronavirus, but they're still against shutting things down here. They think travel restrictions within the UK won't help unless they're 'draconian and fully adhered to', while school closures would have to last weeks to do any good. Instead, they're backing campaigns to encourage people to behave responsibly. They warned that in the run-up to epidemics, before people start dying, there's always quite a lot of scepticism and inaction.

There's still a lot of noise about the reshuffle, which I'm trying to shut out. Gina sent me a firm message, telling me to focus on 'sorting coronavirus'. She's right.

Several of the Wuhan escapees at Arrowe Park went home today, leaving behind touching tributes to the NHS staff who looked after them so well.

FRIDAY 14 FEBRUARY

More Cummings-induced reshuffle fallout. Malicious briefing to the media that Rob Buckland at Justice threw one of his SpAds under the bus to keep his job rather than stand up to Dom and resign, Sajid-style. The SpAd concerned says it's nonsense. Understandably, Buckland, who's a thoroughly decent and mild-mannered type, is very upset. The outgoing SpAd asked if I'd ring Buckland to pacify him, which I did.

The Institute for Government has produced a pleasing little league table of who in government has spent longest in Cabinet. Gove's top, followed by Trade Secretary Liz Truss and me. If you look at continuous service, it's Liz and me, as Gove had a stint on the back benches when Theresa May – not his greatest fan – was in charge.

Jamie has been poached by Oliver Dowden, the new Culture Secretary, as his new SpAd. I'm gutted, but the move suits him. He's going to stay on until I find a replacement.

SATURDAY 15 FEBRUARY

Wuhan has been put into what the Chinese call 'wartime controls', with the authorities going house to house carting sick people off to quarantine centres. Hideous. However bad things get here, I can't see us doing that.

TUESDAY 18 FEBRUARY

PHE says our current approach of tracing all contacts of anyone who's infected is unsustainable. Apparently they can only cope with five new cases a week, which on average will mean 800 contacts. At a push this could be increased to fifty cases, but if we keep using the PHE tracing method it'll be completely hopeless once numbers start multiplying. This is infuriating since only a few weeks ago they told me they had the best system in the world. I've asked for advice on how we could scale up, but I wish they'd told me weeks ago.

There's better progress on other scientific fronts. JVT told me that of the nine confirmed UK cases, we have now sequenced the genome of seven. That means we have the genetic data to understand exactly what this virus is made of, which helps with testing, treatments and of course the vaccine. We are going to trial various antiretrovirals including Lopinavir and Ritonavir to see whether they could be useful. The project is called the Recovery Trial, run by Professor Peter Horby at Oxford. Recruitment starts tomorrow. My role in these trials is to ensure they're funded and protect them from pressure to call the results before they're clinically valid. The scientists can do the rest. JVT is very excited and proud of how fast it's been put together – and rightly so. Patients in China are being given an antimalarial drug called hydroxychloroquine, but there are no trial results of its effectiveness to justify using it here.

I'm still having to spend far too much time on cruise ships. The first 400 or so passengers of the *Diamond Princess* have finally been released. We're reluctantly sending the cavalry to get the Brits home. Raab messaged me a couple of days ago saying other foreign nationals were being rescued by their governments and if we didn't get our act together, our lot would be left behind. He suggested a shared charter with France and Italy, but that was a no-go. I asked the FCO if we'd tried the Americans, and it seems they declined to let us in on their extraction, so we're on our own. I talked to Boris and we agreed we should try to get the Brits to quarantine in Japan, but, perhaps understandably, the Japanese aren't keen.

Work to protect the most vulnerable – now formally called 'shielding' – proceeds at pace. Jenny Harries – who is tough as nails under that soft demeanour – is doing a great job.

Owen Paterson rang this evening asking about Randox. Apparently PHE is still refusing to engage. 'We are losing time,' he said, sounding understandably irritated. Given the situation we're in, it's ludicrous PHE isn't biting the hand off anyone offering help.

I got straight on the phone to PHE again to find out what is going on. It turns out they still haven't sent Randox what they need, despite me instructing them to do so three weeks ago. I'm furious and losing confidence in the organisation's ability to do anything at the urgency and scale required. Frustratingly, I don't have the power to enforce anything directly, even in a crisis, because of PHE's independence. I have to either persuade them or take the responsibility off them altogether.

A rare semi-night off this evening as I shlepped to the O2 in Greenwich for the Brit Awards. Inevitably I pitched up late because of work and missed the dinner. I was seated next to Ronnie Wood and told him I was ravenous. He looked at me rather pityingly and growled something about me obviously needing a pick-me-up. Reaching into his bag, he pulled out a package covered in tinfoil and started unwrapping it. I was already looking pretty pale due to lack of sleep and food;

now I was properly freaking out. Even for a Rolling Stone, Ronnie had a reputation as a hell-raiser, and I was thinking 'oh shit' as I wondered what substance he was about to produce with the cameras all around us. After some further rummaging around, with a grand flourish, he finally unveiled… a Babybel. It turned out that he has young twins and always carries some of the little cheeses with him in case they get peckish. It was exactly what I needed.

Cummings is hassling me again about Simon Stevens.

'Timing agreed?' he demanded.

No. You've been rumbled on this one.

WEDNESDAY 19 FEBRUARY

More discussions about what's in the battle plan. Are we really going to tell people we might shut schools or whole cities? Yes, I say: we might have to do this, so we have to prepare people, and for something as big as this, better a formal government document than briefings to the media – though with Cummings now engaged, you can never rule that out.

THURSDAY 20 FEBRUARY

The virus continues its global march. There's some evidence that measures to keep people apart in areas where they would normally mingle – on transport, in shops, on the streets etc. – are slowing the outbreak in both China and Hong Kong. The term being used is 'social distancing'.

FRIDAY 21 FEBRUARY

South Korea has reported its first death and has cracked down hard. They've closed kindergartens and community centres, sealed off nursing homes and banned rallies in Seoul. Italy has suddenly gone way further, quarantining 50,000 people in eleven municipalities, now called Red Zones. Schools are shut, sports and cultural events cancelled. Anyone breaching the rules can be fined €206 or get up to three months in prison. Wow! This is in Italy!

There is now enough data from around the world for our experts to modify the worst-case scenario assumptions we had based on flu. Professor Neil Ferguson, the Imperial College modelling supremo, gave his updates today. We'd asked him to look at four specific questions:

1. What proportion of the population could be infected with coronavirus?
2. What proportion of those will develop symptoms?
3. What proportion of the symptomatic will need hospital care?
4. And how many will need respiratory support?

His preliminary assumption is that 80 per cent of the population get infected. Of those, 50 per cent get sick, and, of those, 4 per cent go to hospital for an average of six to ten days. He thinks a quarter of hospital patients could need ventilators, which would create a massive supply issue. NHS hospitals aren't generally full of ventilators – normally only a small minority of patients have serious breathing problems.

The estimated death rate is very tentative but could be around 2.5 per cent.

All of this assumes we don't take any mitigation measures and that there are no treatments or vaccines, but the numbers still look horrible. No matter how fast we accelerate vaccines, there's no hope they'll be ready in time. So far, all the data seems to be pointing to the worst-case scenario, though I keep telling myself it's early days.

Amid all this, one of my colleagues sent me the details of a truly hideous non-Covid case involving one of his constituents, whose medical notes were mixed up by the hospital with someone of the same name. She was perfectly well mentally but sectioned in error and given electric shock therapy. Scandalously, she is now struggling to get her medical notes corrected, let alone win an apology. Jeez. It's truly astonishing and just awful. Blunders like this should *never* happen and we *must* improve transparency when there are mistakes.

SATURDAY 22 FEBRUARY

Thirty British and two Irish citizens from the *Diamond Princess* arrived at the Boscombe Down MoD base in Wiltshire and were bussed straight up to Arrowe Park. No horsemen in sight this time. We've now quarantined a total of 273 people from four flights. After the initial pandemonium on Merseyside, the system is working well.

SUNDAY 23 FEBRUARY

Took a call from a very agitated-sounding Jens Spahn, who told me about the news on TV about Italy. I checked my phone to see extraordinary aerial footage of ghost towns. Places that should be buzzing are now eerily lifeless, with everyone locked indoors. Italy's the new focus of the virus. It's now had 150 or so cases and three deaths. They even closed Venice carnival early, with police ordering revellers off the streets.

Meanwhile four of the *Diamond Princess* passengers have tested positive. I feel vindicated about going hard on quarantine. If we'd just let them disperse after bringing them back to the UK, who knows whether they would have stayed at home? Then we'd have had multiple super-spreaders. We've moved them from Arrowe Park into one of our designated coronavirus hospitals in Liverpool. The rest will be swabbed relentlessly till the end of their quarantine. I'm taking no chances.

I spent much of the day battling to get money for our manifesto commitments. Apparently the Treasury has been quibbling over the 'evidence' for our request. I reminded Steve Barclay, who replaced Rishi as the Chief Secretary to the Treasury and is responsible for the government's purse strings, that the Budget is less than three weeks away. Later I spoke to Rishi, who was much more receptive and seemed keen to get things sorted. Unless I keep up the pressure, all those extra hospitals and nurses we announced in such a blaze of publicity during the election campaign just won't materialise.

MONDAY 24 FEBRUARY

Cummings has finally realised that Brexit is no longer the big story and turned his attention to coronavirus. To show he means business, he's organising a daily 8 a.m. meeting in No. 10 for SpAds and officials, but in an act of total idiocy he's timed it so that it clashes with my morning meeting and involves many of the same people. He's made it very clear that he expects this to be the 'decision-making meeting' while everything else is just going through the motions. He has a complete contempt for elected politicians – the Prime Minister included – who he thinks just get in the way of the godlike technocrats he believes should run everything. (He used to call MPs 'flying monkeys' and absolutely relished his 2019 purge of Remainer MPs.)

His power grab has created immediate practical problems. I don't want to insist my team get into the office an hour earlier so we can hold our meeting ahead of his. I also don't want everyone to have to repeat meetings when they're so busy. But Cummings won't come to my meeting and won't have ministers to his. Meanwhile the Prof feels pulled in all directions. He says he will try to do both and then attend a third with the PM. What a farce. I told him it's vital he attends No. 10 meetings to make sure they don't decide anything mad, which is a very real possibility, especially since Cummings is in the habit of inviting a random selection of people according to his whims, including a revolving cast of professors, often statisticians, whom he hero-worships. My SpAds come back in despair.

Cummings and I both went to Exeter College at Oxford University, though he's a few years older than I am, so we didn't overlap. After I left, my old tutor had the idea of introducing us, as he thought we were both free-thinking Conservatives and might get on. It didn't work. While I put teamwork first, Cummings is very much a lone wolf, who makes no secret of his disdain for most other people. His contempt for anyone he considers less intelligent than he is means he has no qualms about burning anyone. When we were at Education together, he saw David Cameron's No. 10 as a nursery staffed by idiots who on no account should be listened to. His whole schtick was that departments should do their own thing. His view, emphasised at every opportunity, was that No. 10 only ever created trouble and should be bypassed and left out of the loop at all costs. Naturally now he's in No. 10 his theory of government has reversed. He dreams of nuking the entire Whitehall system and putting his beloved technocratic philosopher kings in charge of building something out of the ruins. Scratch the surface and it's just an old-fashioned power trip. He doesn't have the subtlety needed to be an effective chief of staff. His destructive approach might have helped get Brexit through but is not a way to run things in a real-world crisis. We need clear lines of accountability – but he hates that because then they wouldn't run to him.

TUESDAY 25 FEBRUARY

Another repatriation headache brewing in Tenerife, where hundreds of British tourists are stuck in a hotel that's gone into quarantine. Police are guarding the four-star Costa Adeje Palace hotel, and nobody is allowed to leave, after a visiting Italian doctor tested positive for the virus. Turns out he came from Lombardy, where the outbreak is still raging. I'm now adamant that we stop these repatriations: we can't become the travel agent of last resort.

Home Secretary Priti Patel is stressing there could be riots if we go too hard on social restrictions. In every COBRA meeting, the Home Office talks about the work they're doing to ensure we are ready if there's a massive backlash and people literally take to the streets or just systematically ignore the rules. My view is that this is very unlikely: people are understandably getting scared and by and large will do what they're asked.

Owen Paterson is getting increasingly grumpy that PHE isn't giving Randox what it needs to develop a test. 'It's now nineteen days since PHE last contacted Randox at your request,' he huffed. I get why he's so cross. Gordon Sanghera is having the same sort of problems. Why? Because certain senior public health officials are absolutely allergic to anything involving the private sector. Evidently they'd rather risk lives than set aside these ideological objections. I must bust through this. It's absurd.

THURSDAY 27 FEBRUARY

Owen messaged to say PHE has now outright refused Randox's request for samples. I've put it on the agenda for tomorrow's big meeting to instruct them to go ahead with all companies who need samples – and set a date. No such sniffiness from the Chinese, who are snapping up the company's services. If this attitude towards our life sciences continues, we're stuffed.

More cheerfully, I had a great breakfast with former presidential hopeful Jeb Bush and a group of newly elected MPs. I've got to know Jeb quite well over the years, initially through Michael Gove as fellow education reformers. Son and brother to former Presidents, Jeb is thoughtful, incisive and, at 6ft 3in., towers over me. He's a big fan of British politics ('PMQs – I love that show!'), so I put together a breakfast of a dozen or so new Tory backbenchers in a small hotel near Westminster to talk about the future of the liberal right. A whole hour away from dealing with the pandemic was such a relief.

Predictably, we're under heavy pressure to use the RAF to evacuate Tenerife. Having slept on it, I'm still adamant we don't. I phoned Shapps, nervous that he'd want to push it, but he totally agrees and sounded relieved that we see eye to eye. The FCO folded in too, and as if by magic a big headache went away. We told people there would be no more rescue flights. Somewhat to my surprise, everyone seemed to just accept it. Amazing!

Back home there's been a major outbreak at a Nike conference in Edinburgh, where at least twenty-five people are thought to have contracted the virus. Health Protection Scotland are going to do full contact tracing for everyone who tested positive there. The Scottish government is being really prickly. I get the impression that Scottish Health Secretary Jeane Freeman sees me as some awful English Tory rather than an ally in a joint battle to prevent a pandemic. We can't afford this kind of divisive nonsense.

In my red box tonight was a copy of the draft battle plan I commissioned. The team has basically pulled together everything we need to do to be ready. It sets out that we might have to lock down, close schools and have everyone in a household with a case isolate at home. It's an extraordinary document, but it's completely necessary for getting people ready for what might have to happen.

In terms of the government machine, the hardest part may be dealing with the devolved administrations. Given that we're one country, I think it's nuts that they are going to take their own lead on domestic public health policy. That kind of devolution is all very well for something like fighting obesity, but not for a pandemic. Unfortunately, there's not much I can do about it: they have these powers, all set out in the 1984 Act. Back then, the decision takers would have been the Secretaries of State for Scotland, Wales and Northern Ireland, all sitting in the same Cabinet. Now it's the devolved governments. Those who framed the Act could not have foreseen what's happening now, but it's deeply frustrating.

After much negotiation, my team managed to get them to back my joint action plan – as long as we put the emblems of Scotland, Wales and Northern Ireland on the front of the document. Eye roll. If that's what it takes to keep them on board, fine. I respect the fact that health services are devolved, but a pandemic does not respect boundaries no matter how historic.

In the plan we've set out scenarios ranging from mild pandemic to 'severe prolonged pandemic as experienced in 1918'. Measures will need to be mixed and matched depending on the course the virus takes. At the peak, a fifth of the workforce could be off sick. This will have knock-on effects, such as the police potentially having to focus only on serious crime. The plan says life should continue 'as normally as possible', though of course it's impossible to say yet how normal this 'normally' will be. It also sets out stark new powers to allow 'medical professionals, public health professionals and the police to … detain and direct individuals in quarantined areas at risk or suspected of having the virus'. This is harsh stuff, but the powers already exist in Scotland and my Arrowe Park experience tells me it's needed.

The plan also identifies what we need to do to protect the NHS, including getting retired medics back into service and making sure that people who don't need to be in hospital can leave. Penny Mordaunt, Cabinet Office Minister responsible for policy on handling deaths, decided to include the precautions from the exercise two weeks ago: that councils need to review their capacity in morgues and crematoriums to deal with a possible increase in bodies.

Perhaps unsurprisingly, given the shocking nature of the content, it's been a huge effort to get No. 10 to agree to publish the document. Thankfully they're now on board. We need to publish next week or it will be too late.

FRIDAY 28 FEBRUARY

Ben Wallace is still being bombarded with requests for the RAF to ferry around Covid patients and is getting cross. This morning No. 10 asked him to fly a single individual from Northern Ireland to Newcastle for testing. He said no. Quite right too. There's no reason why the patient couldn't be tested and treated in Northern Ireland. The RAF is not some kind of private jet service.

Today the sad news of the first British death from Covid: a man who'd been on the *Diamond Princess*. He died in Japan, but I feel it's a wake-up call for the UK.

We've also confirmed the first case of the virus passed on inside the UK. The patient is a man from Surrey – from Jeremy Hunt's constituency in fact – who hadn't been abroad at all in the recent past.

While I get more and more worried, No. 10 are still trying to protect the PM from saying anything publicly about the virus. The Downing Street machine has been pushing back all week on him chairing a COBRA, so I decided to short-circuit them and called him direct. We really need his authority now. When he returned my call, I was in a classroom at Burton End primary school in my West Suffolk constituency. The kids got very excited when I looked at the screen and said, 'I'm sorry, it's the Prime Minister. I have to speak to him.'

'Boris,' I said, 'you've got to show you're engaged on this. You have to chair a COBRA and we have to end the stupid ban on going on the *Today* programme.'

A few minutes later, I got a call from No. 10 asking me to return to London immediately for a formal meeting. On my way back to Downing Street, feeling like a broken record, I pushed for an immediate

COBRA. Once again I was rebuffed and told we needed to give the secretariat time to get the correct papers ready etc. etc. Unnecessary red tape, meaning it will have to wait until Monday. However, I did succeed in persuading the boss to give a short interview at No. 10 this evening underlining that the virus is 'the government's top priority'. Progress.

I was feeling quite good about all this when, to my dismay, I heard a colleague on the airwaves revealing contingency plans to set up a morgue in Hyde Park. Crikey. While I'm very anxious that people take the threat of the virus seriously, we don't need to scare them with visions of corpses piling up everywhere.

SATURDAY 29 FEBRUARY

I woke to a text from Oliver Letwin saying he thinks we need to close the borders: all air and seaports. Despite having worked with him incredibly closely when he ran the Cabinet Office under David Cameron, I'd hardly spoken to him since he was unceremoniously booted out of the Commons last year in the Cummings purge of Remainer rebels. I was pleased to hear from him. He's seen his fair share of crises and is far shrewder than his public image, so I was interested to hear his thoughts.

'Would you still take that view if you knew it was contrary to epidemiological advice?' I asked. Basically, yes: he called me immediately, telling me in no uncertain terms that we needed to get on with it.

At heart Letwin is a Tory loyalist who's not in the business of making life unnecessarily difficult for the government, despite the way he was treated. His advice troubled me. I asked the Prof, who knows Letwin from Ebola days, to call him to explain why he's still advising against closing the borders, which seemed the best way of dealing with it, not least since I have my own doubts about whether the experts are right.

We've had three more confirmed cases, taking the total to twenty-three. Two had travelled back from Italy recently and the third from Asia. So far we've administered a total of 10,483 tests, but PHE's capacity is still growing far too slowly. Incredibly frustrating.

Later I was at a friend's wedding at Shakespeare's Globe theatre, by the Thames. I hate being out of contact at the best of times, but this was in an underground room with no mobile reception, which was seriously stressful. I kept having to dart upstairs and look at my phone to check nothing drastic had happened, not least because I'm doing the morning media round tomorrow.

One message was from the Prof, warning me that there have been a series of new cases, including a British doctor who caught it while overseas. His colleagues have all been taken off duty. Luckily he hasn't been seeing patients.

MARCH 2020

David Cameron texted, saying I needed to explain in more detail why we aren't already introducing restrictions we say we might need soon. He's got a point. I told him that it's down to clinical advice – which is that we shouldn't go too soon for fear that people will only put up with measures for so long – and the fact that what we'll have to do is so huge. If your child's school is going to be closed, if you can't see your family and friends or go out for a drink or a meal, you need to prepare yourself psychologically as well as practically. I did my best to get this across on the Sunday media round, using my slot on *Sophy Ridge* and *Andrew Marr* to talk about the action plan we're releasing tomorrow. (We're avoiding using the term 'battle plan', which is probably a good thing – although I think some wartime allusions are valuable.) It's a balancing act. When I talked to Marr off air before the show, he seemed very worried about the virus and said he just wanted to get as much information to viewers as possible. When we went live, the questions weren't easy, but they were respectful and straight. The news headlines are that we might lock down whole cities. It's shocking but true, and I think Marr himself was pretty taken aback. This is why we have to tell people now: to get them ready.

Meanwhile we're telling everyone to wash their hands more frequently and for longer and encouraging parents to get their kids to sing 'happy birthday' twice while they're washing, to make sure they do it for long enough. I've been delivering the happy birthday recommendation with my usual enthusiasm, but what I really wanted people to sing was the national anthem. Sadly, I was overruled by the system – who exactly I'll never know – as the collective view seems to be that happy birthday is 'less divisive'. I'd love to know who actually made this decision. Since when is the national anthem controversial? Sigh.

Our case total has hit thirty-nine, three of them contacts of an already identified case, meaning there's clear transmission now. We've also had more positive tests in travellers coming back from Italy.

Meanwhile another pathetic response from PHE on why private testing is being held up. They now claim everything depends on systems that local NHS labs can use 'with the least disruption' and 'without the need for further equipment purchase'. What? We're going to have to purchase masses of additional equipment! They have no idea how big this is going to be – and they're meant to be the public health outfit. The blame game between PHE and the NHS is exhausting and there's absolutely no acknowledgement of the role the private sector can play in expanding testing quickly. It's maddening. What's worse is they ignore direct instructions to go faster – and being technically independent of ministers, they can do that. I'm increasingly thinking that we need to take the task off them.

MONDAY 2 MARCH
The PM chaired his first COBRA on coronavirus at 9 a.m. The main room and side rooms were packed to the rafters with ministers, officials and SpAds. The key business was signing off the action plan, which the civil service turned around in record time. I spent the afternoon ringing round newspaper editors to pre-brief them in confidence. They were all spectacularly reasonable and knew they had a part to play in getting us through this crisis.

After COBRA there was a lot of discussion about handshaking.

Should we still be doing it? The clinical advice is that it doesn't make any difference. David Halpern thinks the best way to change behaviour is to suggest a substitute. Japanese-style bows? Indian namaste? Bumping elbows? Not sure which but sounds a good idea.

I had another call with Tedros. We discussed how the UK might be able to help the WHO. I urged him to declare a global pandemic – a major step up from a PHEIC – but he demurred. He thinks containment is working in China and the whole situation 'might still be OK'. Seriously? Has he seen Italy? I got the impression that he may welcome the pressure, as it strengthens his hand dealing with the Chinese. Meanwhile Patrick Vallance reckons there's a roughly one in five chance of the reasonable worst-case scenario happening here. Even though he doesn't have the data to give more than an impression, that is still alarmingly high. Tedros appears to be complacent about the scale of the threat we face.

TUESDAY 3 MARCH

My natural style is highly enthusiastic and positive, prompting my old boss George Osborne to liken me to Tigger from Winnie the Pooh, saying there are too many Eeyores in Westminster. I couldn't agree more – there are – but I know I have to change my tone now. I have to respond in a way that fits the seriousness of the situation, but it's not easy. I believe it's vital to play it straight with people, even if I the way I talk grates with them a little. This is not a time for rhetorical flourishes.

I headed over to No. 10 to brief Cabinet on our plans, then helped prep the PM for the big launch. The plan was to have Vallance and the Prof standing at lecterns beside him in the oak-panelled dining room. Something this important needs the stamp of prime ministerial authority, bolstered by his top scientific wingmen. I sat in the front row next to Neil Ferguson, who coughed a few times throughout the hour-long event. It's now impossible to hear anyone cough without instantly thinking of the virus. I shuffled away in my seat – not that a few centimetres would make any difference if he did have Covid.

It's already clear that the hardest judgements will be where the scientific advice is most ambiguous. There's still no consensus on the handshaking thing. Before the press conference, Cummings was adamant we should advise against it. Lee Cain, once a *Mirror* journalist and now Boris's director of communications, argued that we can't advise against handshaking without saying what we would do instead, and then we'll be parodied for whatever we suggest. The scientists say it doesn't really matter. I don't have a strong view but pointed out that whatever we advised, we'd obviously have to do ourselves, and I'm not sure I want to go round bowing at people. In the end, the boss decided to go along with continuing handshaking. Unfortunately, when the anticipated question came, he was a little over-enthusiastic, gushing about recently visiting a hospital where there were 'actually a few coronavirus patients' and he 'shook hands with everybody'. He obviously didn't really mean everybody. But unfortunately, that's what he said.

This was far from ideal, especially as Cummings casually informed us a few hours later that the boss 'thinks he might be coming down with some sort of flu'. Apparently the PM has been bumbling around Downing Street asking people for paracetamol.

'Be prepared for the PM telling the Cabinet that he thinks he's got corona, so that will be the story,' Cummings said. Crikey.

'Ideally he would not do that,' said Jack Doyle, the Prime Minister's press secretary, with commendable sangfroid. Apparently Boris had said, only half in jest, that he'd probably caught the virus when he was shaking hands with everyone on the hospital visit.

'My humour radar is off – is this a joke?' asked one of my team.

'Um, sadly not,' I replied, though it had got me thinking. What would we do if he did go down? Can the system cope in the crisis if the boss is suddenly out of the picture? I don't want to appear over-enthusiastic about the idea, so I'll ask Wormald to check Sedwill has a plan.

When I got back to the department, they told me that SAGE had updated the reasonable worst-case scenario with the latest international data and reduced the maximum number of deaths from 820,000 to a still horrific 520,000 out of 53.5 million people showing symptoms.

Around 390,000 may be in critical care with such bad breathing problems they need ventilators. These numbers are huge – there's no way the NHS could cope.

One major problem with our forecasting is that the NHS can't seem to answer the question 'How many beds have you got?' Every time I ask them, I get a different version of 'I don't know'. This is hopeless. They explain that there's lots of different ways to answer the question: fully staffed beds? Emergency beds? Recuperation beds? At what time of day? I said to tell us the numbers according to the different definitions – and then we can work out which definition is the most useful. But it doesn't really matter because it's an order of magnitude lower than 390,000 on any measure.

Late this evening Simon Stevens circulated a worrying confidential alert saying that one of the twenty-two new cases identified is a man at Withington Community Hospital who was already seriously ill in the ICU with cancer and diabetes. He's now in a critical condition and needs to be moved to another hospital because the unit has to be decontaminated. As many as thirty-six doctors and nurses who have been looking after him have been sent home to self-isolate. There's a similar problem with an elderly lady at King's College Hospital in south London. She needs to be transferred elsewhere but may not survive the journey. This is just a foretaste of the crises hospitals will soon face on a daily basis. Staff availability is going to be at least as big a problem as beds.

Helen Whately is worried about preparations in care homes, messaging me this afternoon saying that there is a 'growing nervousness' about the capacity of the system to cope. She's been rooting around for any existing pandemic contingency plans in the sector and has only found two: Hertfordshire and Essex.

'My opinion is that they are inadequate,' she told me bluntly. She says Robert Jenrick, the Communities Secretary, has 'similar concerns'.

'The Essex document says providers are required by the CQC [Care Quality Commission] to have plans in place to provide safe care in the event of a pandemic. And, during a flu pandemic, directors of adult social services need to know the effectiveness of providers' plans, emerging risks and capacity to meet demand. That's basically it. Their plan,' she reported gloomily.

It's nowhere near good enough.

'Can you possibly put some serious drive into getting them to a credible position?' I replied. Seems to me we need to do a lot of work here.

She says it's taken her a fortnight just to find these two solitary documents and get a meeting in the diary with the chief social worker (tomorrow).

'You're right. It needs a rocket under it,' she said.

At least there's no more talk of Boris being ill. Hopefully he found some paracetamol, which is in increasingly short supply. In a disturbing sign of the kind of pandemic protectionism we may be about to see, India has just banned the export of certain key ingredients for painkillers. Steve Oldfield, who's in charge of NHS supplies, has been doing an industry ring-round to check what stocks we have. Steve was brought in to prepare for Brexit, and thanks to his work we have an exceptionally good understanding of what medicines we have in the country and what the supply chains look like. There's no immediate issue – he says we have around 500 million paracetamol – but we'll need to keep a very close eye.

WEDNESDAY 4 MARCH

My comms team thinks we need to reinforce the handwashing message and suggested I make a demonstration video. Chipping in, Jim Bethell helpfully suggested I do it 'singing something'.

'Maybe "What do you sing when you wash your hands?" can be a thing. Can we recruit influencers to support it?' he enthused.

Warming to his theme, he revealed – without apparent embarrassment – that he sings the Human League classic 'Don't You Want Me Baby?' when he washes his hands.

I made a mental note never to go to the bathroom at the same time as him. Thank God for Jamie, who quickly killed the idea, pointing out – not quite in these words – that I'd look a complete tit and it will just get parodied.

NHS England has declared coronavirus their highest grade of emergency, a Level 4 alert. It means Simon Stevens – still very much in post, despite Cummings's best efforts – takes command of all health service resources in England. Guidance for hospitals tells them to 'assume they will need to look after Covid-19 cases in due course'. Everyone in intensive care with respiratory infections must now be tested. There will be too many patients to treat on specialist Covid units, so we've said people can be cared for in wider infectious disease wards. Italy, which is a fair way ahead of us on the curve of their epidemic, is to close all schools and universities, while Germany has declared an epidemic and has shifted from containment to mitigation.

Cummings has been stuck at home today throwing up from what he described as a 'toddler bug'. I was rigorously on-message, telling him to self-isolate if necessary.

THURSDAY 5 MARCH

First UK deaths – a horrible landmark. Thank God we have a carefully set out protocol in place, managed by my lead crisis official Emma Reed, for how to handle such sensitive news. The death we announced was a woman in her seventies who had been in and out of hospital with various conditions. She tested positive for the virus, although we don't yet know whether it was the direct cause of her death. Later in the day a man in his eighties died in Milton Keynes. He had recently returned from a cruise.

At a Commons hearing, the Prof said that we may soon need to move from 'contain' to 'delay', banning large events, closing schools and working from home. SAGE is advising us to plan for that in one to two weeks.

I don't attend SAGE, but the Prof, who co-chairs the meetings with Patrick Vallance, gives me a run-through of the key points so I don't have to wait for the official minutes. What I value most from him is unedited, crystal-clear advice on what the very best scientific evidence says.

I'm worried that there are moves afoot to suspend Parliament because of the risk of MPs and staff getting infected. I'm completely opposed to this idea: we can't just shut down democratic accountability in this way. Parliament sat right through the Second World War. We're not closing because of a virus. I called the Leader of the House of Commons, Jacob Rees-Mogg, who strongly agreed. He and I talked about how to head it off at the pass and he's going to discuss with the Speaker.

Helen Whately says PPE supply to care homes is 'still all over the place'. I told her we have to get PPE to wherever it's needed, not just hospitals. The challenge is logistics. The supply chain company that delivers PPE has never seen so much demand and they're really struggling.

In the evening, I went to do *Question Time* in Tunbridge Wells. The non-political panellist was Dr Xand van Tulleken, the daytime TV doctor and health celeb. My children know him from the CBBC series *Operation Ouch!* We did a selfie video in the green room before the show and he very generously told the kids I was doing a great job and that they should listen to their dad's advice. Praise indeed and kind of him. Here's hoping they listen to Dr Xand – not holding my breath! I took the opportunity to ask his professional opinion on handshaking. He made an excellent point, which I think is the answer to this conundrum. He said he'd moved to the elbow bump because, even though there's no evidence either way about handshaking passing it on, it's a reminder not to get too close and that things aren't normal. After the press conference screw-up on this on Tuesday, I think that's wise.

FRIDAY 6 MARCH
Nadine Dorries might have the virus. She rang to tell me she's taken herself into isolation and has been feeling 'a bit peaky' since yesterday. She's very worried, and to be honest so am I, not least because yesterday she went to a No. 10 reception to mark International Women's Day. Boris and Carrie, who is pregnant, were there, as was Liz Truss.

A Health Minister going down with the virus and infecting other key government figures would not be ideal.

It reinforces the urgency of developing a vaccine and getting testing going properly. Alok Sharma, the Business Secretary, and I have found another £46 million from our various science budgets for research to accelerate vaccines and rapid tests. The private sector is going to be critical. Our technical team have started talking to Vallance, Halpern and PHE about an app to help people avoid coming into contact with anyone carrying the virus. They'll report back early next week on what may be possible. Doubtless other countries will be looking into this too: it's simply not realistic for quangos to track and contact millions of people without a serious upgrade in technology.

Meanwhile there's another cruise ship in trouble. This one's called the *Grand Princess* and is languishing off the coast of San Francisco with more than 100 British people on board. There have been twenty-one positive tests so far, though we don't know how many of those are our nationals. Haunted by the saga over the *Diamond Princess*, the Americans are keen to dispatch our lot back to Britain forthwith. The two Emmas are getting exasperated by cruise ships.

I'm thrilled that the PM has signed off David Williams's promotion to Second Permanent Secretary at the department. I stood over Boris in his little study in No. 10 to make sure it happened. This means we won't let our manifesto comments and other essential non-Covid work slacken off.

SATURDAY 7 MARCH

There's a crisis looming with ventilators. We have nowhere near enough. It would be great to boost domestic manufacture, but these are not machines that any old company can knock out: they're seriously sophisticated bits of medical kit. They also need to be operated by trained staff, otherwise they can do more harm than good. If the worst comes to the worst, we may need to put out advice on how to care for a critically ill relative at home, a terrifying prospect for most people. I'm thinking of announcing a competition to encourage businesses to come up with innovative ways of making ventilators quickly. Companies love this kind of challenge. I ran it past Simon Stevens, who seemed keen.

International travel is near enough grinding to a halt, yet somehow there are still a lot of planes in the sky. I was wondering why it seemed to be business as usual up there. It turns out that airlines are flying empty planes around Europe to make sure they don't lose their landing slots, because of some ridiculous EU 'use it or lose it' rule which we automatically adopted post-Brexit. So while we bang on about the importance of net zero, we have a load of aircraft with no passengers in their usual holding patterns over our cities belching out carbon emissions just so they can still land in their normal spots when all this is over. Ridiculous. It's not my area, so I spoke to Grant Shapps and raised it with Cummings.

Cummings replied that the PM's attitude would be that this is an emergency and we should do what we think is best, not worry about EU rules that have clear negative effects in such a crisis. He's asked Grant to 'consider', which in Cummings-speak means 'sort it out pronto'.

I took a few hours off today and thought it would be fun to take the kids to Planet Laser in Bury St Edmunds for a bit of light relief. It involves charging around in the dark in a 'battle suit' firing lasers at other players. I was looking forward to forgetting about coronavirus for an hour or so, but no such luck: it turned out that one of the games is called Infection. Every time a player's laser hit one of the other players, they would get 'infected' with a disease. In between attempts to dodge the fictional virus, I kept having to dart out of the arena to respond to urgent messages about the real one. Weird.

Later I had a constructive chat with Jeane Freeman, who despite my earlier misgivings was sensible enough. Coordinating our response with the devolved administrations is going to be critical, and we agreed that I should go up there soon to discuss in person.

Sporting bodies are starting to cancel overseas fixtures. Ireland v.

Italy in the Six Nations, due this weekend, has already been canned. Next month's Chinese Grand Prix is also kaput, as are football matches in northern Italy. Experts here still aren't recommending it, which meant that Boris and Carrie went to the England v. Wales game at Twickenham. England just squeaked a three-point win.

SUNDAY 8 MARCH

People have started panic buying. They're loading up their shopping trolleys with things like pasta, long-life milk and loo roll. As the Cabinet minister in charge of food, George Eustice has been doing his best to calm things down, telling people that nothing is running out and there's no need to stockpile, but there's a risk that even talking about it makes it worse. We roped Vallance in to reinforce the message, but I'm not sure it worked. I get where people are coming from. There's a pandemic looming and who knows how long it will last or what will happen? Hoarding loo roll is entirely rational behaviour. When the shit's hitting the fan in every other respect, who wants to be down to their last square? It all reminds me of when Mervyn King was Governor of the Bank of England and described withdrawing cash from a bank in the banking crisis as 'rational' – an accurate answer to an impossible question that was both entirely correct and incredibly counterproductive at the same time. Feeling a bit sheepish, we checked through our kitchen cupboards at home, and while we didn't do anything to exacerbate what's being called #toiletpapercrisis on social media, we did order a huge sack of rice.

In a very minor victory, this evening I successfully killed off what would have been a very unhelpful *Daily Mail* front page tomorrow. Sounding slightly panicked, Jamie messaged me saying they were planning to run something completely 'batshit' calling for temperature screening of every single passenger arriving from Italy. I got straight on the phone to the editor Geordie Greig and told him that SAGE has specifically told us NOT to do this, not only because it would require colossal resources but because it would be a total waste of time due to the long incubation period. If we need to stop travel, we will stop travel. Geordie's very reasonable and thankfully saw sense. The media are being very responsible at the moment.

MONDAY 9 MARCH

Jim Bethell's appointment finally came through as my Lords Minister. He's been the whip for a year now and done a brilliant job. I got the appointment over the line after talking to Boris direct. Having someone of Jim's calibre with full ministerial authority will be a real boost – and the team love him. We celebrated with a quick cup of tea and briefing with Chris Wormald. So much to do.

The financial markets are getting spooked. No surprise that the expectation is that we're heading for a global recession. The FTSE dropped nearly 8 per cent, its biggest one-day fall since 2008. Rishi and I talked about the economy. It's the bond market that I'm most worried about. The old Clinton-era joke that there's nothing to fear more than the bond market is true again. So long as the Bank of England can buy bonds through quantitative easing to cover the huge amount we're going to have to borrow, we'll be fine, but there's a limit to how long that can go on – and there'll be one hell of a mopping-up exercise afterwards.

The *Evening Standard* splashed that we're going to shut down London. I've no idea where they got the story, but it's not massively wide of the mark. All the same, it's not ideal at this point and will have contributed to the jittery markets. Of course we're thinking about it – London is ahead of the rest of the country in terms of cases – but we're not there yet.

At another Downing Street press conference, the Prof warned that within the next ten to fourteen days the government will advise anyone who has even mild symptoms to self-isolate for a week. For now, the number of cases is still so low that it's very unlikely a cough equals coronavirus, but it won't be long before that changes.

The FCO has advised against all but essential travel to Italy after Giuseppe Conte, the Prime Minister, extended the lockdown over the weekend to cover the whole of the Lombardy region and fourteen northern provinces beyond. At the same time as we've banned people flying out to infected areas, there are thousands coming back from the very same places. We can't stop Brits coming home, but I don't think we're doing enough to make sure they're not bringing the disease with them.

In my box this evening was a scientific briefing containing a dire warning about how bad hospital bed shortages could get. It suggests the NHS could have a deficit of 150,000 beds and 9,000 ICU spaces. Stark.

TUESDAY 10 MARCH

Nadine has the virus. She rang me around 9 p.m. this evening to tell me she's tested positive. Her voice was trembling and I don't really blame her: it's such an unknown quantity. Most of all she was worried about her mum, who lives with her, as she knows how dangerous it is for elderly people. I told her to look after herself and not to worry about work and tried to reassure her that she'll be fine – but really, who knows?

Her ninth-floor office has been sealed off as if it's some kind of crime scene and PHE's contact tracers are trying to find anyone she's seen since developing symptoms. Luckily I'm in the clear. Thank God she started self-isolating a few days ago.

I called No. 10, then Jamie, to stress that it will be a really big story and we agreed to announce the news tomorrow in as calm as possible a way, so as not to cause panic. Unfortunately, our carefully laid plans were fairly swiftly derailed by Steve Swinford at *The Times*, who got wind of the story and is running it on the front page tomorrow. A Health Minister getting Covid is going to make everyone at Westminster extremely nervy.

Health Secretaries are usually tightly contained to NHS and care matters, but this pandemic is starting to drag me into all sorts of unexpected fields of government. We're getting a load of flak for allowing outdoor events to go ahead. Gatherings of 1,000 people or more have been banned in seven German states, including Berlin, and there are variations on the theme across Europe. In Ireland, they've even cancelled parades for St Patrick's Day next week. Scotland is considering going it alone and banning large gatherings. That would immediately scupper the UK-wide approach we are trying to follow and Boris will hate it.

The problem is that SAGE is not yet in favour. It's a classic political bind, stuck between the intuitively obvious and the scientific advice – not for the first time. The central scientific argument is that large events aren't actually where most infections are passed on, and if we lock down too early we may not be able to sustain it. Plus, these are huge decisions with massive cost, intrusion and pain: the sort no one wants to take. But we've said we're going to be guided by the science, so that's that. There's been a lot of speculation about the Cheltenham Festival, which usually attracts several hundred thousand people over three days, with a large Irish contingent. It's not our call – it's DCMS (Department for Digital, Culture, Media and Sport) territory – and based on PHE advice they've decided it's going ahead as planned.

When it comes to older people, the science is unambiguous: we're now advising anyone over seventy to be extremely careful. When I explained this to MPs, Theresa May cornered me afterwards and quietly asked me if I'm 'deliberately targeting older people'. I had to explain that it's not me targeting these people – it's the virus!

The readout from SAGE was sobering. They now estimate that the UK probably has 5,000–10,000 cases, up to twenty times the recorded figure. Transmission is well under way both in hospitals and beyond. Analysing samples is a research priority, and the scientists are as frustrated as I am at PHE's sloth. I've instructed Duncan Selbie, the chief executive, to produce plans for how he will get testing up from 1,000 tests a week to 10,000. He says he gets it. I don't care who does these tests – just that they're fast and accurate.

The latest modelling suggests the UK is four to five weeks behind Italy but on a similar curve, meaning that without effective mitigation, the peak is probably ten to fourteen weeks away.

The panic buying is spreading to pharmacies. A friend who's on maternity leave texted me at lunchtime today saying there was 'pandemonium' in Boots. Apparently people are stripping the shelves bare of antibacterial handwash and going to the till repeatedly to get round limits on purchases. She said the shop was almost out of paracetamol as well. Retailers need to get a grip before we run short of basic items.

I got home at a reasonable hour – about 8 p.m. After a quick supper I went to my home office to work through the box. I love that room, especially the deep burgundy colour, which makes it feel like a cocoon. I've got everything I need set out on a lovely old refurbished teak school science bench. It's important to me: I spend a lot of time in there.

WEDNESDAY 11 MARCH

Budget Day. Poor Rishi – this should have been his big moment, but the whole thing was completely overshadowed by Covid, and his Budget already feels out of date. It's obvious that the pandemic is going to have a massive economic impact. He's already put £12 billion into fighting the virus, with more to come. There is support for businesses hit by virus restrictions; a guarantee of statutory sick pay for anyone isolating; and more money for the NHS, which he promised would get 'whatever resources it needs' to get us through the crisis. I saw him just after he'd given the statement, and said I was sorry Covid had overshadowed his big day. To his great credit, he wasn't remotely bothered, being much more worried about the economy than his ego. It reminds me of a conversation I had with him just before the reshuffle, when there was a rumour one or the other of us would be asked to take over a new Business and Infrastructure Department. I said I'd rather stay at Health. He said he'd rather stay as Chief Secretary to the Treasury – a behind-the-scenes but powerful job. Neither of us had any idea he'd come out of the reshuffle as Chancellor. It was only two weeks ago, but it feels like an age.

Tedros finally declared Covid a global pandemic, the first ever caused by a coronavirus. The packed stands at Cheltenham aren't ideal, not to mention tonight's Champions League game at Anfield between Liverpool and Atletico Madrid, with thousands of fans flying in from Spain. Needless to say, we are getting grief. Some people seem to blame me personally for the virus, which is weird. If the scientific advice wasn't clear, we might think about the tricky optics and take a political decision to ban these kinds of events. As it is, the advice is unchanged and it's emphatic.

At 7 p.m. I updated the Commons on our response to the WHO announcement. I was able to confirm we're keeping Parliament open, with modifications to the way we work to make it as safe as possible. Jacob and I have been sorting this out behind the scenes. The Speaker is understandably worried, especially after Nadine's positive test, but there are sensible things we can do, such as cancelling visitors. He agreed with us that it's vital democracy keeps functioning. I asked the Prof to phone him to advise on risks and precautions. Thank God his predecessor as Speaker John Bercow isn't in charge or there would be all sorts of grandstanding and histrionics.

After my statement I went to No. 10 to see the PM. On my way into his office, I passed Cummings, who was sitting at his desk a couple of yards from the door to the PM's outer office. He looked ashen-faced. 'Have you seen the latest modelling?' he asked me. 'Yes,' I replied. 'And it matches what we're seeing on the ground and in the hospitals.' As a self-confessed data obsessive, he seemed genuinely shocked. Perhaps the machine will finally swing into action. Now Cummings is finally concentrating on what data we do have – as I've been doing for weeks – he can see what we're dealing with.

Boris is going to hold a press conference tomorrow. The media is obsessing over whether he's been in close contact with Nadine and therefore could have caught Covid. He says not, so Whitty has confirmed he doesn't have to self-isolate.

With things deteriorating like this, I should feel terrible, but I realised tonight that I was feeling something else: relief, because others are finally grasping the seriousness of the situation. It no longer feels as if it's all on my shoulders. It seems a lifetime ago that I stood there at PMQs aghast because Covid wasn't mentioned once.

THURSDAY 12 MARCH

The Prof called early to say we need to raise the risk level from moderate to high. He thinks we now need to move from the 'contain' phase to 'delay'. He's been talking to the Scottish, Welsh and Northern Irish CMOs and they all agree. The plan is to announce it at a press conference.

The Prof was very straight with me and my team about what this means for us personally. 'We're all going to get infected,' he said. 'It's just a matter of whether that happens before or after we have a vaccine.'

Afterwards, I went to No. 10 to help the PM draft his words. He was attacking the keyboard – thump, thump, thud – amending the draft he'd been served up by the civil service. He added more of a warning of dark days ahead and injected more empathy, but there was no gloss to put on it.

'I must level with you, the British public: many more families are going to lose loved ones before their time,' is what he said. Chilling words. Boris finds the upbeat so much easier, so I really felt for him as he tried to get the tone right. That said, he loves to imagine himself as his hero Churchill, and this is our war. In a classic verbal flourish, he declared that the aim is to 'squash that sombrero' – i.e. flatten the rising curve of cases.

While the Prime Minister was standing before the nation declaring we're doing everything possible to save lives, PHE has advised we stop all contact tracing. They've basically given up, overwhelmed by the number of cases. They claim the growth in tests and contact tracers can never rise exponentially, as cases will, and there's now so much spread that contact tracing isn't worth the effort. Their estimates of how many people are needed to do the job are all based on carrying on exactly as before. Infuriating! What we need to do is not abandon the mission but mechanise the process – like Henry Ford did to car building.

After the press conference we had a debrief in the PM's study next to the Cabinet Room. We talked about the likely need for as many as 300,000 ventilators. Without the slightest hint of embarrassment,

Simon Stevens pitched my idea from the weekend of a national ventilator challenge, as if he'd come up with it himself. I maintained a poker
face, but I wasn't thrilled. Anyway, what's important is the boss loved it
so we're going to make it happen.

On the way back from Downing Street I called Simon, resisting the
temptation to comment on his brazen intellectual property heist. I had
more important business. For weeks I've been pushing him to expand
NHS capacity. He says that the pandemic is likely to hit the NHS
workforce very hard, meaning there won't be enough staff to expand
the number of beds – so there's no point trying to scale up. I've been
sceptical of this argument throughout and have decided to overrule.
Staff ratios will have to be stretched thinner than anyone can imagine.
Of course that brings massive problems, but it's far better than the alternative of turning sick people away from hospital. We cannot have
what happened in Italy. To give him his due, he agreed straight away
and said he'd come back to me pronto with a plan.

Over the next twenty-four hours I've got some fairly urgent diplomacy to do with the devolved governments. I'm keenly aware that
Scotland's First Minister Nicola Sturgeon will not be able to resist
trying to exploit the pandemic to further the cause of Scottish independence, so we need as much amicable cooperation as possible.
Given the delicate politics, Zoom isn't going to cut it, so the RAF will
taxi me and my team around the country in twenty-four hours. This
evening we flew up to Edinburgh for the first leg of the tour, taking
off from RAF Northolt at dusk for a late-night meeting with Jeane.
When we eventually got to the Scottish health ministry, she did the
whole 'polite but distant' thing. I didn't exactly feel welcomed, re-
inforcing my suspicions that she has as many antibodies as the rest
of the SNP to any visiting Tories from Westminster. The atmosphere
was particularly gloomy because Scotland had just had its first Covid
death. She said she appreciated the visit to meet in person but told me
frankly that there's only so much she can do to keep the politics out of
it because working with Nicola Sturgeon isn't always straightforward.
Who knew?!

FRIDAY 13 MARCH

I woke up for the dawn flight to Belfast in an Edinburgh airport hotel that felt like a ghost ship. When we landed, we discovered our media strategy in disarray after Patrick Vallance mentioned herd immunity on the radio. He and the Prof have generally been doing a sterling job on the airwaves, but this morning it all went awry. Quite apart from sounding more suited to farm animals, 'herd immunity' is shorthand for 'let it rip'. And we are very definitely *not* just letting the virus run its course. Quite the reverse: everything we're doing is about delaying the spread so the NHS can cope and so we can buy time for vaccines and treatments to kick in and save lives.

I called the PM and told him that we would have to do some very rapid backpedalling, then rang Patrick, who promised to do his best to repair the damage.

In Belfast, I met Robin Swann, the Ulster Unionist Health Secretary at Stormont. Despite his spectacularly dour demeanour – he has a face like a clay mask – he has a wicked sense of humour, cracking jokes without the hint of a smile, just the tiniest glimmer of a twinkle in his eyes. An honour to Ulster stereotypes. We had a useful discussion about intensive care in Northern Ireland, which like so much else is coloured by Northern Ireland politics. Because the NHS there has none of the most specialised intensive care beds, patients with the very highest needs are usually flown to Newcastle for treatment. Sinn Féin, of course, want them to be treated in Dublin instead. Robin and I talked about how to head off this nonsense. I already liked Robin from our calls and I could tell we were going to get along well.

Finally I headed to Cardiff to meet Vaughan Gething, Labour Health Minister for Wales. At all these events, the chief medical officers for each part of the UK have all been in the room, each hugely impressive in their own right. I immediately took to Vaughan, who was spectacularly indiscreet. I imagine our politics are closer to each other's than his to his party leader in either the UK or Wales.

I borrowed Vaughan's office for a call with my fellow G7 Health Ministers. Everyone sounded terrified, especially my charming Italian opposite number, Roberto Speranza. Pre-pandemic, Roberto was wonderfully laid-back on every call I ever had with him. Even after the virus began taking hold, he always sounded chilled. Not today. Even the American who chaired the meeting, Alex Azar, who's previously been very sanguine, was shocked at the way things are developing in hospitals over there. Previously very formal, you could hear the fear in his trembling voice. Thanks to Trump, we are missing American leadership in this global crisis.

For me, it was a bit like group therapy: we're all going through the same thing. What I find funny is how much each minister lived up to their national stereotypes. Roberto, a charmer, was the classic Italian. Jens was very direct and to the point; the classic cool, efficient German. Patty Hajdu, from Canada, wanted to bring people together. Katsunobu Katō of Japan was polite and very formal.

Later the Prof talked me through SAGE's latest discussions. The committee thinks there are far more cases here than previously believed, and that household isolation and shielding of the elderly should come in sooner rather than later, even though there are trade-offs, like the effect on people's mental health. SAGE now thinks far heavier measures may be needed to make sure case numbers stay within NHS capacity. They are examining options.

They are still unanimous in warning against trying to eliminate the virus altogether, as all measures will have to be lifted one day and the main effect would be to create a second peak, which they believe is a strong possibility in China. You can't lock down for ever. The race is truly on between the vaccine and the virus.

It's extraordinary how detailed the advice on practicalities gets. The scientists reckon a safe distance for people to stay away from each another is two metres. This is well beyond the maximum range droplets can travel in a normal conversation, even if there's the odd sneeze or cough. There's no evidence that avoiding handshakes removes the risk of infection, but they now acknowledge that it's a minor sacrifice and worth advising against as a signal: the Dr Xand principle. Much more important, they say, is handwashing and avoiding touching the eyes, nose and mouth in case of infection from a contaminated surface.

The wider world is moving faster than the scientists. The Premier League has suspended games, the London Marathon has been postponed and various summer music festivals are falling by the wayside. Our polling shows there's lots of public concern over the UK not doing things other countries are, such as banning big events, which 73 per cent of people now support. The lesson I draw from all this? Get cracking. People are onside.

Simon Stevens called to propose postponing all non-urgent operations from 15 April to free up 30,000 beds. This really hammers home what's coming. All those people waiting for surgery – many in pain – will now be deferred. He says frail elderly patients who don't need urgent treatment need to be discharged, either to their home or to care homes. He's spoken to the Prime Minister about it and is determined to make it happen. Simon Stevens and Boris go way back – they were at university together – and so he has a direct line to the PM when he wants to use it. He's generally pretty good about not overusing it, but when he really wants something to happen, he does. The NHS is now doing all it can to increase bed numbers and keep them above the projected figure for peak infections, which the rest of the country is going to be making incredible sacrifices to keep as low as possible. Simon is also making progress on my instruction to build emergency hospitals and will update me tomorrow.

I went to bed as I had started the day: listening to a scientist talking about herd immunity on the BBC. This time, it was Graham Medley, a professor at Imperial, who told *Newsnight*, 'We're going to have to generate what we call herd immunity... and the only way of developing that in the absence of a vaccine is for the majority of the population to become infected.'

'No, no, *no!*' I shouted. 'That is *not* what we're "generating".' Fortunately, the kids were fast asleep, because I probably sounded a bit unhinged, but *I will not have half a million people die on my watch.*

I'm all in favour of open debate, but this media blundering by government advisers who aren't expert communicators threatens our crucial public health messaging and will be scaring the living daylights out of people. We have to stamp on it.

In high dudgeon, I rang Patrick to ask him to get them to stop. 'They're either inside the tent or not!' I said, trying to sound calm. I told the team to line up a media round for Sunday and an article in a national newspaper: we've got to grip the narrative.

I'm conscious of how knackered and overworked the whole team are. Today they accidentally sent out a 'Dear colleague' letter to MPs that was only supposed to be a draft and was still being worked on. I didn't get cross – I have a very strong belief that leadership requires a no-blame culture in which the question in response to an error is 'How do we fix it?', not 'Who is to blame?' Everyone's working their absolute hardest and mistakes will be made. What matters most is we learn and don't repeat them. So I messaged my private office and SpAds, appealing to them to have an evening off, before realising it was already past 10 p.m.

Before I finally crashed out, Nadine rang. She's OK but has infected both her daughter and her 84-year-old mum. Fuck.

SATURDAY 14 MARCH

Lockdown is coming. There's more terrible data, all pointing to our reasonable worst-case scenario of 500,000 deaths becoming a reality unless we step in hard and fast. Today there were 342 new confirmed cases, taking the total over 1,000, to 1,140. In just three days, the numbers have doubled. Yesterday, eleven more people died, taking the total to twenty-one. They all had serious underlying health problems, but that will not be the case for long. The rest of Europe is clearly moving into a totally new phase. Italy has been locked down since Tuesday, and Poland is about to lock down for two weeks. France is closing all non-essential venues from midnight tonight and Spain has ordered everyone to stay at home from Monday. Germany has cancelled all unnecessary events.

People here can feel it coming. The streets are empty. Folk are cancelling engagements. Retailers released a joint letter asking people not to buy more than they need, as panic buying continues.

While I was mulling all this over, I took a call from Adam Atashzai, who used to work for Cameron in Downing Street. 'Matt, if you're going to really go for this herd immunity strategy, you've really got to get out there and explain it,' he said.

No! Herd immunity is *not* our strategy and *never has been*! As I feared, scientists' cack-handed attempts to explain a technical concept have lit a wildfire. Now people are confused. Clarity is critical at a time like this. As the US pollster Frank Luntz says, what matters is not what you say but what people hear. I put the phone down feeling unsettled.

At 10 a.m. I went to Downing Street to talk to the PM and others about the looming lockdown decision. Rishi, Whitty, Vallance, Cummings and Lee Cain were all there, looking grim-faced. Vallance told everyone that while we had thought we were four weeks behind Italy on the epidemic curve, we now think it's two. Disaster. It means there's no time to lose.

We wrestled with all the issues. What measures? How long? Would people comply? Are we doing enough to make sure the NHS can cope? Should we keep construction open? What about public transport? No one has done this before, so there is no playbook. Sitting in the Cabinet Room, we were all struggling to get our heads round the enormity of what we were discussing – taking decisions that none of us thought we'd ever have to take, all the while knowing this was only the beginning.

We went through each area based on some huge A3 spreadsheets the Cabinet Office had prepared. Boris set out the case for and against each option. Whitty and Vallance talked through the science. Rishi, Boris and I debated the options, and Cummings intervened whenever he thought things were going off track.

After everyone had had their say, we collectively made the decision: to close large swathes of society. We went over the proposals – how to do it and what would be shut – and gave instructions for the civil service to work up the details ahead of another meeting at 5 p.m. to-morrow to finalise.

As I left the meeting and walked back towards the famous No. 10 front door, I phoned Boris. I wanted to tell him we had made the right decision – and reassure him that this was absolutely necessary. He picked up the phone and said, 'Matt, why don't you come back into my office?'

So I turned on my heels and walked back to the smaller study next to the Cabinet Room, where I found him sitting at his polished ma-hogany desk with Cummings, Cain and private office staff. Cummings had a whiteboard full of numbers flowing from cases to hospitalisa-tions to deaths – with predictions with question marks next to them and then a chart depicting hospital capacity. The figures on the white-board were familiar. He was doing exactly what I'd called Boris to do: hammering home the point that this has to happen. We have to keep the number of hospitalisations below the NHS limit – and that means lockdown.

Afterwards, head still spinning, I went back to the office to work on a piece for tomorrow's *Sunday Telegraph*, killing off the herd immu-nity story and setting the scene for Monday. I agreed the newspaper piece with Cummings and talked to Boris about exactly how to phrase it on TV tomorrow morning.

Meanwhile David Halpern has finally managed to get PHE round the table with private testing companies at No. 10. It's due to happen on Wednesday. I am pushing this very hard and I hope it will provide the jolt we need for the testing programme. There's a new machine developed by Roche that can handle 5,000 tests a day, the same as our current daily total for England. I'm told PHE is showing some interest, which is a turn up for the books.

Simon Stevens called about hospital capacity. Some absolute genius has had the idea of converting the ExCel Centre into an overflow hospital. Stevens, who doesn't seem to be claiming the credit on this occasion, has put a team onto it. He says London hospitals are already starting to 'run hot'. We can't act soon enough.

SUNDAY 15 MARCH

I woke at 5.30 a.m., going over in my head everything that I needed to convey on this morning's media round to hammer home the points in the *Sunday Telegraph* article. 'I've got to sound urgent but measured,' I thought to myself, knowing that there was a very real prospect that I would sound either too matter-of-fact or too Doomsday. Pacing around the subterranean green room at BBC Broadcasting House, I repeated the key line over and over with Gina and Jamie: 'We'll stop at nothing to fight the virus.' This is the single most important message to get across.

I didn't go into much detail, but I wanted to ensure elderly people and the vulnerable are ready. 'Quite soon, anybody over the age of seventy is going to be asked to stay inside their house for up to four months,' I said.

Though I'm more optimistic than the scientists about how people will behave, I also warned that we will introduce powers enabling us to enforce quarantine if necessary. The most striking thing was that after my media round, there was no pushback at all. People are frightened. They just seem to accept it.

Restaurant bookings are crashing and West End theatres are starting to cancel shows: the Old Vic made the first big move today, ending its current run two weeks early.

The international shutdown is also intensifying. The White House has extended a ban on flights from the EU to cover us as well, and our Foreign Office has advised against all but essential travel to Spain and the US.

This was the backdrop to the 5 p.m. meeting to agree the details of the announcement tomorrow. No one's calling it a lockdown, but that's essentially what it is.

Before going in I spoke to Chris Whitty. We're worried that the individual measures we discussed yesterday morning aren't enough. It's as much about people's behaviour as the specifics.

So at 5 p.m. I sat in the Cabinet Room, opposite the Prime Minister with my back to the window and the spring sunshine, and said words

I'll never forget: 'Prime Minister, we are going to have to tell everyone to stop all unnecessary social contact.'

Boris shifted in his seat, looking uncomfortable. 'Well, you better go out and tell them, then,' he replied. I stared at him, slightly open-mouthed. I'd be happy to of course, but really? Doesn't this need to come from their Prime Minister? He's never liked being the bearer of bad news. In this instant, clearly his instinct was to shy away. Maybe he could see the look on my face – he is very good at reading a room – and recovered himself pretty fast. By the end of the meeting, we'd agreed to the package of restrictions, and that the Prime Minister – not the Health Secretary – would advise everyone to end all unnecessary social contact for the foreseeable future. Although it's a relief to be taking these essential steps, it still feels surreal and I still can't believe we are doing it.

MONDAY 16 MARCH

So this is it. Today we came down hard and life is going to be very, very different.

Just after 3 p.m. we had a COBRA meeting to get formal agreement on what we're doing and make sure all the devolved administrations were on board. There's always a risk that Sturgeon will cause difficulties, no matter how serious the subject, but on this occasion there was remarkable unanimity. The only debate was over precise timings: Simon wanted a couple of days to get the NHS 111 system ready to answer questions from the public, but the PM did not want to hang around.

Once everyone formally signed the package off, Cummings, Cain, Whitty and I went into Boris's study overlooking the Downing Street garden and finessed the message he was going to give in a televised press conference. We huddled around the PM, making suggestions as he bashed away at his keyboard, muttering to himself then accepting, rejecting or improving our various ideas. Then, at 5 p.m., it was time. Looking as grave as he ever has, Boris stood in front of the cameras and warned the nation that without drastic action, we will lose control of the spread of the virus. Rattling off the list of new measures, he told the elderly and vulnerable they are going to have to stay at home, and even avoid contact while at home, for twelve weeks. For now, we're not closing schools, but SAGE is very worried about the situation and will review over the next couple of days.

Afterwards, I dashed over to the Commons to make a statement at 6 p.m., acknowledging that what we are doing 'will change the ordinary lives of everyone in this country'. I went into more detail about some of the things the PM had less opportunity to explain, like our planned increase in testing, which has grown, albeit agonisingly, to 5,000 a day and will go up to 10,000, then much further as private sector growth kicks in. I outlined the emergency Coronavirus Bill we're bringing to Parliament on Thursday. This will give us the power to take control of essential services – for example public transport – if they judder to a halt because so many staff have Covid.

My Labour shadow Jonathan Ashworth asked about schools, which I said would stay open, though I told him the situation is under continuous review.

Given all the panic buying and the supply chain issues that seem inevitable as we tell people to stay at home, one question is whether we need to include the ability to introduce food rationing in the emergency Coronavirus Bill. Rees-Mogg, who's on the Bill team, is sceptical, pointing out that as soon as people get wind of it, they'll rush to the supermarkets and load up their trolleys with everything they can get, thus making matters even worse. He has a point.

Neil Ferguson has been in and out of Downing Street helping them focus on numbers. The paper he put out today in coordination with No. 10 suggests we could face 250,000 deaths even with measures to mitigate the pandemic. He's a lot more pessimistic than I am about timeframes for a vaccine, while publicly acknowledging that this is our likely way out.

The NHS is facing an extraordinary test. Earlier today we met in my office to go through what will have to be done to maximise the chance of it coping. Nadine passed on an update from a trust clinical director that nursing shortages are going through the roof because of the number of people self-isolating. Managers are being inundated with calls from staff about whether they should come into work, given the new guidance. Many are staying away just to be on the safe side. They want to do the responsible thing, but it's a hell of a dilemma. Should they stay away to minimise risk or should they go in as staff are desperately needed? Simon Stevens seconded Nadine's info, saying we need urgent clarity on exactly which staff are or aren't supposed to be off work.

'Hospitals will start running short of people tomorrow,' he said.

'Tonight,' Nadine corrected.

Everything comes back to expanding testing. Unless staff can find out whether they're infected and know they need to take off work, Stevens said shortages 'will cripple services almost immediately in some parts of the country'.

It was obvious from the questions I was asked in Parliament that we have a problem with not telling pubs and restaurants to close. Unless we mandate closure, they can't claim anything on insurance. If we don't sort this fast, thousands of businesses will collapse. I came into politics to help businesses grow and protect them from what happened to my family business when I was growing up. It's sickening to be doing the exact opposite, but we have no choice.

Given the incubation period, it will be at least two weeks before we know whether any of this is going to work.

TUESDAY 17 MARCH

My special advisers came back from the 8 a.m. meeting in Downing Street open-mouthed after Cummings told them most decisions don't need PM sign-off any more. He says that if they're easy and no one disagrees, just do it. From the ultimate control freak, this is quite something.

At Cabinet, Rishi presented his plan for £330 billion in loan guarantees. I've been used to big figures since my Bank of England days, but a third of a trillion is more than anyone's ever thrown at a problem.

Wow. Rishi also proposed £20 billion in outright grants and tax cuts for companies at immediate risk of collapse. Who would have thought that the Tory Party would preside over the biggest programme of state intervention in the economy since 2008? Unlike almost any other economic crisis, this hardship is directly driven by our own policies to save lives, so it's only right and fair to put policies in place to help people through.

The point is that liberal individualism is a great political philosophy – probably the most successful in the history of mankind – but no use in a pandemic, when the problem is essentially communitarian, stemming from the fact that we all catch the same disease because we're all human. Anyway, Rishi got Cabinet's full support. As Boris put it, 'We must act like any wartime government and do whatever it takes to support our economy.'

Later a senior civil servant came over from the Cabinet Office, charged with getting agreement across government for what's going in the emergency Bill. I've worked with him on a host of projects and he's a first-rate generalist classic civil servant, but he nonetheless took some time to adjust to the notion that this new legislation needs to be drawn up and enacted right away. I was not at my most patient best, and our exchange quickly became somewhat heated as I told him in no uncertain terms that we can't delay, and that if any departments don't get their act together by Thursday, we'll have to publish the Bill anyway. There are some measures I simply won't countenance – like a bonkers proposal from the Ministry of Justice to let prisoners out, as they'd be easier to manage if they're not in prison. Yes really: they actually thought this might be a goer.

I was emphasising this point so hard that all of a sudden my chair could take the strain no longer and ripped, tipping me unceremoniously onto the floor. Humiliating as it was, it broke the ice, and the stony-faced mandarin finally cracked a smile. After that, we came to an agreement pretty swiftly.

Continuing to work through the practicalities, Steve Oldfield updated me on the huge stocks of PPE in a warehouse in the north-west:

a billion items. Just one problem – we can't get it out. It turns out that when they laid down the PPE stockpile in the 2000s, no one thought about the circumstances under which we might need it, i.e. an emergency, in which time is of the essence. It's in a huge storage unit which only has one door. Ergo, only one lorry can pull up at a time. Shame nobody looked at Amazon's warehouses for inspiration – they have dozens of lorry bays. What a classic government fail.

Lack of doors notwithstanding, we have a real moral responsibility to sort this out. It's about protecting everyone who is putting their own health at risk to look after others. I called Ben Wallace to ask if the army can help get this stuff out to hospitals, and he was immediately on board. Overnight 150 trusts had PPE shipments and I'm promised that by the end of the week all trusts will have had at least one delivery. Care homes are desperate, and I've insisted they also each get a load. It doesn't matter if they are private businesses: it's an emergency and we need to do our best to protect everyone in the country.

As instructed, Steve and his team have been buying from abroad. He told me our plodding procurement processes are a massive hindrance. The rules say they have to buy at the bottom quartile of the market, which in normal times is vital for value for money, but prices are shooting up and we are losing deals. I told Steve to throw everything at it. 'Anything out there – you buy it. Identify it and buy it. We need tiger teams across China seeking and buying the PPE we will need.' How ironic that only a few weeks ago we sent a plane load of our own PPE to… China. The right thing to do at the time, and only a tiny quantity in the grand scheme of things, but if we'd known what was coming, we might not have been as generous.

We are at least finally making significant progress on testing. David Halpern plus Will Warr, the health policy lead in No. 10, organised a crunch meeting with potential testing providers, with PHE, NHS officials and everyone else we needed in the room to make things happen. Boris opened the meeting, stressing the importance of the mission, and then passed to me to chair. I listened to the private testing companies describing all the barriers they face to expanding their capacity. It was a sorry tale.

I am lucky to have so many allies on this challenge. Sir John Bell, the dynamic Oxford professor of medicine who oversees the university's links with government, also sees expansion of testing as critical and talked about a world in which mass DIY testing will be available on demand and it'll be perfectly normal to get up in the morning and do a coronavirus test before going to work. During the meeting PHE was completely unable to give a convincing plan for scaling up exponentially. I just don't think they're capable of thinking coherently about industrial scale or private sector involvement, so I took an executive decision and announced there and then that I'd take responsibility for the testing programme away from them. The Department of Health will now take the lead. PHE officials in the room graciously let it go without a fight: they were probably relieved. We agreed that they and the NHS should carry on expanding as much lab capacity as they can, but we will also set up a mass-scale testing programme, alongside the existing system, for antigen tests, another for antibody tests and a strand for surveys to find out how many people have it and have had it. We designed these four 'pillars' in the room and allocated initial responsibility for each.

The PM turned to me and asked who was going to be in charge: we need someone to pull the strands together. 'James Bethell, as our Life Sciences Minister,' I replied.

Bethell, who obviously had no idea this was coming as I'd only just thought of it myself, looked a bit shocked, but he's more than capable.

Away from Westminster, the cruise ship saga continues. A vessel called the MS *Braemar* with Brits on board has now been drifting around the Caribbean for weeks, begging every port it can find to let it in. The ship still has full internet access and the poor folk who've been confined to their cabins as the vessel floats around aimlessly have quite rightly been hassling their MPs to help get them out. The MPs in turn have been on my back, demanding I do what I can to get their constituents home. Finally, the Cubans let it dock and have now given the Foreign Office permission to fly British passengers home. This really shouldn't be my problem – it's an FCO thing – but Raab's department doesn't seem able to cope with high-speed events, so Emma Dean has been handling it. At least the FCO has finally advised against all non-essential international travel – not exactly before time...

It was my son's twelfth birthday today, almost all of which I missed. My family is already paying a heavy price for this crisis. After the testing meeting, I rushed home and just managed to give him a big hug before he went to sleep.

WEDNESDAY 18 MARCH

Sometimes this whole business just comes and whacks you in the face. Our death toll has now passed 100, with thirty-two deaths in a single day. Tonight I was sitting on the edge of the bath at home and looking at that number, thirty-two, and I just couldn't believe the magnitude of it. It's going to get much worse.

My long years of training and working in economics mean I see the similarities between epidemics and economics; I see the behaviour of individuals at the scale of whole societies. I understand concepts like exponential growth, so I can picture where we are on the curve and how steep it's going to get. Translate those statistics into people's lives and it's clear to me what lies ahead. It's obvious that we have to do more.

This morning Boris proposed we shut all schools. He'd decided not to try to wait until the Easter holidays and not to keep certain year groups open: to shut straight away. I didn't demur, and we discussed the crucial concern of the impact on the NHS and other core services if staff have to stay at home to look after their children. The solution we've come up with is to keep schools very partially open for the most vulnerable kids and the children of key workers.

At lunchtime I joined the PM at PMQs. The deserted House of Commons feels very weird now: still functioning, but so quiet. How completely different to a month ago, when everyone was packed in, cheerfully asking about anything other than Covid. It's all Covid now.

Then Boris talked to Cabinet about schools. I supported him. Given the level of disruption closures will cause, I was expecting a lot of flak, but nobody objected. We also discussed what to do about public transport. Stopping Tubes, buses and trains would be a disaster for the NHS and other essential workers because they wouldn't be able to get in, but doing nothing risks making the whole situation worse and will cost an absolute fortune. It's a massive problem, with no obvious solution. Unusually, I didn't have a strong view. Grant can sort that one.

Thank goodness there's some promising news on testing. Oxford University scientists based in China have developed a new rapid test for the virus, which can produce results in half an hour – a quarter of the time it currently takes. They're now exploring quickfire devices that could be used in places like airports and even, potentially, by people in their own homes. They're planning to get the tests validated in the UK.

Slightly worryingly, Neil Ferguson has Covid symptoms and is self-isolating. I was right to be worried about his coughing when I sat next to him at No. 10 the other day. So far I don't have any symptoms and nor do any of the family, but it's a bit unsettling.

Later I borrowed a room in the Cabinet Office for our first COBRA by teleconference, a prospect I wasn't exactly savouring after the farcical experience of giving interviews on Skype. To my surprise, this time everything worked, though it's fair to say that some colleagues are adapting to the world of online meetings better than others. During an extremely important discussion about shielding the vulnerable, I struggled to keep a straight face as the Work and Pensions Secretary Thérèse Coffey – who must have thought she had switched off her camera – lay back in her chair, chomping on a sandwich. Meanwhile Robert Buckland was clearly watching on his phone – he kept slipping down the screen, then eventually disappearing, before suddenly popping up again, presumably having repositioned his mobile on some kind of stand.

Another challenge is making sure our MPs are onside. To that end, I went to speak to the 1922 Committee of Tory backbenchers in the cavernous Committee Room 14 in the Commons. As well as keeping them in the loop, I wanted to gauge the mood and try to get a sense of how constituents are reacting. The main feedback was about small businesses facing collapse. Colleagues are clearly feeling the heat. They do, however, know that we're in uncharted waters, so there was no real dissent over our strategy. I'd approached the encounter with some trepidation and emerged feeling relieved: it was very pragmatic and can-do.

The political world is now taking a deep dive in epidemiology and the Prof is getting annoyed with everyone asking him what he thinks of the latest interesting titbit they've read in the media, whether it's about blood groups and Covid, the effect on pregnancy or whatever. He messaged today asking us all to stop using the 'very small CMO team' as a 'fact-checker for every media medical story except the really big ones'. People have got into the habit of bombarding him with links to the latest *Guardian* or *Spectator* article and asking him for his authoritative view. He was characteristically diplomatic but rightly says it's not the best use of his time.

Nadine, as ever in the vanguard of the epidemic, says she's lost her sense of smell and taste and everyone she's infected has got the same thing. Strange: that's not one of the official symptoms. I'll ask the Prof to see if we need to add it to the list.

THURSDAY 19 MARCH

The scenes coming out of Italy are shocking. In the town of Bergamo, they've run out of morgue capacity to store bodies. TV bulletins are full of gruesome images of convoys of military lorries carting corpses away and hospital wards crammed with wheezing, gasping patients on beds, stretchers and chairs as they wait their turn. Hospitals in Bergamo look very modern and efficient, but they've run out of beds in intensive care units, relegating patients to trolleys and floors. All too many are going to die. The exhausted staff, sweating in their PPE, are doing their best, but it's clearly a desperate battle. Watching this stuff, I am filled with dread and a huge sense of responsibility. It is a chilling illustration of what we could face here if we mess this up. Italy as a whole has now recorded more deaths than China.

As planned, we published the Coronavirus Bill, which gives the government extraordinary scope to curtail individual freedoms for the common good. It's spectacularly unconservative, and I'm acutely conscious of how controversial it could be. For a full two years we'll have the authority to take sweeping steps to protect public health, issuing diktats that would be unthinkable in normal times. We will have the power to restrict or ban public gatherings, control or suspend public transport, order businesses to close, temporarily detain those suspected of being infected, suspend ports and airports, close education, enrol medical students and retired health workers back into the NHS, relax some regulations to ease the burden on hospitals and take direct control of how bodies are dealt with, all switched on and off according to medical and scientific advice. The reaction to publication was astonishingly positive. Even those who hate it merely argued that it shouldn't be for two years but a shorter time. A massive relief.

There is a very faint glimmer of optimism in China, which has reported zero new infections contracted locally, the first day it's been able to do that – though who knows whether the figures are to be believed.

I was on *Question Time* this evening in Weston-super-Mare. I took Gina, who's brilliant at the art of communicating in a way that people actually hear. As someone immersed in policy, I've got a tendency to end up sounding too technical. Gina's question is always: but what are you *really* trying to say to the people watching?

It seemed to go pretty well. There was an impressive scientist called Professor Tom Solomon from Liverpool University, who suggested he'd like to observe what was going on in the department to write it up for history – for next time. Good idea. I made a note to talk to Chris Wormald about that.

In the car on the way back, I called my Australian opposite number,

Greg Hunt. He's a wonderful, straight-talking Aussie. We're both crick-et fans and joke about the trouble that brings. He talked me through the approach they're taking: aiming to be as tough as possible at the borders in the hope of avoiding a lockdown. They are feeling quite lucky at how few cases they have had relative to Europe. A little bell of doubt rang in my ear. I finally got home at around 1 a.m.

FRIDAY 20 MARCH

Rishi has unveiled his biggest bazooka yet. He's calling it 'furlough' – clever to use a word that's unfamiliar in the UK.

I was on my way out of a COBRA meeting at the time, and as I walked through No. 10 to the car waiting outside the famous black door, I saw Rishi was giving his statement and paused to watch. I hadn't been involved in the details of the scheme. When I heard we're going to be paying 80 per cent of people's salaries, I thought, 'Christ, that's generous.'

This evening's press conference was another huge moment. The PM instructed pubs and all hospitality to close from tonight.

I'm trying to be sensible about getting enough sleep – there's no nat-ural cut-off point in a situation like this. Unless I'm strict with myself, I know I'll end up going to bed later and later and getting up earlier and earlier, and it still won't be enough to feel I'm on top of everything. As we headed to yet another meeting in No. 10 today, Chris Wormald had a quiet chat with me in the lift. 'You know, Matt,' he said, 'this isn't going to be short. It's going to last for months.' This focused my mind on practicalities for the weeks ahead. A family friend kindly offered me the use of his flat, which just happens to be really near the office. Convenient as this would be, if I base myself there, I'll never see the family – and as Chris says, there's no end date to this. I've decided not to take it and will use the time travelling in to work to make calls and do paperwork. The roads are empty now anyway.

It seems extraordinary, but PHE still can't reach a conclusion on asymptomatic transmission. Plenty of people have tested positive without showing symptoms, but there is still no definite evidence of them passing the virus on to other people, so they won't officially advise that it's possible. I find this infuriating.

I saw another side to Thérèse Coffey today. She is known for being quietly effective, but today she was on fire. During a long meeting about how we link NHS and benefits data to identify and contact those most vulnerable to Covid, she became increasingly exasperated by all the objections and excuses. The lawyers raised GDPR; NHS Digital said they don't give patient information to DWP for fear people will stop going to the doctor; and the IT people said it was all too difficult. On and on it went, all problems and no solutions. I sat in semi-silent despair, trying to suppress a growing desire to shake them. This will soon be a life-or-death matter for thousands and thousands of vulnerable people! Thérèse sat there quite quietly, her face getting progressively redder until finally she exploded, thumping the table, deconstructing each of the objections, and telling them in no uncertain terms that we absolutely *have* to get this done, so they'd better crack on. I was shocked – and impressed.

We're properly cranking up testing now. My goal is for a new national testing service that combines the public and private sectors: we have got to break out of PHE cottage-industry mode. In another great national effort, I'm trying to encourage former doctors and nurses to come back to work for the NHS, a bit like mobilising reserves in wartime. I issued a big public call to everyone who could return to apply. There is a vast reservoir of talent and experience: we'd be crazy to waste it. One of the most important things will be ensuring the system doesn't put petty bureaucratic obstacles in the way of getting people back.

SATURDAY 21 MARCH

The PPE problem drags on. Jamie sidled up to me in the department today, bearing an expression that I knew meant bad news. Brandishing his mobile phone, he showed me some pictures of nurses at Northwick Park Hospital in north London clad in bin liners because there are no PPE gowns. My heart sank. It's completely unacceptable. Naturally we're being accused of sending these brave NHS staff to their potential doom by not giving them the protection they need. The absurdity of the situation is that we actually have enough – we just can't get it out of the damn warehouse. Thankfully the Cabinet Office has now published new guidance saying we can use emergency procurement to buy what we need. This will shorten the process from months to weeks, though the truth is that we only have days.

I spent much of today trying to sort out who is going to enforce the closure of pubs and restaurants. Cummings showed a surprising level of interest, revealing that his family owned a nightclub called Klute in Durham for thirty years. He said the threat of clubs or pubs losing their licence would be a far more effective stick than fines.

'Lose your licence, you're fucked… getting it back is a nightmare,' he said animatedly.

Weekends count for nothing now. Today was another full day in the office, albeit the car came at 9.15 a.m., not 7.30 a.m. I am not complaining – it is an enormous privilege as well as an immense responsibility to be navigating this crisis – but it is hard on my family and my team.

Meanwhile case numbers just keep getting worse. Within days, we are going to have to pull all our remaining levers and put the whole country into full lockdown.

Just about the only good news is on our push to get people to rejoin the NHS. Some 4,000 nurses and 500 doctors have signed up in the first twenty-four hours! Amazing.

SUNDAY 22 MARCH
Following Thérèse's explosion – and thanks to a lot of hard work – we've managed to identify 1.5 million of the most vulnerable people who should now stay at home for twelve weeks. This is the single most effective step we can take to save lives. Rob Jenrick and I are writing to them all, a letter we have to get just right. The people who receive it will be worried, and the prospect of loneliness will be very daunting for many. At the same time, we are working up support – food and medicine deliveries – for those stuck at home. When I saw the first

draft, it was hideously bureaucratic: Whitehall at its worst. We had a strict Royal Mail deadline, so I sat up rewriting the wretched thing past my midnight bedtime deadline, trying to inject as much humanity and empathy as I could.

The army is doing a great job on PPE delivery. Now I've seen what they can do, I want to get them involved in the proposed ExCel Centre temporary hospital. The PM is keen. Meanwhile there's an idiotic situation with workplace canteens. With a few exceptions – hospitals, care homes, schools, prisons etc. – we ordered them all to close. Unfortunately, Jenrick's department forgot to include police canteens in the list of exemptions, meaning that officers who use their own staff canteens are technically breaking the law. We're doing a hasty rewrite.

Then in the afternoon I went from the department to another crunch meeting in Downing Street. We went through all the data: what we know about the number of cases and the reports from hospitals. None of it is good. Throw in the facts that businesses actually want a legal lockdown (not just a strongly worded advisory one) and the public are also strongly in favour, and it's all pointing one way.

The Prime Minister weighed up all the options in the room. He's famous for this and sometimes does it out loud, so it's impossible to know in the middle of the meeting where he's going to end up. It's his way of making big decisions. In the end it was straightforward and we unanimously agreed to a formal lockdown as soon as possible. We sent the civil service team off to work out the details overnight for a full-blown legal lockdown and we will formalise the details tomorrow. We've got to throw everything at this.

MONDAY 23 MARCH

A totemic day, in which the Prime Minister instructed everybody to stay at home: no longer guidance but a legal obligation. In the history of this country, there has never been anything like it.

Most of the day was occupied preparing the details of the announcement. Once a decision like this becomes legal, all the details about the boundaries of the rules become extremely complicated very quickly – and cock-ups like the police canteens become inevitable. And these rules will affect every single person in the country.

I met Ben Wallace about military support. The 20,000-strong Covid Support Force starts work today and they're going to have a command post in our department. Demand for PPE continues to skyrocket and our distribution system is collapsing, so the MoD's logistics teams are going to get involved.

On my way back from the Ministry of Defence I got the latest data, and it was terrible. More than 300 people have now died with Covid – up from fifty just a week ago. That figure is going to multiply and multiply. The R number is now 2.6 to 2.8 – much higher than anticipated – and the number of hospital patients is doubling every three to four days. Alarmingly, London could run out of beds within the next ten days.

Then in the afternoon I had to go to an almost empty House of Commons to take the Coronavirus Bill through. When I'd called Labour in to look at the draft, Baroness Shami Chakrabarti from the Lords was very tough, suggesting some of the rules needed hardening up, which came as a surprise given her background as the head of the civil liberties pressure group Liberty. So I took her comments on board, and there was no dissent in Parliament – even to these most draconian of powers. Quite simply, people – including politicians – are frightened. There were – rightly – questions asked about detail, and how long these powers will last, but Parliament really came together, as it so often does in moments of crisis.

Straight from the Commons to the COBRA, called for 5 p.m., to take the legal lockdown decision formally, and to get the buy-in of key political figures – London Mayor Sadiq Khan, Nicola Sturgeon and representatives from Wales and Northern Ireland. My main goal was to ensure that everybody understood what we were doing, i.e. legally enforcing restrictions we've already announced. If anything, Sadiq was even more gung-ho. He wanted it all to come into force tonight – and the PM agreed. It meant a scramble, but the team was able to get the legals in place in time.

So, at 8.30 p.m., the Prime Minister gave his address to the nation.

'From this evening, I must give the British people a very simple instruction: you must stay at home' was how he put it.

The instructions will stay in force initially for three weeks, but I think everyone realises it will be longer.

Boris rammed home the message that we must prevent the NHS from being overwhelmed. This is how everyone can contribute to saving thousands of lives. The broadcast ended with the catchphrase that will appear on all our publicity material and at the daily government press conferences: 'Stay home, protect the NHS, save lives.' I think Lee Cain, the PM's director of comms, came up with it. He has a real talent for that kind of direct and punchy message.

Along with the new rules, we announced an avalanche of other state interventions, including nationalising all the rail franchises for at least six months to stop operators going bust. Meanwhile the Foreign Office is advising all British nationals abroad to come home ASAP. If they don't get on a flight fast, they risk getting stuck as other countries close their borders.

In my own household, we're trying to adjust to family life without school. It's a massive deal. I found an old computer in the attic and have set it up for our youngest, though I'm not sure how online school is going to work for a six-year-old. We're only just getting started and with me largely absent it's tough on the family.

TUESDAY 24 MARCH

Steven Dick, our deputy ambassador to Hungary, has died in Budapest. He tested positive a week ago and was feeling fine. Now he is gone. I worked closely with him when he was my head of strategy at DCMS and I remember him as a cheerful, bright, optimistic man, just the kind of guy I click with. He was also a consummate professional and only thirty-seven. It is a real shock. I read about it in the paper and it really hit me – Steven was younger than me and has died from this. Who is it going to get next?

We've had to give a lot of thought to how each of us in government works and who actually goes into the office. How can we justify coming in at all, when we've been telling everyone else to work from home if they can? But the number of decisions ministers have to make at high speed and the number of meetings we need to inform these decisions mean we can't practically manage the pandemic from home. As for civil servants, Chris Wormald has been going through staff lists, working out who really needs to be here.

My government driver Louise fetched me at home in Queen's Park as usual this morning. I was intrigued to see what the streets of London would be like. It was extraordinary. Instead of the usual 45-minute drag, we cruised to Victoria Street in under twenty minutes. Driving down Park Lane there wasn't a single other car on the road – not one. I sat in the back of the car feeling almost sick. All I could think was: *What have we done?*

I arrived at the office to discover that workmen had been in overnight. On the floor were eleven yellow blobs, each two metres apart. I had my blob where my chair was and there were others spaced out round the table for meetings. According to our own rules, we will all have to stay on these blobs as if they have a force field round them. There's also a line of blobs two metres apart in the corridor outside my private secretary's office where officials stand waiting for me so they can come in with questions and updates between meetings. My three SpAds are usually packed into a windowless office the size of a cupboard. That's not going to work now. My office is absurdly large, so I'm going to have one of the walls moved so they can have more space. I tried standing on one of the blobs and felt pretty silly, but this is what we're asking people to do – as if they're in the transporter room where Scotty beams up the crew on the *Starship Enterprise*. My rules, so I'd better get used to it.

As we're no longer allowing non-passholders into the building, we'll be doing a lot by video conference. Some of these meetings are going to involve dozens of people, so the tech needs to work. In an illustration of Whitehall's standard performance on these things, one of the two big screens on my office wall has been dead for months. Every so often, some earnest-looking IT person appears at my door, saying they've come to fix it. Each and every time, half an hour or so later, they slope away, looking defeated. If anyone can revive it before the end of the pandemic, I'll be very surprised. Whitehall being Whitehall, officials tried to insist on developing our own in-house video conferencing software, claiming it was necessary for 'security'. I pushed back, and we'll just use Zoom.

Later on I went to the ExCel Centre to see how they're getting on. It's coming together so fast. When China built a hospital in ten days, I thought we could never match it, but here we are: on track for nine days. Crucially, the building already had electricity, plumbing, ventilation and even the cubicles normally used as stalls at trade shows. The plan is to build several others across the country. They're going to be called Nightingale hospitals. The ExCel will have capacity for 4,000 patients, with troops doing the fit-out in record time. I hope they won't be needed, but it's reassuring to know the capacity will be there.

I've been talking to Rishi about the construction industry. In the debates over the weekend, we decided to keep it open – shutting it down would be a huge hit to the economy, and the work is mostly outdoors. He and I are looking at this crisis from different viewpoints. He's rightly desperate to limit the impact on the economy, while I'm trying to save lives. What that means is that if we both agree on something, it's probably the right thing to do. It helps that he's from an NHS family, and my family ran a small business, so we each see the other's point of view. When I got back to the office, I noticed that the building site over the road had fallen silent. Funny to think that we have been so worried people won't follow the rules, yet they are going even further than we intended.

This evening it was finally my turn to front the daily Downing Street press conference. I was flanked by Jenny Harries and Professor Stephen Powis, national medical director of NHS England. We gathered to prep in Thatcher's old study, where Jack Doyle went through all the tricky questions we might face. I was unusually nervous as I walked across the hall, past the famous staircase and into the oak-panelled dining room, knowing that more or less the whole nation would be watching. After all, we'd just banned them from doing almost anything else. Jenny and Steve went first, and I took a breath. I thought to myself, 'Just talk as if you're talking to Dad: a highly intelligent non-expert.' The main business was to launch our new NHS Volunteers scheme. Like our call for ventilators, it is very much in the spirit of a national mission. The idea is to sign up 250,000 volunteers to help people who are shielding. They'll be doing things like delivering food and medicine, taking people to appointments and, crucially, just giving them a call to see how they're doing and if they feel like having a chat. I love these national missions. So many people want to help.

Oxford's vaccine research has got off to a flying start. The project uses the same technology as a vaccine they developed for Ebola. They started tests a few days ago, with human trials likely to begin in a month or two. This is phenomenal.

I received a plaintive message from Seb James, CEO of Boots, who said fit and healthy staff are failing to show up for their shifts, citing 'government guidance'. This is alarming: we're going to need pharmacies operating at full strength. I am also sick of the ongoing Whitehall battle over GDPR. Thérèse and I have made it crystal clear that the overriding public emergency takes priority over data sharing. We've started sending the letters to people about shielding, but the NHS is still refusing to give the Cabinet Office and DWP the details they need to do the follow-up. I have now explicitly overruled the data concern/excuse, issuing a direct ministerial instruction for the NHS to send names, addresses, NHS numbers, postcodes and any other information required to the Cabinet Office so they can hold the database of shielded people. The Cabinet Office, whose officials are also kicking off, should then share it with councils and the DWP. Seriously: this is about saving lives, and people already think one part of government should be able to talk to another.

WEDNESDAY 25 MARCH

Prince Charles has Covid. What a leveller this is. I hope he's OK. My thoughts immediately turned to the Queen. What if she gets it? When did he last see her?

Two doctors have also just died from the virus, a tragic reminder of how exposed all our NHS staff are to the virus. One was a GP; the other, a surgeon. Both had moved here from abroad to work in the NHS. The news has hit the NHS hard. To be honest, I'm not feeling great myself. Being only forty-one, if I do get it, I should be fine, but there are no guarantees. And I don't have time to be ill right now.

The response to our call for NHS Volunteers has been absolutely staggering. By this afternoon, an unbelievable 405,000 people had signed up, way more than we were expecting.

The Prof is pivotal. People seem to like his calm, reassuring manner and that intense way he has of looking at you with total concentration, like you're the only person in the world. We need to make the most of this public respect, so I asked him to do a social media clip repeating the key mantras, like 'Always try to stay two metres apart', in his most authoritative voice. He finds recording these sorts of things terribly embarrassing but appreciates it's part of the job.

My super-carefully worded letter to everyone we think needs to shield has finally started to arrive. A university friend got in touch to say something must be wrong because he's as fit as a fiddle but he'd got a letter. A few exchanges of messages later and we worked out it must be because he had a heart op five years ago. Although he'd made a great recovery, anyone with a heart operation in the past five years is on the list. I was actually encouraged to hear from him: although he was a borderline case, the fact that he got a letter shows the system is working. Another recipient was a very senior Conservative Party colleague – someone who's dealt with plenty of crises. He should have known better than to collar me in high dudgeon, taking offence.

'Are you telling me I'm too feeble to do my job?' he puffed.

I tried to soothe his ruffled feathers, saying it was a standard-issue letter, you're more than capable, at the height of your powers etc., but I'm not sure I was very convincing. It shows just how emotionally people react to being told that, on the best clinical evidence we have, they're particularly vulnerable to this thing. I fear there will be a lot of messenger-shooting to come.

The Coronavirus Act received royal assent today, giving formal legal authority across the UK to all the measures we have introduced. The police will have the power to use 'reasonable force' to make sure people do what they're told. By way of example, there are now 500 officers on the rail network to deter unnecessary travel. Parliament has also shut early for Easter recess to give time for all the necessary safety works to be put in place so it can keep doing its proper job while minimising infection for staff and members.

Boris called Michael Gove and me in to talk ventilators. He wants Michael to pick it up, given all the procurement people are actually based in the Cabinet Office. In meetings, Michael likes to ask what he calls his 'daft laddie' questions – the really basic ones that nobody else dares articulate for fear of sounding stupid. Adopting his most innocent expression, Michael eyeballs officials and asks questions like 'Where are most ventilators made?' and 'Have we asked car manufacturers to help?' It's a slight guilty pleasure seeing how it rattles them.

Our competition is proving a mixed blessing. Some participants are a little over-enthusiastic. James Dyson, the vacuum manufacturer, has been contacting numerous people in high places to ensure he has a prominent role. He's continually on the phone, including to Boris, pushing to take part. He's an amazing innovator and engineer and he's completely right to turn to this – after all, we put out the call – but it's becoming awkward. Plus, existing ventilator manufacturers are extremely sniffy about anyone else muscling in, stressing that these machines are hugely sensitive and can kill people if the calibrations are wrong. My view is that the competitive tension is a good thing. Michael texted asking to talk urgently about what to do about Dyson. It's a fine line between enthusiasm and getting in the way.

I've been running on adrenaline for weeks now and generally doing fine, but for the first time today I was really flagging. I just felt exhausted. Nadine, who has made a good recovery, was leaving our weekly ministers' team meeting when she heard me cough. She told me I should get a Covid test. My private office was brilliant and immediately made the arrangements. Just a few hours later, the Queen's nurse, no less, came to test me in my office. She wore heavy-duty PPE and pushed a swab down my throat. I braced myself like I was at the dentist and tried to feel grateful that I was able to have a test when we still don't have nearly enough to go round.

Today Boris declared that we'll go from 5,000 to 10,000 tests per day. Then, plucking figures out of nowhere, he declared that we'll go from 25,000 'hopefully very soon up to 250,000 per day'. Sharp intake of breath on my part. I like the ambition and his optimism, but even by my 'glass half full' mindset, I'm the one who has to deliver these promises.

THURSDAY 26 MARCH
I was still feeling a bit ropey when I woke up this morning so decided to stay at home. Added to this groggy feeling is the gut-wrenching uncertainty about whether we can stop the spread. We are shooting up the curve with alarming speed – cases are doubling every seventy-two hours – but there are no more levers to pull. Normal life has ground to a more dramatic halt than we expected or even planned for. If we've got R below 1 then the rise in numbers might just stop before the NHS is overwhelmed. If all this still leaves R above 1 then there's nothing more we can do and we're still in exponential territory.

Initial findings from the Office for National Statistics (ONS) show a huge reduction in people's social contacts. Numbers on public transport have plummeted, and very few people are going to parks. Anonymised data from mobile phone companies showing people's movements strongly suggests that the over-65s are staying in one place. This is really encouraging on so many levels and shows what modern analytical technology can do when a crisis requires crashing through the usual bureaucratic hurdles.

Meanwhile SAGE has reported that significantly more men are being admitted to hospital – and dying – than women. Nobody knows why. Spare bed capacity in London is down to about 20 per cent and we're still only at the start. The Nightingale can't come quickly enough.

The modelling is being updated increasingly rapidly to reflect what we're actually experiencing. The peak is now expected in April. A new draft worst-case scenario forecasts 65,000 deaths by September, based on our mitigation measures, with 320,000 people needing hospital treatment. If we lift the measures after six months, another, even bigger peak is likely later in the year with a further 90,000 deaths. These numbers are lower than before, but they are still staggering.

There's conflicting data on the effectiveness of existing treatments. Today France approved the use of hydroxychloroquine. I'm adamant that we don't make hasty decisions based on poor data just because other countries are going down one route or another: everything needs to go through proper scientific clinical trials. The Prof can hardly bring himself to comment.

There's been a classic bureaucratic screw-up with the EU over ventilator procurement. Someone from No. 10 appears to have told LBC Radio that we aren't involved in Brussels' scheme for buying ventilators because we aren't in the EU. Whoever came up with this line clearly forgot that we're still in the transition period, which means we still have access to these things. Evidently they also didn't know that I actually signed something saying we should speak to the EU just to find out what may be on offer. I got my private office onto officials this afternoon to find out what had happened. Initially they claimed that the EU hadn't in fact invited us to join their procurement scheme. A little later they came back somewhat sheepishly and admitted that Brussels did invite us but EU officials sent the invitation to the wrong email inbox. No one in Brussels bothered following up when they didn't get a reply – and nobody this end felt the need to chase. There's a huge media fuss about it, with viewpoints all shaped by positions on Brexit. Brexiteers all blaming EU inefficiency, Remainers all blaming Brexit. What a complete waste of energy.

Self-isolating meant I was indoors for the 'clap for carers' at 8 p.m., an initiative which got everyone out on their doorsteps to show appreciation for NHS and care staff. I clapped as hard as anyone, but in my case out of the window from my red office at home. I found the collective gesture incredibly moving, especially seeing it replicated in other countries: a reminder that we're all in it together as never before.

We've been getting a lot of flak about late reporting of the number of deaths. Inevitably this leads to accusations of a cover-up. The truth? A load of effort is going into getting permission from families before including individuals in the daily figures. Once again, the system is wedded to absurd privacy rules – these poor people have died and their families are being asked to sign consent forms – and there's no privacy angle anyway. It's more gold-plating and completely unsustainable. I gave the instruction to sort it out.

FRIDAY 27 MARCH
A nurse called first thing this morning to say I've got Covid. She was ringing from the lab at St Thomas's Hospital just over the river from Parliament and delivered the news in a pitying tone. I wasn't particularly surprised and I'm certainly not freaking out – I just feel tired and under the weather – but it's not ideal.

I called Jack Doyle in No. 10 to break the news. 'Erm, that's interesting, as we're just about to announce that the PM has tested positive too,' he replied.

'Right,' I gulped, wondering how we're going to handle this. Announcing one of us has gone down with it is unfortunate. Announcing we've both got it – just days after Prince Charles – will give the impression we're dropping like flies.

I hung up and slumped back in my chair, feeling momentarily overwhelmed by the scale of it all. Then I thought I'd better ring Boris. He sounded fine. We agreed that we should both tweet out videos to show that we're in one piece. My effort was very wobbly indeed and at one point I somehow managed to flip the whole thing upside down. Not a stellar performance from a former Minister for Digital. To cap it all, the Prof also has symptoms and is working from home. Losing him too right now would be a disaster.

The press is getting really wound up about the speed of the testing programme. I emphatically share their views, though publicly I can hardly express my frustration.

For all the media furore, we're finally making progress. The Randox test has finally been approved. From next week they'll be doing 1,400 tests a day, using three new hub labs set up for the duration of the pandemic. Unsurprisingly, there's a global shortage of testing kits – including reagents, a vital ingredient of the kits – so we're stepping up procurement wherever we can find supplies. Amazon and Royal Mail are going to help with the logistics and we're expanding NHS and PHE capacity as well as looking at the reliability of new home testing kits, which would be a game changer.

NERVTAG scientists have identified a major increase in outbreaks in care homes – 239 new clusters in the past seven days. This is a big worry. Some of the most vulnerable people in the country live in care homes, and we must also avoid the sort of situation we saw in Spain where all the residents of one institution died because all the staff went home. There are no easy answers.

SATURDAY 28 MARCH

Two hundred and sixty deaths announced today, taking the number of fatalities past 1,000. Another awful milestone. I feel terrible. Worse is the fact that we still have no evidence that the lockdown is having any impact. My rational brain tells me that because of the incubation period it's just too soon to tell, but if everything we've done doesn't turn the worm, we're on for half a million dead.

News that Boris and I both have Covid has gone global. I've had messages from people around the world, including some I haven't heard from in years. My poor daughter has been inundated with people telling her they saw her dad on TikTok.

The testing data is looking promising at last. We've hit our target of 10,000 a day for the first time on the way to 25,000: a good start.

Boris is definitely under the weather now. No. 10 warned my team that decisions may not be as quick as they usually are because the PM 'is feeling a bit shattered'.

Meanwhile Donna Kinnair, the RCN chief executive, is on the warpath. She's complained that the new guidance on PPE doesn't give enough priority to staff doing home visits, some of whom are being refused kit even when they ask. I get on incredibly well with Donna, who's very professional behind the scenes and has been helping the department with PPE. There's absolutely no way we can afford to fall out right now. I talked to the NHS chief nursing officer Ruth May, who's been leading on it and is going to try to broker a solution – but it must recognise the real-world constraints on supply. We can't magic this out of thin air.

As if to prove the point, the devolved administrations, usually so determined to do things their own way, are coming to us appealing for supplies. In Wales, the testing contract seems to have fallen through, and the Scots want PPE and 200 ventilators. I instructed the team to get packages together for them and Northern Ireland. 'Make a thing of sending them with great big Union Jacks on the boxes,' I instructed, meaning it. Nothing wrong with proclaiming the benefits of the union.

SUNDAY 29 MARCH

Boris is doing video calls from the flat and looks pretty sweaty. I've suggested that he writes to every household in England – that's 30 million addresses – warning things will 'get worse before they get better', which might equally apply to him. Given the way this is going, I feel we need to prepare the nation psychologically for the possibility of long-term restrictions. Privately, Jenny Harries told me today it could be six months before life can return to 'normal'.

During Zoom meetings today I've done my best to seem cheerful, but the truth is I'm also going downhill. My throat hurts so much that I can't swallow and I can't eat or drink. Beyond that I don't feel that bad – just lethargic – but the pain in my throat is intense. It's hugely frustrating when there's so much to do. Martha has also got it, along with our daughter and our live-in au pair.

Meanwhile there are still dire supply issues with PPE. The BMA is going nuts, issuing a load of shroud-waving statements claiming hospitals and GP practices face 'life-threatening shortages'. It's not as if I think it's acceptable: it's not! There's just no quick fix, as BMA leaders know full well. Almost overnight, PPE has gone from a fairly specialist item to required kit for every single person working in clinics, hospitals and care homes. When the whole world is after it, it simply isn't possible to get as much as we need as fast as it's required.

There's a meme going round on social media, complete with the HM government and NHS logos, claiming Simon Stevens is banning the sale of alcohol from today 'after his team have discovered that the toxin lowers immunity'. It's sufficiently realistic for Simon to have felt the need to issue an internal clarification. 'For the avoidance of doubt, we have not introduced prohibition tonight,' he said reassuringly.

Ed Taylor in my office now spends virtually all his time trying to sort out numbers: tests, cases and deaths. Gathering data from all over the country, checking it's correct and then publishing it in a timely fashion is horrendously complicated. The figures have to be spot on or we'll be crucified. The NHS told Ed that almost 7,000 tests were done yesterday when the correct figure was in fact over 10,000. At least it's in the right direction, but we cannot afford to make these kinds of blunders.

Throat burning, I found myself dealing with an enormous pile of other problems: how to handle the terrible story of an ENT doctor who died of coronavirus after three weeks in ICU; an order of ventilators due to be delivered shortly but which turns out not to be coming; and instructing Simon Stevens to come down hard on Imperial College Trust in London after they stupidly declared that they'll restrict ventilators to patients who are 'reasonably certain' to survive; not to mention Jenrick mangling the latest PPE numbers at tonight's press conference, meaning we had to delete one of my tweets – at 1.30 a.m. All in all, just an averagely quiet coronavirus Sunday.

MONDAY 30 MARCH

Boris and I seem to be on the same trajectory with the virus: ill but still working. Cummings has now joined the club and is self-isolating with symptoms. My SpAd Emma has also gone down with it.

Encouragingly, Vallance says there are early signs that social distancing is making a difference. I have been desperate for any snippet of evidence and am hugely relieved. Transmission of the virus within the community is thought to be decreasing, and hospital admission data suggests cases are not rising as fast as before. I have a plot of the daily cases and deaths on a spreadsheet, and I watch the shape of the curve like a hawk.

We've had more updates from SAGE on the reasonable worst-case scenario. The projection now is for 50,000 deaths, peaking in April, with a slow decline after that. If people don't generally abide by the rules, the worst week will be the one starting 6 April, when as many as 2,700 people may die. That's about a thousand more than the average number of deaths per week in England from all causes. If people do follow the rules, the peak will be this week with an expected 1,900 deaths. I'm trying not to tempt fate by letting myself hope that we could soon be over the worst. Happily, ICU capacity is not yet overwhelmed, even in London.

Just as I was allowing myself to feel a bit more cheerful, I received a very unwelcome call from Steve Oldfield, informing me, in essence, that the PPE supply chain has blown up. He told me that the government-owned company that gets supplies to hospitals across the NHS has effectively collapsed. The increase in demand for PPE was so enormous that they couldn't fulfil it. This is a total disaster. I'm absolutely furious that the people who are meant to be experts in logistics have been unable to cope because there are too many actual logistics. The real question of course is how to fix it. We're bringing it all in house – Steve will have to do it, and we need to find some amazing people to get it sorted.

It's another massive task landed on my plate. In just a few days, we've gone from having a company that supplies 250 hospitals with small amounts of PPE and specialist equipment, to unprecedented demand from 56,000 GPs, dentists, all the care homes. Steve told me that we do still have stockpiles of kit. It's depleting, and we've been buying more from China, but the immediate problem is still lorry access to our storage facility in the north-west. Funnily enough, nobody has been able to magic up any extra entrances, so we're still stuck with single lorryloads at a time. Hats off to those who bought a billion items of PPE all those years ago – I just wish they'd put more thought into getting it out. Worse, it turns out a load of it is now out of date, and some kit bought over a decade ago doesn't conform to the latest standards. Then there's a batch which is actually still usable but has the wrong 'best before' date on it. How we will persuade people to use that is anyone's guess.

In a weird but predictable unintended consequence of the lockdown, the number of people having accidents at home has rocketed. Hospitals are now under pressure from people who've burned themselves baking, fallen off bikes, twisted an ankle trying to roller skate in the house etc. One of our MPs messaged saying his mother fell and broke her arm yesterday (no acrobatics being attempted at the time) and was told by the hospital that they couldn't operate because they don't have the staff.

At the same time, an amazing 730,000 people have now joined NHS Volunteers – way more than we know what to do with. The hard part will be matching enthusiasm to need.

With so much on my plate, we've got to pull more people in. Chris Wormald told me I'm effectively the CEO of the whole effort. He meant it as a compliment, but it's a problem. Testing, vaccines, PPE, ventilators – right across the board we need strong leaders to take these huge projects on. I rang Boris to discuss. He keeps talking about Max Beaverbrook, brought in by Churchill during the war effort to bang the table and make things happen. 'We need our Beaverbrooks,' Boris shouted, not sounding as ill as I'd feared. I agree. The civil service are working at full capacity, and we need a different skillset: strong mission-driven leadership. That can be found in all parts of the economy – but the private sector often has more. The very best people often have both private and public sector experience. We're looking for those who can get stuff done in a hurry.

I told the team that when I get back to the office next week, I want new language about 'a war against this virus, a war in which the whole of humanity is on the same side'. My team is usually pretty quick to puncture my pomposity. Diplomatically, they let this one pass.

Dyson's enthusiasm notwithstanding, we are still desperate for ventilators and need to issue another appeal to industry. Word from No. 10 is that Boris is too sick to front it, which is worrying. I still can't drink anything, but I'm otherwise fine.

TUESDAY 31 MARCH

I felt much better when I woke up this morning and was able to get down lots of fluids. Unfortunately, the same can't be said for Boris. He doesn't look any worse but is still hacking his way through meetings.

A letter in the French newspaper *Le Monde* signed by hospital officials across Europe, including the CEO of Guy's and St Thomas's, warned that supplies of the anaesthesia drugs curare and propofol – used for the most severe cases of Covid – will soon start to run out in the worst-affected areas. Even our hospitals with the largest reserves will run short in two weeks' time. The good news is that we stockpiled these drugs in case of transport problems under a no-deal Brexit. The bad news is we are using them up fast and the worm still hasn't turned – cases are still going up. Meanwhile the global debate over hydroxychloroquine is intensifying. It has now been approved as a treatment in France, though with very tight restrictions. President Macron is being harassed by a YouTube celebrity doctor in Marseilles to make it far more widely available. In the States, Trump has recommended taking it in a cocktail with the antibiotic azithromycin. Here, my ministers are being bombarded with messages saying we should be using it. I held the line, saying we're running a big trial and we'll go as fast as the science allows.

In addition to the pressure over ventilators and PPE, I'm being hammered on testing. Why haven't we hit our 25,000 target? How come the Germans are so far ahead? Are we misleading the public about reagent shortages? I'm feeling increasingly defensive on this one. The fact is we're building a national diagnostic capability from nothing and it's moving extremely fast. There are global shortages of these reagent chemicals – of course there are! The boss at Roche, the biggest company in this area worldwide, has said the supply chain just can't keep pace, but that doesn't cut any ice. Lobby hacks are hard-wired to cast everything as the UK government's fault.

Amid all this, Cummings's morning meetings have turned into a shambles. I can't say I'm shocked. The feedback is that no one really knows who's meant to be talking about what, to whom, or indeed whether they're supposed to be at that meeting or the one an hour later. We can't have our most senior people tied up for two hours in the mornings like this.

'If No. 10 want grown-up meetings, they have to organise them properly,' I told my team grumpily. Managing No. 10 is a massive and extremely frustrating part of my job.

APRIL 2020

Final day in my own personal lockdown. I'm feeling fine now and keen to get back to the office and put the final touches on a new testing target, which I want to announce tomorrow.

We've already carried out 153,000 tests, more than any other European country except Germany and Italy – pretty impressive when you think about how little capacity we had at the start.

Part of the announcement is about bringing in outside organisations like Boots and Amazon to deliver tests, expanding our testing efforts and answering a critical question: what proportion of the population have had the virus? This is central to when and how we come out of lockdown. If there's a high level of immunity in the population, we'll be in much better shape. If not, there's no way out without a vaccine.

I also need to be at the podium. Alok took the press conference today and got absolutely pummelled on testing. I felt incredibly sorry for him: all he did was robotically repeat our scripted lines to take, which is what No. 10 asked of him. It was so painful to watch that I wanted to switch off after five minutes. I knew he wouldn't gaffe – he's totally reliable like that – but understandably, given that this isn't his beat, he just couldn't deal with detailed questions. Putting him in that position wasn't fair and I felt guilty that I wasn't leading on it.

Roberto Speranza has extended lockdown in Italy, and COP 26, which was supposed to take place in Glasgow this autumn, has been postponed to 2021. Thank goodness for that. People are beginning to realise we're in it for the long haul. I was weirdly upset when I heard that Wimbledon has been cancelled for the first time since the war. I thought of all those wooden plaques in sports clubs across the country which have gaps for the war years and will now have another gap due to the pandemic.

This evening Boris posted a video he took of himself in No. 10. Bad move: he looked so ropey. He talked about it being a 'sad day' with a record 563 deaths then tried to reassure people that he's OK, saying that despite being 'sequestered' in No. 10 he's still in constant touch with his officials. Not his most convincing performance.

THURSDAY 2 APRIL

Normal hostilities are beginning to resume in the press. They've been unusually supportive these past few weeks, doing their bit to pull together during a time of national crisis etc., but the fragile consensus over our response is beginning to splinter. The *Daily Mail* broke first, running a highly critical piece about not having enough tests. Privately, they're right of course, and Geordie Greig was decent enough to call me to say he knows we had to start from scratch and that I'm on it.

The WHO has said again today that 'there has been no documented asymptomatic transmission'. It's infuriating as it's obvious there is, but the formal scientific advice just isn't there. We do not have time for these bureaucratic processes.

The rest of my day was dominated by the big testing target announcement. Unusually, I was nervous: lives depend on me pulling this off. Some people have said it's too politically risky to tie myself to a big target when I don't know if we can hit it. Forget it. I'm prepared to put my career on the line to make it happen.

After a quick and distracted breakfast, I was driven to the office for 7.30 a.m. It was great to be back, and everyone clapped me in – much to my embarrassment. At 8.30 the PM's morning meeting took place in the Cabinet Room as usual – only without him.

The place was deserted. Normally the corridors buzz with staff hurrying from one room to another. So much business gets done bumping into people on their way between meetings. Today: nothing. It was unsettling.

Boris appeared on screen, looking dishevelled and frankly knackered. He was coughing badly and doesn't seem to be improving. He was also extremely grumpy about the state of testing, firing out all sorts of ideas for speeding things up.

Back from Downing Street, I wanted to double-triple-check my target is achievable and asked Kristen McLeod, the newly appointed lead official on testing, to come and see me.

'How many tests can we do by the end of the month?' I asked.

'120,000,' she replied.

I asked: if we set a 100,000 target, would we hit it? 'We can hit it,' she said, 'but I can't promise for certain.' That much is obvious, but it will focus minds.

Then it was into drafting and rehearsing my speech, with me pacing up and down the room trying to get the tone exactly right as I practised my lines. Gina sat on the sidelines, urging me to sound 'more human'. I found the whole process agonising, trying not to sound too flat while avoiding sounding glib. The team is so worried about my propensity to make off-the-cuff remarks to try to lighten the mood that they've written a huge sign saying 'NO JOKES' and stuck it to the wall in their office.

As we ran through my speech again and again, Gina became increasingly agitated. She didn't think I'd nailed it. She was right. We only just finalised the words before I went over to Downing Street.

We did a last-minute run-through of the script in the Thatcher Room on the first floor of No. 10, the great lady's portrait looming over us. Walking into the press conference, I knew what I had to do, but I was still worried about stumbling over the numbers of people who have died and somehow seeming disrespectful.

In the end the questions from the media were almost all straightforward and thoughtful and we got the message across.

The hardest bit was being asked what we've got wrong. Politicians can't win with this question. Whatever you say, the press has a field day. So I went against everything I've learned and just answered the question without fear of the consequences, saying we could have brought in the economic package a bit quicker. It was pretty innocuous and didn't get much pickup, except from Rishi's people, who took it very personally. Liam Booth-Smith, his super-bright adviser, called my team and went absolutely tonto. I don't want to damage relations with Rishi, who I rate and like, so I'll buy him something nice to apologise. In truth I should have given a frank answer about something I was responsible for – like that we haven't got the private sector ramping up testing fast enough – but in the heat of the moment I couldn't come up with something that was both true and wouldn't have caused all sorts of complications afterwards. Not my finest hour.

I went straight from the press conference to see Rishi. The internal door between No. 10 and No. 11 is always open, as is a second set of doors to No. 12, once the home of the whips, until Tony Blair turned it into the comms operation. Disturbingly, I found that door sealed off with a plastic sheet: apparently everyone who normally works there has Covid.

I turned right into the Chancellor's study, a room I know well, having spent many hours in there with Rishi's predecessors, first George Osborne, then Philip Hammond and then Sajid Javid. It's the most private of studies, with twin back-to-back doors to prevent anyone overhearing, accidentally or otherwise. The pair of us talked about the pressures we're under. He's got to get the furlough scheme up and running in a matter of days. He asked how I'm sleeping. 'Fine,' I replied truthfully. I'm not lying in bed tossing and turning, because each day I know I've done everything I possibly can. Of course, given that there's no playbook to this, we are making mistakes, but there are also signs we're getting the virus under control, and the work on the vaccine is progressing. I know I'm giving this my best shot and my conscience is clear. I certainly couldn't ask my team or the NHS to give any more.

Rishi congratulated me on my testing target, or 'BHAG' – meaning 'Big Hairy Audacious Goal' – as he put it. He loves all that American business-school speak, having done an MBA at Stanford and spent years working in California.

'I need to galvanise the system,' I told him. I may live to regret it, but at least I'm holding myself accountable. Always anxious to think the worst of people, Cummings has accused me of doing it for PR reasons.

At today's press conference, I also tackled the issue of Premier League footballers' wages – a hot topic because some clubs are taking advantage of the furlough scheme. My view is that everybody needs to play their part in this national effort – including multi-millionaire players.

My intervention didn't go down well with everyone. Former Man Utd and England right-back turned TV pundit Gary Neville tweeted that I have a 'f**** cheek', before going into a bizarre rant wrongly stating that I can't even get NHS staff tested. Evidently I touched a nerve, as he then insisted Premier League stars are working on some vague plan to support people affected by the pandemic.

Emerging from Downing Street feeling dazed and relieved, I called the SpAds to see how it had all gone down. Encouragingly, Jamie thought I'd 'completely nailed it'.

Sadly, there was no time to sit back feeling pleased with myself, as I had to head to Uxbridge – the PM's constituency – to do *Question Time*. On the way I stopped for food in a windswept housing estate. There wasn't a soul in sight. The only shop open in this little parade was the pizza delivery store. I sat in the back of the car thinking how end-of-days it felt to be out and about.

The other panellists were Yvette Cooper for Labour; Donna Kinnair, head of the RCN; and John Sentamu, Archbishop of York.

Sentamu, appearing via Zoom from York, told me about a rabbi friend of his whose wife had died of natural causes – not Covid. They'd

been married for over fifty years, yet he didn't attend the funeral because he was elderly and followed the 'stay at home' instruction to the
letter. I was shocked and moved: we never meant people to go this
far. Of course they should attend a spouse's funeral. After the show, I
immediately contacted my private office telling them that we have to
issue clearer guidance on funerals.

En route home I called Boris, who was not sounding good. 'I think
I'll stay in quarantine for the weekend and come back on Monday,' he
rasped. 'You'll have to hold the fort until then.'

He did at least manage to haul himself onto the steps of No. 10 to do
the clap for carers this evening.

Before I collapsed into bed, one of the team rang to run me through
what happened at the latest SAGE meeting. We've managed to avoid
the NHS becoming overwhelmed in London, a huge achievement.
They say that by 13 April they should know whether everything we've
done has proven effective or whether 'further interventions' might be
needed. Like what, exactly? Every public place is completely deserted.
Here's hoping none of the hardliners are getting ideas from Peru and
Panama, where they've just announced gender-based curfews: men
allowed out three days a week, women three days and no one on Sundays. Imagine trying that here.

SAGE also says, with spectacular understatement, that there's a risk
that lifting restrictions too early 'could lead to a second wave of exponential epidemic growth ... requiring measures to be re-imposed'. No
kidding.

While we battle this at home, worldwide reported cases have gone
past 1 million, and reported deaths have hit 50,000. According to the
Prof, these figures are pretty much meaningless. He says nobody can
record case numbers accurately and very few countries will be chart-
ing deaths as meticulously as we are. We will only ever know the true
facts a long time afterwards.

Simon Stevens is keen to release essential hospital capacity and has
been pushing for guidance on how to discharge elderly patients who
can be cared for just as well in other settings. Negative tests won't be

required prior to transfers/admissions into care homes. The tragic but honest truth is we don't have enough testing capacity to check anyway. It's an utter nightmare, but it's the reality. Under the circumstances, we must make sure that anyone going from a hospital into a care home is kept away from other residents. We have put this in the guidance, although we have precious few levers to ensure it happens. I hope it is followed. The decision has been very difficult. If we keep people in hospital, the NHS will be overrun. There are no simple solutions to this, because people are at risk if they stay in hospital too, but a decision had to be made – no matter how hard. If only we had more tests.

FRIDAY 3 APRIL

A thirteen-year-old boy who died from Covid was buried without any mourners today, lowered into the ground by four men in hazmat suits. His parents weren't even at the graveside because they were self-isolating. I felt almost physically sick reading it as my own boy, just a year younger, slept peacefully in the room next door. To lose a child is the worst thing that could ever happen. Not to be there to lay him to rest is unimaginable. It doesn't matter that this was never our intention. I must sort it out.

Boris is still in bad shape and has decided to stay out of circulation longer than strictly required by the protocols, as he still has a temperature. I called him this morning and told him about the thirteen-year-old and he was shocked and upset. He tries not to let on, but he is actually a very emotional man… He's still working incredibly hard, coughing through the call. He's very worried about looking feeble and hates any sympathy.

'A general's job is to show strength, not weakness,' he told me ruefully.

Against all the odds, the Nightingale hospital at the ExCel Centre is ready. Between them, the NHS, the armed forces and some outstanding private sector contractors pulled it off, creating a 500-bed hospital in just nine days – quicker than the Chinese. No one believed we could do it. I headed over for the official opening but had to stop en route to settle a ridiculous debate over what to do with prisoners.

Because of the challenges associated with social distancing in jails, this issue has been rumbling on for weeks. A few weeks ago, officials told me Justice Secretary Rob Buckland wanted to release thousands of non-violent prisoners to take the pressure off the system. I've always been against it and keep writing 'NO' in large letters on submissions asking me to sign it off. It's obvious the public won't wear it. Yet the idea keeps going back and forth on paper. After about the third iteration I called Rob, who to my astonishment told me he'd been advised that I was the one who wanted to release them. As for him, he wasn't nearly as enthusiastic about the idea as my officials had made out. Do they not think we talk to each other?

Unfortunately, this still wasn't the end of the matter. Clearly someone in Whitehall still thought it was a good plan and kept pushing it, to the point that the PM asked to talk to us both. The only slot we could find in the diary was while I was on the way to open the Nightingale. So this afternoon I found myself sitting in the back of the car in a car park outside the ExCel Centre, making my views crystal clear.

'We cannot lock up literally everyone in the country except prisoners, who we instead release!' I spluttered. The argument was dragging on, and I was on a deadline to Zoom Prince Charles for the formal opening. Eventually I explained to the PM that I really had to go. Commendably, he concluded that we absolutely did not want to release prisoners. They are mostly young. If they have to spend more time in their cells due to staff shortages, so be it. If there are particularly vulnerable individuals, they can always be isolated on Covid-free wings. Ye Gods.

That matter settled, I took a deep breath and headed into the new hospital for a tour. I can't ever remember having such mixed feelings: elation at a job extraordinarily well done; anguish at the idea that it might soon be full of people fighting for their lives. Once you're on a ventilator the chance of survival is only about 50:50. Surveying the scene, all I could think was, 'Half the people who end up in these beds won't get out alive.' There aren't even any loos for patients, because none of them will be conscious. If they recover, they'll be taken back to normal hospitals, so they will never know they were there.

The opening was meticulously choreographed, with all the key people who made it happen standing outside on marked spots two metres apart. I gave a short speech and then introduced Prince Charles, who was appearing in his first ever public Zoom. To the astonishment of almost everyone, all the technology worked, and the opening went smoothly.

With Boris still struggling, I took the Downing Street press conference again, this time with JVT at my side. What people watching on TV won't have realised is just how short he is, because we got him to stand on what we call a Sarkozy box – the Whitehall term for a plinth that's sometimes used to make people look taller when they're standing at a podium.

'You're a wonderful man but not blessed in the height department. It's that or heels,' I told him cheerfully. He messaged me just after 11 p.m., having watched the press conference back, to say that both he and his wife Karen loved his new look.

I only realised it when I got back from isolating at home, but the staff of my private office have all been working eighteen-hour days too. Natasha, who runs the show, has now decided to put them on a shift system. We'll hire in some more support, then half the team will work 6 a.m. to 6 p.m.; the other half will work 11 a.m. to 11 p.m. They are unbelievably dedicated to the cause. I've been trying to think of a way to show some appreciation and came up with the idea of bringing a different private secretary to each of the Downing Street press conferences. (I always take someone with me in case of last-minute checking or printing.) Most have never been into the building, despite working in the heart of government. Today I took Cindy, one of the newest members of the team, and managed to take a picture of her beaming from ear to ear as she walked up the main staircase past the famous pictures of all the Prime Ministers on the wall. Although I've had the privilege of being in No. 10 countless times, that thrill never wears off.

This evening Nadine Dorries alerted me to a story in the American press about hydroxychloroquine, which thousands of doctors now believe is the best available treatment for Covid. In the UK, it's used to treat rheumatoid arthritis and lupus. I got straight onto Jim Bethell, who says we're already buying, though naturally there's a scramble. JVT is working out allocations between patient groups in a way that doesn't undermine our clinical trials, because it's too early to say whether it works.

Around the world, leaders are turning inwards. China has asked foreign diplomats to stay out of Beijing until 15 May. Trump has invoked the Defense Production Act to halt the export of masks and other PPE. It's hardly surprising: the US has confirmed 32,000 cases in one day, a new record. The breakdown of international cooperation just when we need it most is another sign of the enormity of this thing.

The US Centers for Disease Control (CDC) today released the first solid evidence showing that asymptomatic transmission is occurring. I've been banging on about this for weeks, but the advice I have been getting has all pointed towards asymptomatic transmission being unlikely. PHE is re-investigating. I should have pushed this much harder.

SATURDAY 4 APRIL

Carrie has Covid. She's heavily pregnant, which probably makes the symptoms feel a hundred times worse. What an awful year for her and Boris, who is now being accused by unnamed 'sources' in the media of 'stubbornly refusing to stop working'. There is growing muttering that he's jeopardising his own recovery by failing to rest. True.

Meanwhile President Trump has randomly and dangerously declared that hydroxychloroquine is an effective treatment for Covid, despite a total absence of the evidence required for such a statement. What does he know that JVT doesn't? I am despairing. What an awful, awful man.

Every day I check case numbers obsessively, hoping to see that the worm has turned. Every day I'm disappointed.

SUNDAY 5 APRIL

A *cri de cœur* from Helen Whately, who is under massive pressure over PPE shortages in care homes. 'It is still all over the place,' she said.

Apparently she is getting contradictory information from officials, who can't seem to answer any questions about supplies. 'There is only so long I can keep saying to the social care sector that we're working on it without losing all credibility,' she said miserably. I promised to do everything I can.

On the morning media round, I did my best to make Boris sound in better shape than he is.

'I've been talking to him every day, several times a day,' I said truthfully, adding that he's very much got his hand on the tiller. I admitted that he's still running a temperature but stressed that he's in good spirits.

After *Marr*, I found myself in the BBC green room with Keir Starmer, who took over as Labour leader yesterday. What odd circumstances in which to become Leader of the Opposition.

'At least Jeremy Corbyn becoming PM and destroying the country can come off my worry list,' I told him cheerfully.

'Happy to lighten your load,' he replied.

Scientists, politicians and journalists are beginning to ask more searching questions about the origins of the virus. The wet market theory is now looking less credible than what goes on behind closed doors at a virology laboratory in Wuhan. It just so happens that there's a leading coronavirus research facility in the exact same place that this nightmare began. More than a bit suspicious, no?

Assuming nobody intended to cause such a catastrophe, it strikes me as possible that Chinese scientists discovered the virus in the wild, took a sample to examine in the lab and then let it escape as a result of poor biosecurity. Though the international consensus and the government's position is that the virus originated at the Wuhan wet market, I remain sceptical. There must be a full investigation into what happened.

This evening, the Queen gave a special coronavirus address to the nation and Commonwealth. As always, Her Majesty struck exactly the right note, conjuring up Vera Lynn's wartime classic when she said that together, we will beat this thing – and meet again.

I was just about to go to bed when my phone rang for the umpteenth time. It was almost out of charge and I had to crouch on the floor by a socket to take the call. It was Mark Sedwill, who informed me, in a very matter-of-fact tone, that the Prime Minister was on his way to St Thomas's Hospital 'as a precautionary step', because his symptoms are not getting any better.

'We all need to rally round' was the crux of the message. Sedwill told me that as First Secretary of State, Dominic Raab will lead on key decisions, supported by me, Rishi and Michael Gove – the 'quad'. Shellshocked, I immediately called the others. Raab was already on his way back into the office. He was incredibly grown-up and restrained, making clear that he wasn't going to try to look like he was Prime Minister but instead hold the fort.

The hard part is that Boris is still furiously texting everyone. We agreed a protocol, whereby Raab will take any big decisions to the PM, and the rest of us will back off to give him space to recover.

There is one chink of light on the horizon: Spain has reported a decline in cases for the third day in a row. Maybe the lockdown is going to work after all.

MONDAY 6 APRIL

Boris has been taken into intensive care. Everyone is stunned. I'm told there's a 50:50 chance he'll end up on a ventilator; and if that happens, we know there's a 50:50 chance he will die. Nobody at Westminster can quite believe it's happening.

The minute the news came out, pharma companies started calling my private office with offers of experimental drugs. Natasha did her best to triage the approaches, separating credible offers from chancers and unhelpful enthusiasts. Anything that sounded as if it might have potential was forwarded to the Prof, who's in touch with the PM's clinical team. Among the many calls was one from the White House. Having failed to get through to me direct, they reached Natasha, who messaged to say that Vice-President Mike Pence wanted to talk to me urgently.

An hour or so after the story came out, I received a text from ITV political editor Robert Peston, who claimed the PM is on considerably more oxygen than is being reported. How on earth did he know about the PM's medical condition?!

Raab is doing a great job of looking like he's not the Prime Minister, which is definitely better than trying to pretend he is. It's a fine line, though: giving an interview with the BBC's Laura Kuenssberg late this evening, he looked very sweaty and not his usual steady self. Here's hoping he's not going down with it too. If that happens, Rishi has apparently been lined up as next in charge.

This is a moment of terrible peril for our country. We all know there's a real chance Boris won't pull through.

Earlier I gave Rishi a box of wine to say sorry for my thoughtless comments at the press conference the other day. He couldn't have been more charming. Sadly, he won't be enjoying it. Turns out he's teetotal. I had no idea. He was extremely gracious about it, and said his dad would enjoy it. I'm mortified, but I hope he appreciated the gesture.

TUESDAY 7 APRIL

I awoke to the news that Boris didn't have to be intubated overnight and seems to be turning a corner. I'm massively, massively relieved and so grateful to the staff at the hospital.

Tomorrow, the Queen is to give another broadcast to try to reassure the nation. Thank God for Her Majesty: a universally respected figure who stands above party politics and embodies everything that is great about the United Kingdom.

Meanwhile JVT is very excited that we've recruited 1,900 patients for the Oxford University Recovery Trial.

'Fastest recruitment for a trial like this in history?' I asked.

'Almost certainly,' he replied.

JVT would never boast, but it's another feather in the cap for British science. Now we can find out if hydroxychloroquine and all the other suggested remedies actually work in practice.

In another positive development, Cambridge University has set up a new testing centre, working with AstraZeneca and GSK. These pharma companies are not big on diagnostics but they're leaning in to help with the national effort. It will begin with 1,000–2,000 a day by mid-April and reach 30,000 by the first week of May. It's a week late for my target, but that's not the point – we are hustling every test we can get.

I asked JVT about a serology survey being done at Porton Down to estimate the proportion of people who've been in contact with the virus. He is chasing. This is absolutely vital info because it will indicate how many people may already be immune.

Later I was given top lines from the SAGE meeting. They'll go so far as to say there's no current evidence that transmission is accelerating, and in fact it may be slowing. ICU admission doubling time is lengthening, especially in London, where it's now 8.8 days. Fingers crossed. NERVTAG have concluded that increased use of masks would have minimal effect in terms of slowing the spread. One finding jumped out at me: it looks like obesity is a significant risk factor. Maybe that is why the PM went downhill. The single biggest risk factor is still age, followed by gender: men are twice as vulnerable as women. Then comes obesity, followed by ethnicity. We've got to publish this, and ensure the debate follows the science. I don't want snippets leaking and being taken out of context.

On the subject of misrepresentation, WhatsApp has said it will introduce limits on forwarding material to combat Covid-related fake news. It's a start but nowhere near enough. If we do manage to develop a vaccine, there's going to be all manner of rubbish circulating on the internet. I've asked officials to set up a meeting with social media companies to firm up their resolve.

WEDNESDAY 8 APRIL

Boris spent a second night in intensive care and is stable and responding to treatment. I worry about him for the sake of the country – losing the PM to Covid would be an absolute disaster in the midst of the biggest challenge for public administration in our times – but, even more,

I worry about losing a close colleague and friend. When you spend time with Boris, it's impossible not to like him. He's endlessly funny and engaging and thinks differently and more laterally than anyone I know. This can bring its challenges when straight-line thinking is required, but for grasping the big picture there's no one like him. I feel as if we've been in the metaphorical trenches together and feel sick at the thought that this wretched disease might kill him.

Later today his brother Leo called to tell me that he is sitting up, but they're keeping him in the ICU and off his phone to make sure he doesn't relapse. There has been some suggestion among scientists that Covid patients might benefit from plasma donated by people who have recovered from the disease. Leo joked that Boris started to recover when they told him he'd have to be infused with Nadine's blood.

Raab is very clear that he wants all communication with the boss to go through him. As Boris is an inveterate texter, I doubt that will last, but I'm respecting it for now.

Nobody speaks of it, but there is a 'worst-case scenario' plan for if Boris doesn't pull through. We couldn't possibly have a normal Conservative Party leadership election, so the Cabinet would have to take a quick decision, advise the Queen and rally round. I don't know exactly which part of the 'deep state' formulated this succession plan, who approved it or even if it's written down, but someone's done the thinking and it's pretty sensible. This is the upside to having a flexible constitution: we can somewhat make these thing up as we go along. Thankfully nobody is talking about who might be chosen under such dreadful circumstances. It's not going to come to that.

Amid a global scramble for drugs of all kinds, some of the most basic medicine is becoming hot property. A case in point is paracetamol, which is good at bringing fevers down and recommended for treating the temperature that goes with Covid. We're desperately trying to get hold of more from India. Priti Patel has a direct line into Prime Minister Modi and has been trying to help. His government has approved the export of 2.8 million packs to the UK for over-the-counter sale in pharmacies. High Commission staff in Delhi are now trying to sort out shipping. Hopefully the consignment will come in on a consular flight from Delhi or Goa in the next few days. Next up: 250,000 gowns from Egypt. This sort of hand-to-mouth management of materials is unknown to any government outside wartime.

The second floor of the Department of Health is now the HQ for national testing. It's literally a military operation. While the rest of the building is deserted, it's packed. As I walked onto the main floor this evening, those in uniform stood to attention and saluted. The formality was strangely disconcerting.

The senior officer from the Royal Logistic Corps introduced herself. She has organised everything on strict military lines. There's a map of the UK on an enormous board with movable pieces representing the various testing units. Some of these units can head to hotspots where we have problems. When they're shifted round the board it looks eerily like those pictures of Fighter Command during the Battle of Britain – a very tangible reminder of how many lives are at stake.

There are also clinicians, consultants from Deloitte and a load of civil servants, all dutifully trying to keep their distance from each other. The presence of the army brings an intensity and gravity that galvanises everyone.

Somewhat predictably, the EU's ventilator procurement scheme is proving a flop. A couple of weeks ago we were widely criticised for declining to join. So far, they haven't managed to source a single one.

A fabulous image of the Queen has appeared on the giant screens at Piccadilly Circus, all lit up. Under the picture are quotes from her address to the nation: 'We will meet again.' Looking at it, I felt quite emotional. What we are all going through is quite extraordinary. God save the Queen.

We are running out of more key drugs. Raab says the Americans are aware of our plight and keen to help. He's due to talk to Trump's son-in-law Jared Kushner and asked me for a wish list. I sent him a note to pass to Jared asking for a bunch of things: most importantly, anaesthetics. We also need feeding tubes; around 600 machines for people with kidney failure; 500 blood gas analysers; swabs and reagents for

PCR tests; and a long list of intensive care and Covid medicines: propofol, noradrenaline, suxamethonium, azithromycin and hydroxychloroquine. We still don't know which of these work, but it's vital we have supplies for the clinical trials. I'm praying that Jared and the Americans can bail us out. In the meantime, I'm getting JVT to develop a global shopping list, so the whole Foreign Office can go searching for what we need. I've made it clear this is top priority: if people find out that hospitals are on the brink of running out of life-saving drugs, all hell will break loose. The other priority is of course ventilators. We've ordered 1,500 from American companies but have no idea when or even if they'll be delivered. In an ideal world, we'd like a further 2,500. At the moment the most likely source is China, but our doctors much prefer the better-quality American machines.

THURSDAY 9 APRIL

Boris is out of intensive care! Such great news, though it will be a while before he's out of hospital. Raab now chairs daily meetings. His style is very different to the PM's. One is all detail and no strategy; the other, all strategy and, shall we say, less of the detail. I can't imagine what their exchanges are like when it's just the two of them. Dom has introduced discussions about how to come out of restrictions. It feels very premature. There are tentative signs that the lockdown is working, but it may be a temporary lull. Meanwhile we've recorded 1,030 deaths in the past twenty-four hours alone, the highest figure so far.

Helen Whately messaged to say she's just been sent the first proper data on care home deaths 'and it's not good'. Ominous. Earlier this week there was a Covid major outbreak at a nursing home in Newcastle-under-Lyme, resulting in as many as eleven deaths. Some staff walked out. We must identify precisely how the virus is getting into homes and then spreading within these settings.

On a practical note, the state has never had more transport options at its disposal. Shapps's department sent us a cheerful message, asking if anyone needed any planes or trains. 'Now that we've nationalised virtually all transport, we have lots of people, drivers, cars, vans, railway carriages, helicopters, planes etc. If you have logistical needs, get in touch,' they offered cheerfully. Could come in handy!

Later JVT messaged to tell me that Porton Down has finally been able to give us an indicator of how many people in the UK are likely to have already had the virus. The answer is devastating: just 5 per cent. What this means is that 95 per cent of the country don't have any immunity at all.

'Are you sure it's that low?' I asked anxiously, hoping it was some kind of misprint.

He said it was just a 'ballpark' and was not for public consumption, but yes: the survey just kept coming back with negative tests.

If the proportion of people with antibodies is anywhere near 5 per cent – way below the ridiculous media speculation that 'most' people have had it – and we have 1,000 people a day dying despite lockdown, the logic is that we are not going to be able to lift restrictions until the vaccine has made enough people safe. In my view, it kills off any remaining notion of seeking 'herd immunity'.

I opened my laptop to do the maths myself. So far, 9,692 people have died. Deaths lag cases by about three weeks on average, so even if there were no more infections, at 1,000 a day that will be 30,000 deaths in three weeks' time. That's with 5 per cent of people infected. So without restrictions let's assume, say, half the population get infected (though Chris Whitty thinks 80 per cent is more likely) – that leads to between 300,000 and 500,000 people dead overall. This fits with the worst-case scenario in the early official forecasts. We can't have that.

By contrast, the fastest we could possibly have a vaccine is the end of the year, after which we will need three months to vaccinate the vulnerable. I stared at the figures feeling almost nauseous as the full implications sank in. Basically, we are looking at another year of restrictions. How on earth are we going to tell people that?

The only way through this is to suppress the virus until the vaccine comes good. There is no alternative. And the best way to do that is to get cases right down, then loosen up until R equals 1 and no higher.

There is no time to lose in our quest for a vaccine.

At least today's numbers suggest the epidemic is reaching its peak. Cases, bed occupancy and ICU numbers – which seemed only ever to go up – are now flat. Calls to NHS 111 and 999 appear to have peaked.

So here we are, right at the apex of the deaths. Cases are just starting to top out, and there are signs we really have got R below 1 and the NHS will not be overwhelmed. Now we enter a new phase: how to get it down and keep it down until help arrives.

In other good news, the chief veterinary officer has formally advised that the risk of transmission from felines to humans is low. At least we're not going to have to kill anyone's cat.

FRIDAY 10 APRIL

I talked to the Prof first thing about my fears over the 5 per cent figure. Depressingly, he had reached exactly the same conclusion, with an added factor: winter. He basically thinks we are in this till next spring.

Confirmed deaths worldwide have passed 100,000. The US Federal Reserve has announced a $2.3 trillion programme to help small businesses and state and local government. I thought back to my time at the Bank of England during 9/11, which triggered massive bailouts, but nothing like this.

We now have a 24/7 military operation across the UK to ensure PPE supplies get to the right place. It's a Herculean effort. An army reservist has done an amazing job designing the portal, with the help of people from eBay and NHSX, the health service's digital innovation arm. I've made it clear that people need to treat PPE as the precious resource it is. Meanwhile we're employing tens of thousands of officials to monitor outbreaks and contact everyone who might be carrying the virus with instructions to isolate. Not yet a German-style 'test and trace' system, which is proving effective there, but we're working on it.

JVT told the daily press conference that the lockdown is 'beginning to pay off' but was very cautious.

No word from Raab about the medicines we need, so I chased him up. Jared had got back to him saying they can send us 200 ventilators (am grateful, but it's nowhere near enough!) and will look for more.

SATURDAY 11 APRIL

Great excitement in No. 10 over an initiative in South Korea which involves getting citizens to wear tracker bracelets to monitor adherence to Covid restrictions. Cummings wants to know whether we can issue everyone in the country with one of these devices, which would use sat-nav technology to identify whether people have been in close contact with someone who has Covid. Hmmm. Providing 50 million of these things would be no mean feat and there's a slight 'electronic tag' feel to them. Lockdown-sceptic MPs would go nuts. All the same, we're looking into whether some version of the idea might be possible and have got Apple involved.

Among the many things bothering me is whether we are being too cautious on potential treatments that have not yet been through full trials. I was struck by a list of medicines they're trying in a top US hospital in Houston, including hydroxychloroquine and remdesivir, and asked the Prof whether we could do something similar here. He replied that we must always wait for clinical trials to produce robust evidence. He's right of course. There are now more than 3,000 people in UK trials. We had a discussion about whether we could put out interim guidance for drugs that are still experimental.

'The question I have is whether we have more people going from moderate illness to death because of underuse of some of these treatments which are promising but unproven?' I asked.

He replied that individual doctors can adapt what they give patients but that he would be 'very cautious' about advising clinicians to use treatment in advance of evidence. He says there is usually a burst of enthusiasm followed by all the downsides emerging. He pointed out that there is a growing debate over whether we are actually ventilating too many patients. Apparently many of the new drugs are 'potentially quite high-risk' and may do more harm than good. Fair enough. We have to be responsible.

So far nineteen NHS workers have died of Covid. They have paid the ultimate price. There's zero evidence that any of the deaths were linked to lack of protective gear, but I'm getting a load of flak for saying we should use it carefully. Keir Starmer went so far as to accuse me of 'insulting' staff. What shameless political point scoring! The idea that we need to manage our resources carefully in a crisis shouldn't be controversial. I'm not saying don't use PPE. Far from it – those working in the NHS and in care homes must use it. I want people to be safe. I'm just pleading that we don't waste any as it's becoming increasingly scarce.

I got a lovely supportive message from Oxford history professor Andrew Thompson, thanking me for everything I'm doing. Notes such as this from people I admire really give me a lift.

'The responsibility is great but so too is the motivation,' I replied.

SUNDAY 12 APRIL – EASTER DAY

The PM has left hospital and gone to Chequers. No. 10 says he will be taking a break from work while he recovers. He issued a video statement, wearing a suit and tie, praising the NHS for saving his life and saying that we will win the battle against Covid 'because our NHS is the beating heart of this country. It is the best of this country. It is unconquerable. It is powered by love.' He was clearly very emotional – understandably so, after such a close shave. Carrie also thanked staff and everyone who sent messages of support, admitting that she and the family had been through 'very dark times' last week.

Churches held virtual services for Easter Sunday; the Archbishop of Canterbury conducted his from his kitchen. I took a break from work to tune into one of these services, choosing something from Ireland as all the rest of the family are Catholic. The remainder of the day was spent prepping for tomorrow's Downing Street press conference, which I'll use to talk about the new contact tracing app we're developing. I'm a bit worried I've over-egged it: people are desperate for a silver bullet to end lockdown. This isn't it. Even with widespread testing and tracking I don't think we can keep R below 1 without restrictions.

Unusually, EU Commission President Ursula von der Leyen is being quite helpful, at least in terms of managing expectations. She has suggested that the elderly may need to isolate indefinitely till the vaccine is produced, maybe till the end of year and beyond. It's depressing, but useful to have others saying it.

Meanwhile China has reopened wet markets in Wuhan. Really?

MONDAY 13 APRIL

Helen Whately is frustrated about the policy for discharging elderly patients from hospitals into social care. The NHS urgently needs to clear beds for Covid patients and won't keep people on wards if they're fit for discharge. The problem is that care home managers are highly reluctant to take these vulnerable patients in because of the risk of infection. As Social Care Minister, Helen has repeatedly asked PHE whether these discharges are OK from an infection control point of view. She says the NHS are 'determined not to budge on discharging patients who are fit to discharge'.

'I can see the NHS point. At least they have managed to win the battle of getting patients who are fit for discharge actually out of their hospitals. The important things is that we don't force care homes to take them,' Helen added. Her view is that local authorities should take ultimate responsibility for people who don't need to be in hospital but do need to be quarantined. I've told her to write her preferred solution into the text of the guidance we are putting out. Apparently officials keep deleting her suggestions in favour of their own.

I've been talking to the Oxford vaccine research team about what they need. The lead is Sarah Gilbert, a professor of vaccinology, who's spent the past fifteen years working on novel influenza vaccines. I asked how the government can help at this stage, and the answer is money: she's talking to the research bodies about the £20 million she needs to make progress, but it hasn't come through. I'm horrified that she has had to wade through treacle to get what she and her team require. I told her I'd sort it and got straight onto David Williams, the keeper of the purse. This is total top priority, I told him, and Professor Gilbert needs her cash ASAP so she can get on with the job. Whatever it takes.

TUESDAY 14 APRIL

Cummings is back in Downing Street after two weeks self-isolating and is on the warpath over PPE. He's being extremely aggressive, demanding to know why we have shortages, when it's blatantly obvious that global demand is through the roof. The minute we decided all NHS frontline staff should wear it, there was – entirely predictably – a desperate scramble. The new rule was a tricky judgement: we could have required less, and left people more exposed, which might have been politically easier but would have been the wrong thing to do. He wasn't there when we made this judgement, has no idea about the complexities of the supply chain and is just generally being a massive pain. He's begun personally calling in junior officials, circumventing the usual channels and lines of responsibility because he thinks certain individuals are 'heroes' and can solve everything. The arrogance is breath-taking. Where he's right is that we clearly need someone very good to grip it. I talked to a few of the saner No. 10 people to see if they can come up with some names.

I reflected on how much easier it was to get stuff done when Cummings was stuck at home.

We're still struggling to get each department the data they need to run the shielding operation effectively, so we've drafted in a Beaverbrook-type outsider to sort things out: Chris Townsend, who was commercial director of the London Olympics and – more than any other person – is probably responsible for the decent state of broadband in the UK. I'll never forget meeting him in the Commons shortly after I became Culture Secretary. We went to the Pugin Room – a ridiculously grand tearoom where MPs often take guests – and he ordered two glasses of champagne and told me I should become Prime Minister. He then said, 'In the meantime, what we're doing on broadband isn't nearly good enough. You've got to tell the whole system that we're moving past copper and we're going to deliver full fibre broadband everywhere.' He was right. Between us we galvanised the system and made it happen. Thank God, because if most of the country had rubbish broadband and the digital divide was still as bad as it was five years ago, handling the pandemic would be way, way harder. Imagine how difficult it would be if 10 per cent or even 5 per cent of pupils didn't have a good enough connection for home schooling?

Chris went on to work for Chelsea FC, but he's coming in to bang heads together. Jenrick and the MHCLG (Ministry of Communities and Local Government) are working out how we use the army to deliver food packages to the most vulnerable people, but none of that is possible without all the right data. Hopefully he can kick them into gear.

Dom Raab, Rishi, Michael and I met in the Cabinet Room to discuss what we should say to the PM about continuing restrictions. My view is that we need to hold the virus down until we have a vaccine. Whatever happens, R needs to stay below 1 or the thing will take off – it's a simple consequence of exponential growth. There's no point running 'hot' at a higher level of infections: we should get them right down and hold them down, as the same restrictions will be needed to keep cases level at 1,000 a day as at 10,000 – but with far fewer deaths.

Unfortunately, persuading people about this consequence of exponential growth is not easy. Treasury officials, with their mathematical minds, should get it. But all I'm hearing from them is about opening up as fast as we can. I find this astonishing. Surely they can see that if we loosen restrictions now, we'll just have to come down harder for longer later? You've got to understand the dynamic effects, i.e. what happens down the line. That's what economics is supposed to be all about.

I talked to Jens, who's under the same pressure to reopen. The Germans are thinking of setting a numerical target for daily cases – probably 4,000. I like the idea, because it turns the maths into a number that people can grasp.

We mustn't screw up it up as badly as Trump. I love America, but they're in a complete state, and he's the worst possible leader in this sort of science-based crisis. New York City's death toll has passed 10,000, higher than any European country. Now Trump has announced he will freeze US funding of the WHO for sixty to ninety days while he reviews whether to pull out of the organisation altogether. He thinks

Tedros & co. are ducking the hard questions about what he calls 'the Chinese virus' – and he has a point. If the US were to pull their support completely, it could leave the UK as the biggest funder of the WHO – though at this stage of the pandemic it's pretty much useless. Countries are approaching it as a domestic crisis.

WEDNESDAY 15 APRIL

We're thinking about trialling the new tracing app on the Isle of Wight. It's a neat idea, as the island is self-contained and it's easy to monitor comings and goings.

Bethell messaged to say that if we're going down this route, we'll need 'a Bob Seely strategy', by which he meant that we'll need to figure out how to keep the eccentric local MP onside. He's right: we don't need Bob kicking off.

Bethell also told me to 'keep my head up more' in Zoom meetings. 'When you put your head down, you look, bluntly, a bit grumpy,' he observed. I didn't know I was doing it. Funny how Zoom changes etiquette.

From today, everyone going from hospital into social care will be tested and then isolated while the result comes through. Good. Now there is more capacity, the NHS and CQC are also increasing testing for care home staff and residents amid reports of rising deaths, though we are struggling to get precise figures. Meanwhile I've finally got changes to funerals over the line. Under new guidelines close family will be able to say goodbye to deceased relatives wherever possible. I've personally made sure the new care home guidance is also clear that visits at the end of life should continue.

In more cheerful news, a veteran called Captain Tom Moore is raising money for the NHS by doing laps of his garden with his Zimmer frame. The amount of money donated has reached £7 million. He wants to do 100 laps by his 100th birthday on 30 April. His original aim had been to raise £1,000 by tomorrow. He hit that target by 10 April, just a couple of days into his walk. Then BBC Radio 2 covered the story and it went viral. What an inspiration.

THURSDAY 16 APRIL

Up early to go on the morning media round. A grilling from Nick Robinson on Radio 4, then *Good Morning Britain*. I really like Nick, who is great company, though today he belittled the importance of his role by asking snippy 'gotcha' questions. By contrast, I've only met Piers Morgan once. He didn't seem remotely interested in any answers I gave him and kept launching into absurdly aggressive monologues, like a caricature of himself. What a waste of time.

Raab messaged afterwards saying I've been 'terrific in the toughest of times' and urging me to keep going. 'We can't do it without you,' he said encouragingly. I'm not flagging, but it was nice of him to acknowledge the pressure.

I went from the morning round to the daily meeting, still chaired by Raab. Thankfully I've won the argument about (not) opening up, and we've made the very obvious decision to extend lockdown for 'at least' three weeks. Cabinet Office officials have come up with five 'tests' that must be met before restrictions are eased. This is a classic government device to frame a decision yet to be made. Frankly, everyone knows it will take much longer.

The tests, set out by Raab at the press briefing, are:

1. The NHS is able to provide enough critical care throughout the UK;
2. death rates are falling;
3. infection rates are falling to manageable levels;
4. testing capacity and PPE stocks are sufficient to meet future demand;
5. changes to restrictions would not risk a second peak of infections.

After the morning round, I went to open the Birmingham Nightingale, virtually this time. I gave a heartfelt speech about how amazing the team had been and thanked them for getting the hospital ready, should it be needed. A few minutes later one of my oldest friends sent through a photo of the comical situation I'd been put in, a huge face on a screen looking down on lines of people standing to attention. 'I always feared we'd end up in a 1984 situation, but I never thought you'd be Big Brother,' he joked.

Meanwhile my battle with PHE continues, specifically on testing. Today they told SAGE that they're unable to deliver a community-based testing programme. No kidding! That much is obvious. Just because they're not capable of doing it, doesn't mean nobody else can. My testing team despairs.

A few other key takeaways from SAGE: black people have a higher risk of being admitted to hospital and of death; and a disproportionate number of BAME healthcare workers are dying. We need to find out why. There's still a lot of ambivalence about the benefit of masks.

FRIDAY 17 APRIL
Steve Oldfield sent round an extraordinary snapshot of the PPE procurement push in action. It's a video of a pilot taking a BA 777 passenger plane on a 28-hour round trip to Shanghai to pick up gloves, gowns etc. Every seat has a big box of facemasks lashed to it instead of a passenger and smaller boxes are crammed in all the overhead lockers.

We're setting up a taskforce to coordinate work on vaccines, headed by Vallance and JVT. Sir John Bell, who is the government's life sciences champion in addition to his Oxford professorship, will be a key figure and is going to oversee the university's effort.

Captain Tom's fundraising campaign has hit £20 million. Amazing!

SATURDAY 18 APRIL
Someone's briefed the *Sunday Times* that we're planning to lift lockdown in May, and the paper's splashing it tomorrow. It's complete rubbish and is going to cause no end of grief.

As soon as I saw it on Twitter, I messaged Cummings to say that if this is what Downing Street is planning then we're all finished. New case numbers are not even falling. To my relief, he replied that he's not seen the story and dismissed it as 'total crap'.

'These guys are all just inventing stuff,' he said.

Meanwhile there's a problem with a consignment of PPE we've got coming from Turkey. Apparently the Turkish government has brought in a rule that they can only export two gowns for every one that stays in country. It's infuriating, but I get it. So often in international politics people forget the domestic pressures at the other end. The Turkish government is also feeling the heat on PPE. Imagine the furore if we dispatched a stack of our stuff to Turkey. I messaged Raab saying this will clearly have to be sorted out at a higher level. He agreed and is talking to his counterpart in Ankara, as well as our ambassador.

Hospitals and care homes haven't yet grasped the fact that we're only going to get out of this if we test, test, test. According to figures I received today, the average care home has carried out 0.5 tests, which is exasperating, given how hard we're working to increase capacity. Hospitals are not much better. Former Labour Home Secretary Jacqui Smith, who now chairs the University Hospitals Birmingham NHS Trust, told me they're doing an average of just 130 a day for 22,000 workers, i.e. less than 0.6 per cent of the workforce. Birmingham has one of the country's most modern hospitals, with its own labs and a chair who's pushing the testing programme. If they're doing so little, other hospitals will be doing nothing.

Voters underestimate just how much time and sweat it takes in government to make things happen. You are constantly pushing water uphill. Ministers may think everybody's listening when they issue instructions, but if they sit back and wait for people to follow through, nothing materialises. You can push buttons, pull levers, chivvy, cajole, even threaten, and still policies that everyone solemnly agreed will come to nothing unless relentless pressure is maintained. Tony Blair once said he spent his first term pulling at the levers of government and the second realising they weren't connected to anything. It is exhausting. We are clearly going to have to get much tougher with hospitals and care homes, and if they don't budge, we'll start mandating.

I was still musing on all this in my home office with the TV on in the background when Robert Jenrick hove into view at the Downing

Street press conference. He's a steady hand and I was only half watching as he fielded the usual questions about restrictions, testing, schools etc. He was coming under a bit of pressure on PPE – nothing he couldn't handle – when all of a sudden I heard the word 'Turkey'. I snapped to attention and listened with mounting horror as he gaily announced that eighty-four tonnes of PPE, including 400,000 gowns, were at this very moment winging their way to Britain.

I got straight on the phone to Jamie Njoku-Goodwin asking why we weren't sticking to our standard self-preservation policy, which is not to talk about any foreign consignments of anything Covid-related until it's actually on terra firma.

'What happened?' I demanded, trying not to sound too panicked.

'No. 10 was completely up to speed on the situation. We told them not to use it,' he replied despairingly.

I called Jenrick the minute the press conference was over and he explained that someone in Downing Street had told him about the Turkey consignment just before the conference started. Nobody warned him he couldn't tell anyone, so naturally he mentioned it when he came under pressure. Heaven knows how the Turks will respond.

Hundreds of businesses are approaching the department offering to manufacture this or that and even provide flights. Half the time nobody returns their calls, even with big companies like Primark. The problem is weeding out timewasters and chancers – of which there are many – without missing opportunities. One company with a good product got so pissed off they sold everything to the Scottish NHS. Even the Labour Party are writing in with suggested names of companies and individuals who could help – generally without doing any due diligence on the offers they're putting forward.

SUNDAY 19 APRIL

Update from Raab re. Turkey: the Foreign Minister is going to talk to the Health Minister and escalate it to the President. Jens Spahn texted to offer any help Germany can give us with testing, ICUs and ventilators. He is a real friend to the UK. Meanwhile we have two further flights about to arrive. I instruct the department not to tell anyone until they are in the country.

MONDAY 20 APRIL

Crunch week for hitting my testing target. There's an uncomfortable amount of speculation about my career depending on it. I'd be lying if I said it wasn't an unnecessary and irritating distraction. The PM is supportive, but the Downing Street machine has been useless, presumably because Cummings is itching for me to fail.

I asked Simon Stevens why hospitals are testing so little, and he says they don't want to test too many staff in case too many results come back positive and staff have to go home. What?! That's precisely the point: we *want* staff who are positive to be at home, isolating, not at work, infecting. What an astonishing attitude. I've also got a problem with the MHRA, which won't approve home testing. Companies have developed good home testing kits, but the MHRA seems to be completely against trusting people to administer their own tests. It is exasperating.

I've been in this game long enough to handle so-called colleagues briefing against me, but the sheer volume of 'Matt's job is on the line if he doesn't deliver/Matt's an idiot for setting a completely unrealistic target/only fools set goals they can't achieve' etc. began to get to me this evening.

I confided in my team. They are also exhausted. Allan reminded me why we did this in the first place: not for the sake of achieving a precise number but to force the whole infuriatingly sluggish machine into action. I snapped out of it and told him truthfully that I don't care if this ends my career. It's about doing the right thing in a massive crisis.

Meanwhile the farce over the Turkish PPE continues. Ankara seems ready to release the consignment and Ben Wallace sent an RAF plane to pick it up, only to discover that the seller is trying to renegotiate the price. Thankfully we've got another load coming from Burma, some of which has already arrived. Here's hoping it's up to scratch. We recently

ordered and paid for 200,000 gowns from a Chinese manufacturer –
who sent 20,000.

So far, the Labour Party has behaved quite well, recognising that
it's a national emergency. One exception is Alastair Campbell, who
lost the plot over Brexit and never regained it. He was one of the first
left-wingers to go on the offensive over our handling of the pandemic
and has become increasingly aggressive: all part of a desperate attempt
to remain relevant. His latest screed in some online magazine labels us
a 'Cabinet of Incompetents' and lays into pretty much the whole government with little substance beyond his dislike for our performances
at the Downing Street podium. Apparently something I said provoked
his 'loudest shout at the telly'. What an image. Blair's ageing rottweiler,
once the terror of Westminster journalists, sitting there in his retirement slippers howling at the screen.

His former boss has been a discreet and sometimes helpful adviser. I
rang to ask him how to deal with his old spinner. Tony gave an audible
shrug of the shoulders and told me there was no real way of reining
him in. 'Your problem isn't what Alastair's saying on Twitter,' he said. 'It
doesn't matter. What on earth are you doing spending your time looking at Twitter?' Fair point. I'll leave Campbell to bark at the moon.

Social media really has blown up in the last month. We're now film-
ing more videos than ever before, and with the press conferences and
parliamentary appearances to think about, Allan has said it's taking
up too much of the team's capacity. He's suggested we recruit Asher
Glynn, an eighteen-year-old he met last year who does a lot of political social media, to manage my accounts. I met Asher recently and am
glad to have him on the team.

TUESDAY 21 APRIL

Boris is clearly on the mend and texted me for the first time in a fortnight, complaining about some minor story in the *Telegraph*. ('Ridiculous.') Later he texted again, saying I'm doing a great job. Sadly, not
great enough to conjure up the PPE from Turkey. Our RAF plane is on
the ground, but the shipment has vanished.

Better news on vaccines at least: finally the team at Oxford have commitments for the cash they need and the first human trials begin the day after tomorrow. I've also spoken to Robin Shattock, the Imperial professor working on an mRNA vaccine. He's only a few weeks behind Oxford, and we're giving him all the support he needs to get his vaccine to trials.

Parliament has returned with a maximum of fifty MPs in the Chamber. Everyone else is logging in by Zoom. Meanwhile SAGE has completely changed its tune on masks and now recommends face coverings in enclosed spaces where social distancing is not possible. I think it's the right decision, but explaining such a spectacular U-turn is going to take some serious verbal gymnastics.

WEDNESDAY 22 APRIL

Great news – the Oxford vaccine works on monkeys! Sir John Bell messaged to tell me. He says the chance of it working in humans is now 'way up' and that single-dose efficacy is 'amazing'. There is a huge prize here: the potential to save millions of lives. The upside of being the first country in the world to develop a successful vaccine would be huge. I want to throw everything at it. Sir John's excitement was infectious and the Prof clearly thinks I'm getting a bit carried away. At the Downing Street press conference this evening he struck a much more cautious note than I did, describing the chances of having either a vaccine or good treatments within the next year as 'incredibly small'. He also said it was 'wholly unrealistic' to expect life to return to normal any time soon and that social distancing restrictions are likely to be in place for the rest of the year. Listening to him, my heart sank a bit, but he's right to manage expectations.

At home later I found a note in my box advising me to talk to the pharmaceutical giant Merck about the Oxford vaccine to 'welcome their engagement'. There's a long-standing arrangement between Oxford and the American company, which normally commercialises their drug innovations. According to the briefing I've been given, officials think Merck is the 'most appropriate partner'. They also think we'll need to manufacture overseas to be sure of producing enough. The note says that if we do a deal with Merck, we can 'expect' access rights to the first batches of vaccines.

I looked at the advice with growing disbelief. Why can't we manufacture the vaccine here? And what's with the use of the word 'expect'? Far too vague. If British taxpayers are supporting the development of the vaccine, we will need a binding agreement to give us priority doses when it's ready. The big threat here is Trump's 'America First' attitude. I'm worried about any US company getting their hands on our vaccine. To protect our position, it has to be physically manufactured here.

Increasingly uneasy, I rang Sir John Bell – who has been acting as an interlocutor between the government and all the various scientists and pharma companies trying to develop a vaccine – and told him I've got a bad feeling about the Merck deal. Evidently the best he has been able to extract from them is a gentlemen's agreement that we get first dibs.

That just isn't going to fly. As I told Sir John, if we do this on a handshake, Trump will use the Defense Production Act to get it for America first. Then a British vaccine developed in British labs, with the help of the British taxpayer, will be vaccinating Americans while Brits have to wait. How's that going to go down?

'You'd better line up an alternative,' I said. Sir John replied that he'd already been thinking through options for plan B with Patrick Vallance. 'What about AstraZeneca? They're based in Cambridge, and their chief executive Pascal Soriot is a man I can trust,' he suggested.

'Great, but they'll have to sign up to everything we need,' I replied.

The PM keeps asking, 'Are we through the peak?' Privately, the answer is yes, but we're being ultra-cautious about what we say publicly. SAGE thinks it's too early to relax restrictions anyway: any more socialising could push R back above 1.

THURSDAY 23 APRIL

The first UK patient has been injected with a vaccine in Oxford's Phase 1 human trials, which started today. Another was injected with a control substance. It's a record and an astonishing achievement to take the vaccine to its first clinical trial just over three months after the virus was identified as the cause of the Covid outbreak.

The Oxford team put out an appeal for volunteers to take part and were inundated. Within hours, literally thousands had come forward. Sir John reckons our chances of success are 80 per cent.

It's certainly more cheerful than obsessing about my testing target, which hangs over me every waking hour. Capacity is more than 50,000 a day now, but that leaves a long way to go in a very short time. There are now thirty testing labs across the UK, with more being set up each day, mostly by approved private operators.

All this was whirring around my head when I heard that Trump has suggested injecting people with disinfectant as a potential Covid cure. Chucking around ideas in the manner of a child being asked to speculate on what aliens might eat, he went on to suggest that a 'tremendous hit' of 'heat and light' might also do the trick. White House Covid coordinator Deborah Birx just sat there looking utterly perplexed. A small part of me found it funny – this is the President of the United States. The leader of the free world. A much bigger part of me was horrified. You'd like to think nobody would take these wild suggestions seriously, but around the world doctors are now genuinely having to warn people not to attempt to treat themselves with Cillit Bang.

Alongside the race for the vaccine and my own increasingly frantic effort to hit the testing target, we're putting the infrastructure in place for a national contact tracing system, to be called 'Test and Trace'. It's going to involve hiring at least 18,000 people, including 3,000 medical staff.

Less positively, I've given up on the shipment from Turkey, and the RAF are coming home. The whole episode is an epic example of a comms screw-up evolving into a substantive failure. The big lesson is: never, ever talk about kit until it's in the country.

I was so shredded after my last meeting that I collapsed on the small sofa in my office, flopping my feet over the arm. I was still lying in this undignified position when Wormald came through the door, looking slightly concerned at my crumpled appearance.

'I still feel like I'm running this entire operation,' I said wearily, conscious that it sounded a bit 'me me me'.

'Effectively, you are,' he replied.

I snapped out of it when the PM called, worrying about PPE.

'If NHS workers don't have enough kit, we'll have to answer to their families,' he warned.

He acknowledged that I'm like a one-man War Cabinet right now and wants to get someone else in to manage the PPE situation. I think he was worried I might push back, but I'm hugely relieved. As I said to him, I didn't come into politics to buy PPE. All that matters is that we get as much as we need, fast. He floated the idea of Paul Deighton, the man who essentially organised the London 2012 Olympics. He is exactly the sort of no-nonsense person we need.

Helen Whately is still up against it on care homes. She messaged today appealing to me to try to get NHS England to be more supportive and constructive, given the enormous challenges associated with caring for very frail people in a pandemic. 'Need a shift from battling to get them to help to them coming forward with ideas and offers,' she said, sounding miserable. I told her draw up a list of specific requests and I'll get it to Simon Stevens.

FRIDAY 24 APRIL

Simon Case, former private secretary to Prince William, is back from the Palace to run the Covid response in No. 10. I asked how he was finding it. Frustrating, apparently.

More positively, Paul Deighton has all but signed on the dotted line to run PPE. Quick work.

Downing Street called my office saying I needed to schedule a quick call with the PM. I asked if there was anything I needed to prepare, and it was all very vague: 'Just a catch-up now he's getting better.'

I was looking forward to it, until I switched on Zoom to see the PM at Chequers flanked by Cummings and about a dozen other advisers. Rishi was there, looking sheepish. I realised instantly what was going on: an attempted ambush. There was Cummings, looking shifty, itching to start the interrogation.

Boris opened with some gentle warm-ups, then Cummings started the shelling, subjecting me to a barrage of questions about my department's response: on PPE, testing, NHS capacity, ventilators. Every so often one of the others would pile in. Most of the questions seemed to be based on inaccurate media reports.

It was utterly exhausting, but I've lived this for months now, eighteen hours a day, pretty much every day, so I am on top of every detail.

Boris and Rishi said almost nothing. When they finally ran out of ammunition, I pressed 'Leave Meeting', sat back in my chair, checked my body for shrapnel wounds and saw that I was broadly intact.

Next?

SATURDAY 25 APRIL

My first day in months without any major meetings. The BBC ran a flattering profile of me, including some nice quotes from George Osborne. I messaged him thanking him for bigging me up. 'You are big now and I'm proud of how you're coping and handling yourself', he replied charmingly.

I spent the day at home hanging out with the kids, though I squeezed in a call with Simon Eccles, who's leading on the tech side for the testing rollout. Simon is a gloriously eccentric live-wire who drives a classic Bentley to work. I don't know how he ended up with the Bentley, or one of only eight parking spaces in the departmental car park, but it's impossible not to like him. The tech platform is the rate-limiting factor on the testing expansion, as you can't run a system on any scale from spreadsheets. The good news is he seems confident we can deliver in time to hit my target.

SUNDAY 26 APRIL

Boris is back from Chequers. He spoke to the Queen, and to Trump, who says he 'sounded incredible'. According to Trump, 'It's like the old

Boris, tremendous energy, tremendous drive.' Good news, though I'm bracing myself for a barrage.

Another note about the Merck deal. They're still not offering exclusivity. Officials have also taken on board my worries about Trump, noting 'concern regarding whether Merck would be the most appropriate partner in light of US policy considerations'. I think that's Whitehall speak for 'you can't trust the President'. This is very good progress.

I am running on adrenaline and relishing the challenge, but the stress is beginning to show. It's not only the thinning hairline – today marked my first ever grey hair. I'm sure there will be more where that came from.

MONDAY 27 APRIL

Boris is getting more and more stressed about PPE. 'We are getting hammered in focus groups and polls. Disaster area,' he said anxiously.

I reassured him that we're gripping it and have a plan (aka Deighton).

Two days to go on my testing target. Capacity is expanding just in time. The challenge now is also to ensure there's the right level of demand. Open up eligibility and have too much publicity and either the website will crash or parts of the country will run out within minutes, and people will be told to travel miles for slots. Too little demand and we won't get there. I'm acutely conscious this could be a very public screw-up.

TUESDAY 28 APRIL

I messaged George Osborne first thing saying I could really do with a testing splash in the *Evening Standard*, which he now edits. We have 22,000 spare slots at the drive-through testing centres, and I'm desperate to boost demand. He replied that if I give him some exclusive quotes by 8 a.m. tomorrow and brief the political editor, he'll put it on the front page. Testing capacity has reached 73,000 a day, which is all well and good, but we've only done 43,000 in the past twenty-four hours. 'The facility isn't much good if nobody's using it,' he observed.

Meanwhile SAGE has changed its position on masks, back to essentially 'don't know'. They now say (again) that it would be unreasonable to claim a large benefit. I've decided to say as little as possible on this issue, or I'll look an idiot when they inevitably change their minds again.

Cardiologist Aseem Malhotra has written a piece for the *Telegraph* calling for 'an honest conversation' about the link between obesity and the risk of dying from Covid. He's the guy behind Tom Watson's incredible weight loss. When Tom was Jeremy Corbyn's deputy, he was huge. At one point he weighed twenty-two stone and was on heavy meds for Type 2 diabetes. He once told me he was so fat he thought he was going to die. Then he went on Aseem's 'Pioppi diet' (named after a village in southern Italy where there's an unusually high life expectancy) and lost eight stone in a year. I sent Aseem's article to Boris, saying I thought he had a point.

Boris agrees that we can't duck this issue. He pointed out that many of the NHS staff who have died have been visibly overweight.

'I'm sorry, but it's just true,' he said.

Amid all this, a truly sobering moment when, at 11 a.m., we held a minute's silence for fallen health workers. I stood on my balcony, alone. In St Thomas's Hospital, just in view of my office, NHS staff had striven to save the Prime Minister's life, and succeeded. But not all of them had themselves come through. Now, as the virus just begins to abate, we can be confident the NHS won't be overwhelmed, but some have tragically paid with their lives.

Amid all this, Merck have revealed their hand, and it's not good. After I demanded certainty on priority UK access, they're only prepared to offer an agreement in principle and are refusing to put it in legal text. That's that then: I won't sign it off.

At the same time, Patrick Vallance and the Oxford team have come up with another solution, and it's much better. They've been having parallel discussions with AstraZeneca over the weekend. In less than forty-eight hours, AstraZeneca have signed up to all my demands for exclusive UK access *and* agreed to provide the vaccine to the rest of the world, at cost. It's a spectacularly generous deal. Right now, they are probably the largest pharmaceutical company without a vaccine candidate. They don't have suitable manufacturing facilities themselves, but they do have the experience and capability to make it happen. Everything has moved very fast and they want to announce the deal tomorrow. Alok's wavering, but we agree to go for it before they change their minds. We need a clear undertaking to supply the whole UK population (not just the most vulnerable) and a legally binding commitment to domestic manufacture. If they can deliver that, we should get going.

WEDNESDAY 29 APRIL

Carrie has had a baby boy. Lovely news for her and Boris, but not ideal for my *Evening Standard* splash.

What an extraordinarily intense time Boris and Carrie are having. Brexit, lockdown, nearly dying and now a baby, all within a few weeks. I hope they're all OK and the boss gets some sleep.

MPs have been complaining about the new set-up in Parliament. The voting lobbies are small and airless – exactly the kind of environment in which the virus thrives – so Members are having to queue instead of going through in a big throng. It's taking ages and they're getting upset, so we're introducing electronic voting so people can vote from home. Parliament enters the twenty-first century.

In a surprising development, Cummings sent me a completely helpful and constructive message, saying we need to start planning for how the NHS will get through the winter, assuming 'dark scenarios'. How would we cope with a new Covid surge, particularly if it mutates? What about severe flu coming along at the same time plus some unexpected crisis? As he points out, Test and Trace will be very different once thousands of people with flu are worried they have Covid. He sensibly suggested getting someone really competent to focus purely on a future plan, without being distracted by urgent day-to-day stuff. Cummings at his supportive best can be a real asset. 'Optimism's at a slight discount these days,' he said gloomily, as if he were buying shares.

I'm impatient for progress on the vaccine and called Sarah Gilbert to see how it's going. The system seems intent on us not talking direct, but there's no reason why we should only communicate through officials. I asked her again if there's anything more we can do. What will we regret not doing if we asked ourselves in a year's time? Etc.

The issue is still money. The Treasury agreed to forward £20 million but hasn't done so. I told her I'd chase it up.

I also checked in with the testing team. Whether or not we hit the target, we've galvanised the system. Of course I want to get to the 100,000 figure too, but what's vital is building momentum. One of the most impressive members of the team is a former military commander who has thrown everything at it. There was a last-minute logistical glitch involving some bags needed as part of the lab process. They were stuck in Bristol and needed to be in Manchester. He rang one of his former colleagues from Hereford to get on his motorbike to dispatch them and hey presto – within a matter of hours it was sorted.

What's frustrating is the mismatch between supply and demand. I spent the evening pulling every string I've got, talking to big employers etc., to try to get the word out, before piling into bed, exhausted.

THURSDAY 30 APRIL

Today we hit 81,611 tests. When Boris announced the figure at the press conference later, I could see certain hacks salivating as they did the maths. It's tight. Ben Wallace sent me a really thoughtful message, telling me not to worry if we don't hit the exact figure: the point is that we've forced the system into top gear.

'The awful media are just trying to be negative,' he said.

I did my best to distract myself, helped by a serious internal debate over whether we can now declare that we're past the peak. What we don't want is people relaxing and sending R above 1 again. However, I think we're now safe to do it and Boris agrees. The plan is for him to announce it at tonight's press conference.

Hearing him say it was a strangely emotional moment. I watched with my team around me on the little TV in the corner of my office and all I could think was, 'Thank Christ. The NHS wasn't overwhelmed. We are on the way out.'

All the same, there's still no way back to normality without a vaccine. In our WhatsApp exchange this morning about the target, Ben also asked if we're taking steps to maximise the benefit to the UK if we win the global race to develop a jab – including ensuring that nobody steals the recipe?

'Our adversaries are already trying to steal IP!' he warned.

He didn't elaborate, but prime suspects for stealing the intellectual property must be the Chinese. The irony is that the deal we've done with AstraZeneca will allow anyone to manufacture the vaccine, anywhere in the world, at cost. The Chinese won't need to steal the design – all they'll have to do is pick up the phone and ask for it.

David Spiegelhalter, a Cambridge statistics professor, has written an excellent piece for *The Guardian*, putting our Covid mortality figures in perspective. We are frequently accused of having some of the highest death rates in the world, but a lot is down to the way figures are collated. I've always been adamant that we should be as transparent as possible about how many people are dying, which means that anyone who dies having tested positive for Covid is counted. Obviously this exaggerates the figures, because it includes a significant number of people who actually died of cancer, cardiac arrest or a fall and just happened also to have Covid. If we didn't count these cases, doubtless we'd be accused of some kind of cover-up. In any case, identifying and classifying cause of death is a complicated science. Our approach means we have far higher figures than many comparator countries, which some people never stop going on about. Spiegelhalter argues that trying to compile league tables at this stage is pointless. We need to wait a year or two for it all to come out in the wash.

Encouragingly, hospital admissions are now declining consistently across the country. Survival rates for ventilated patients are also improving relative to the start of the pandemic, and most people are still sticking to social distancing measures. All this is great, as is Tom Moore's incredible fundraising effort. It's his 100th birthday today. He'd drummed up £33 million for the NHS by the time his JustGiving page closed last night. Amazing.

MAY 2020

FRIDAY 1 MAY

We did it, and with a very comfortable margin. 122,347 tests! Let the naysayers put that in their pipe and smoke it! George Osborne messaged me at the crack of dawn, saying his political team at the *Standard* had picked up from their own sources that we'd hit the target and asking me to confirm.

I told him truthfully that I couldn't, because I didn't know myself. I spent the next few hours on absolute tenterhooks.

Normally I don't get the data until 2 p.m. and we publish the daily stats at 4 p.m. Today it came in dribs and drabs, first from our new network of Lighthouse Laboratories (38,645, way above their target), then home tests (27,497 – way more than I thought possible), then from the NHS and PHE, which delivered 34,807 between them. Throw in tests carried out in Scotland, Wales and Northern Ireland, and we more than made it. Whichever way you measure it, we smashed the target.

Heading over to Downing Street with Jim to do the daily press conference, I was elated. It has been an enormous team effort and I'm so proud of them, though I was conscious that it would not be remotely appropriate to look or sound triumphant, under the circumstances. Nonetheless, I'd be lying if I didn't say I enjoyed my moment, given how desperately certain people were willing me to fail. Even Tedros tweeted congratulations. ('Together, my friend @MattHancock!')

The news was way too late for the *Evening Standard* front page, which meant Osborne had to run a bit of a mishmash of a Covid story. This morning he tried to bounce me into giving him the testing figures by threatening to run a front-page story criticising our record on testing instead if I didn't play ball.

'We'll go with Starmer's interview with us calling on you to do more,' he said bluntly.

'More testing?' I replied.

'Yes. 250k,' he answered. Seriously? That is our policy anyway! 100,000 was just the first step. Labour have no idea how hard this is and just carp from the sidelines.

'Is that the best line he's given you?' I asked scornfully.

'His bigger call is on tracking,' George replied. Apparently Starmer thinks we're not throwing enough at it.

I told him it would be ridiculous to run this lame critique.

'Give me something better…' he replied mischievously.

His transformation from former Chancellor of the Exchequer to ruthless newspaper editor has been quite something to behold.

SATURDAY 2 MAY

I chased JVT for an update on the Oxford vaccine. He said 601 people have now been injected in trials and that side effects aren't causing concern. He expects a readout on immunity in about three weeks.

Boris and Carrie are naming their baby son Wilfred Lawrie Nicholas. They chose Nicholas in gratitude to two of the respiratory doctors who saved the PM's life: Dr Nick Price and Professor Nick Hart. Nice touch.

SUNDAY 3 MAY

Boris thinks Australia's decision to cut itself off from the world might be the way forward for the UK. He messaged me mid-morning, saying he'd just had a 'depressing' conversation with Aussie Prime Minister Scott Morrison, who is preparing to lift restrictions Down Under.

They are among the most urbanised in the world, with huge exposure to China, yet are about to restart sport and reopen theatres, art galleries and cafes.

He was clearly very exercised, listing all the things they've achieved – like keeping manufacturing going throughout – and noting that unlike us they closed the border to China the minute this thing started, and didn't get indirect infections like we did. He admits that Morrison is probably bigging up his own government's record but says we're going to have to explain why they've only lost 100 people to Covid, whereas we are losing thousands.

'A prize for the best 100-word explanation for why the UK has 28,000 deaths and Australia has 100,' he said, laying down the gauntlet to me, Cummings, Vallance and the Prof.

I consulted Jamie.

'Hot weather and lots of BBQs?' he suggested helpfully, pointing out that coronaviruses are seasonal and Australia may have been lucky with the time of year.

I got straight back on the phone to the boss.

'Coronaviruses are seasonal and don't transmit as much outdoors. It is striking that no part of the southern hemisphere has seen such a significant outbreak,' I said confidently.

This seemed to do the trick, as Boris replied that I (or rather, Jamie) had got the prize, the nature of which he says will be 'determined later'.

At least we've got one up on the French. David Cameron's old chief of staff Ed Llewellyn, now our man in Paris, messaged the boss this evening to say that the Élysée has 'reverse ferreted' on plans to quarantine anyone who crosses the Channel for up to thirty days (!). This would have been a massive problem for truckers and would have crippled supply chains. Thank goodness Macron has seen sense.

The truth is that we still haven't figured out what to do about travel. Raab, Shapps and Sunak all want to keep the borders open. Crucially, they're supported by the Prof. On the other side, Priti Patel and I are in favour of far tougher measures, as is Boris, especially after half an hour listening to Scott Morrison gloating.

MONDAY 4 MAY

Deighton is doing a great job on PPE, which has spurred me on to find more 'Beaverbrooks', most pressingly to head up testing and to lead on vaccines. After thinking it over, Boris suggested Kate Bingham for vaccines. She's a formidable venture capitalist with a background in the pharmaceutical industry and will be ideal. When I called her to sound her out, she sounded excited but wary, not least because it will mean abandoning her day job and pretty much everything else in her life for the next six months. Laying it on thick, I told her – truthfully – that her country needs her and that this will be the most important job of her life. By 7 p.m. she was asking for my email address so she could send me her thoughts on terms of reference for the role. The plan is to put Dido Harding in charge of testing, another great fit. I've known Dido on and off for years – I first met her when she was CEO of TalkTalk and I was responsible for cyber security and have worked very closely with her as chair of NHS Improvement. Like me, she is also an amateur jockey. She's a ball of no-nonsense energy and will really grip contact tracing efforts.

Tonight Pfizer announced that it began human trials in the US yesterday for a potential coronavirus vaccine in collaboration with the German company BioNTech. There are hundreds of vaccine projects and we need to be on top of them all. Kate's appointment can't come soon enough.

The pilot of Test and Trace has opened on the Isle of Wight, with the app designed in-house by NHSX. There's been a sniffy response from the devolved administrations, who seem to think they can come up with something better. As part of her relentless campaign to differentiate herself, Nicola Sturgeon is now pursuing a zero-Covid strategy, loftily declaring that Scotland is 'in a strong position to eliminate the Covid-19 virus'. It's against all clinical advice, which is clear that zero Covid is impossible to achieve: Sturgeon will only be delaying the inevitable. Tonight she announced a 'summer push to elimination', a policy which has about as much hope of working as Chairman Mao's attempt to eliminate starlings by getting the Chinese population to bang pots and pans. Much as I'm sure Nicola would love to build a Trump-style wall between her fiefdom and the rest of Great Britain, we're all in this together – and I'm certainly not turning us into a hermit kingdom.

One person who's clearly not keen on a hermit lifestyle is Neil Ferguson, the man who probably gave me Covid during a Downing Street press conference. I don't hold this against him, obviously, but nor was I particularly sympathetic when I heard he'd been caught breaking the rules. He's issued a grovelling apology, claiming he thought he was immune from the virus because he's already had it, but it was obvious he couldn't continue to act as a government adviser, and he's resigned from SAGE.

The global death toll has now passed 250,000, a horrendous milestone. Our own official death toll has overtaken Italy's, making us the worst-affected country in Europe – at least in theory. In return for preferring to overstate rather than understate our figures, we will of course be hammered. While it will be painful, we owe it to the people of this country to be completely transparent – even when others aren't. I'm confident history will show this in time, but until then we just have to know we're doing the right thing and ride out the criticism.

WEDNESDAY 6 MAY

Any doubts I might have had about Kate's enthusiasm for the vaccine job were dispelled when I opened my email inbox this morning to find she'd already sent her terms. Since this is going to be pro bono, it's completely reasonable that she sets out exactly what she's prepared to do.

She wants to be accountable direct to the PM, which is no skin off my nose, and she needs a clear budget, instead of the current muddle involving a split budget with BEIS (the Department for Business, Energy and Industrial Strategy). My overriding objective is to ensure Cummings isn't anywhere near it, because all he'll do is screw it up.

I got drawn into commenting on the Ferguson thing. I told Sky I was astonished when I found out he'd breached the rules, given his position. Nor is he the only one. Scotland's chief medical officer was also in hot water for flitting back and forth to a second home. Together we made these rules: it totally undermines all our messaging if we're seen to break them.

THURSDAY 7 MAY

Just as I'd feared, Cummings is trying to meddle with the Bingham appointment and has spent the past twenty-four hours trying to amend her terms of reference. It makes no difference to me because the team brings all the vaccine decisions to me anyway, and I'm on a formal board to sign off anything big. He's also interfering in the Dido appointment and is trying to engineer things so that she reports to him – a ridiculous suggestion. After twenty-four hours of painful back and forth with No. 10, Dido and I just agreed that in practice she'll report to me and together we'll report to Boris, no matter how much Cummings may mess things up. The confused lines of accountability he's trying to create – just to expand his own power base – make life so much harder for the people trying to run the system.

While we were ironing out these details, scientists at Porton Down finished evaluating antibody tests developed by Roche. They're happy with them. The tests allow people to find out if they've already had the virus, meaning they may have some natural immunity. Roche's production plant is in Germany and has a deal with the German government to provide a large number of tests. I rang Jens, who said there would be enough for both countries. I told him we think 15 per cent of the London population have been infected and are keen to see if we're right.

There are still well over 400 people a day dying, a terrible figure, though way lower than the peak. The PM wants to give everyone some hope and will announce the first cautious steps out of lockdown on Sunday.

Clearly his mates with country houses have been bending his ear, because he's particularly exercised about village cricket.

'Surely village cricket could be played while obeying social distancing??' he asked the Prof.

'I suspect the tea/beer afterwards is a much greater hazard than the minimal risk of the game. Maybe bowlers could use alcohol gel between overs?' the Prof suggested helpfully.

FRIDAY 8 MAY

I occasionally appear on Chris Evans's breakfast show on Virgin Radio. It's my favourite part of the morning broadcast round – his politeness gets far more out of me than the headbanging monologues of Piers Morgan ever will. This time he persuaded me to part with my pride and joy: a Newcastle Utd shirt signed by the whole team. I grew up near Chester, but I've been a fan of Newcastle since I was a teenager, when my Geordie uncle Dave used to take me to Boxing Day games between Newcastle and Man Utd. Chris wanted it for an online auction to raise cash for a voluntary sewing group that makes non-surgical scrubs for NHS staff. I could hardly think of a better cause, so I reluctantly let it go. It sold for £1,850, my small contribution to an auction that raised a magnificent £600,000. Chris did a great job of drumming up donations from showbiz mates including Ant and Dec and Rod Stewart.

I messaged Jens to say we should talk about a proposal from our French counterpart, Olivier Véran, for a UK, Germany, Italy, France tie-up so we can each get access to whatever vaccine wins the race. I suggested we invite the Dutch too, as I've been working with their Deputy Prime Minister on vaccine manufacture and they are well advanced. International cooperation is going to be at a premium. Jens didn't reply immediately, which was strange as it's something he's been interested in. I hope he hasn't been sat on by Angela Merkel.

Wales has extended its lockdown for a further three weeks, just as Australia announces a three-step plan for businesses to reopen. Down Under, gatherings of up to 100 people and interstate travel will be allowed before the end of July. Boris's competitive instinct is going to make this one tricky, given his friendship with Scott Morrison.

SATURDAY 9 MAY

Trouble brewing with the French. Boris has received an email from Macron urging him not to make French travellers to the UK quarantine. Clearly the President does not want to face the wrath of French truckers if they are forced to spend two weeks in the Premier Inn every time they cross the Channel, or deal with a backlash from the handful of businessmen still using the Eurostar to commute to London.

'De facto, we are talking here about the few remaining travellers and some lorry drivers who will be exempt anyway, so it's a matter of communication,' he said adding – somewhat ominously – that if we go down the quarantine route, he would 'have to reciprocate'.

He made clear that he has no intention of imposing quarantine on other travellers within the Schengen area, only for the UK in Europe, which would – as he put it – 'not create a good messaging'. What he meant is that it would look like another Brexit bust-up. His breezy sign off ('Amitiés, Emmanuel') did not disguise the threat. Suffice to say there are divisions over how to handle this one. Vallance and the Prof had SAGE advice saying that quarantine only makes sense if you keep out travellers from countries with a higher transmission rate than ours. But given that France has opened its borders to the rest of Europe, if we exempt France we're effectively opening ourselves up to the whole continent, which Lee Cain doesn't think will go down well with voters.

'Quarantine surely an essential part of any exit strategy... Public will think (rightly) we are potty. Overwhelming support for tougher action at our borders!!' was his summary.

As the day wore on, the whole thing turned into a bit of a mess, with Gove trying to smooth things over with the Élysée general secretary, Alexis Kohler, while Priti did the exact opposite, telling the French Interior Minister that we were indeed going to pull up the drawbridge. Rail Minister Chris Heaton-Harris was so stressed out that he WhatsApped the boss warning that if we go ahead and close the border, 'it will blow apart French/UK relations'.

'The French, bless them, helped UK citizens avoid this fourteen-day issue when entering the EU. It could also be the straw that breaks the camel's back for Eurostar, who are currently refusing help financially,' he told Boris. As of tonight, it's unclear how this one will play out.

The *Mail on Sunday* are running a hatchet job on me tomorrow, clearly briefed by Cummings. I can just imagine his self-satisfied smirk when he sees the 'PM loses trust in Hancock' headline. It's so low grade and obvious. I'm cracking on with the job.

SUNDAY 10 MAY

The top line in the *Mail on Sunday* piece is that I told the PM to 'give me a break'. What it doesn't say is that Cummings had been showing him manufactured pictures of PPE shortages from Momentum supporters on Twitter, and even pictures from Spain, which was obviously infuriating.

Ben Wallace sent a nice message, labelling it a 'nasty drive-by'.

'For what it's worth, I think you've done a pretty good job in an unprecedented event,' he said kindly, adding that he can't imagine those who briefed the story managing anything. He observes that the boss is surrounded by some pretty unpleasant people these days, who are only trying to divert attention from their own failures.

More importantly, the PM announced a 'conditional plan' for easing lockdown, which will allow people to take unlimited outdoor exercise and go back to the office if they can't work from home, avoiding public transport if at all possible. BEIS wanted certainty; the Treasury wanted to ditch all measures; and I wanted to make sure we get case numbers down and keep them that way. We all agreed that the common goal is to minimise infections until the vaccine comes good, though the Treasury is generally much more gung-ho about risking a temporary spike to get the economy going again.

In a pre-recorded broadcast at 7 p.m., the PM said lockdown has prevented this country from being 'engulfed' by what could have been a 'catastrophe' – though at 'colossal cost to our way of life'. He described the new plan as 'the first sketch of a road map for reopening society'.

The R number is now 0.5–0.9, but we must keep it below 1, so the reopening has to be very cautious.

If infections don't start spiking again as a result of our first set of measures, we can move to Step 2, the phased reopening of schools, starting with reception and years 1 and 6, on 1 June at the earliest, after half-term. The plan is for secondary pupils facing exams next year to get at least some time with their teachers before the holidays.

In Step 3, from July, some hospitality will start to reopen. Soon, anyone flying into the UK will be quarantined, though there's no date for this. The PM asked me to call round the Cabinet before the formal meeting, while he squared the devolveds. There was no dissent.

The PM road-tested a new slogan: 'Stay alert, control the virus and save lives'. Not exactly catchy.

MONDAY 11 MAY

Labour's kicking off about our dealings with Randox after *The Guardian* ran a ridiculous story suggesting we awarded them a £133 million contract 'unopposed'. The opposition is making great play of Owen Paterson's role as an adviser to the company, painting it as 'contracts to cronies'. It is totally unreasonable. It's an emergency! Of course we could not spend months putting everything out to tender in the normal way. There are existing emergency rules for rapid procurement, operated by the civil service. Randox is the UK's largest existing testing company and has a long and impressive track record of delivering the kind of services we needed. Given this expertise, they were obviously an important option for the expansion of testing. The injustice of the accusations really gets to me. Everyone concerned has been doing all they can to expand testing capacity. The call to action was not just about Randox but to all UK potential testing capacity. To imply otherwise is completely wrong. We're not choosing between companies here – we're buying from whoever can credibly supply what's needed. I make no apology for getting Randox involved – they saved lives. To avoid all dealings with the UK's largest laboratory diagnostics company because a paid consultant had mentioned their services would have been absurd and a dereliction of duty.

TUESDAY 12 MAY

Signs that the Tory press is turning against us. The latest attack comes from *Telegraph* columnist Ambrose Evans-Pritchard, who's labelled our handling of Covid 'a very British disaster'. The PM knows Ambrose from his own *Telegraph* days and says he's overexcitable, but he's clearly ruminating about this damning assessment. Ambrose is a libertarian arguing for a stronger lockdown, so his critique is all over the place – but the boss is unsettled. Cummings and I let it go – no point winding him up by getting defensive.

Speaking of Cummings, he's suddenly very enthusiastic about the potential benefits of Vitamin D. While we wait for a vaccine, we've got to make the most of what we already have and there are some indicators that Vitamin D may have preventative effects. Cummings thinks we could give it to literally everyone.

'We could just pay Amazon to distribute it free to the entire population. No admin required,' he suggested. Warming to his theme, he said a 'back of fag packet' calculation points to it costing two to three quid per person, 'so £200m cost – peanuts in current situation. Apart from Covid, would have some other mild positive effects.'

He points out that the army already gives Vitamin D to healthy soldiers, with no evidence of side effects.

'I like it,' Boris replied.

Just one downside: there's no clinical evidence of effectiveness. So the Prof is against.

Over the next ten days, the entire population of Wuhan will be made to take Covid tests. The reach of the Chinese state never ceases to amaze.

WEDNESDAY 13 MAY

Secret Downing Street meeting to talk about the way deaths are counted. I say secret because nobody asked me about it and I only found out through the Prof – it's a Cummings initiative. No. 10 seems to have twigged that the existing system makes our record seem much worse than it is. I'm not sure what Cummings wants and he hasn't communicated with me about it, so I doubt anything will change. In principle, I'm up for changing the way we count deaths, as the existing system exaggerates the numbers, but I'm not going to do anything this important without checking with Boris. Dom's unilateral attempt to oust Simon Stevens taught me he doesn't speak for the boss.

THURSDAY 14 MAY

We need new voices out to defend our record in care homes, where there are still high numbers of Covid deaths, which are almost never just about Covid. People don't understand the grim realities in these settings. Even the BBC's Laura Kuenssberg, who is very sharp, seems to have no idea about the number of deaths in these settings in normal times.

'She thinks it's all a disaster and doesn't get the complexities,' I told the Prof gloomily. He's suggested we find a 'sensible GP' to provide some context.

It is true that the number of deaths in care homes is terrible – a constant anxiety. It is of no consolation that the situation is even worse in Scotland or many countries in Europe. People are starting to blame us for discharging elderly people from hospital into residential settings without testing them properly, before we introduced strict rules. The evidence simply doesn't bear that out: care home outbreaks rose sharply long after we had enough tests to put that right. We urgently need to identify precisely what's going on here. Jenny Harries thinks it's likely to be staff movements, but I don't want to say so publicly. Carers are going to heroic lengths to support these vulnerable elderly people. The last thing I want to do is damage their morale.

The ONS has released results of a survey on prevalence of the virus. It estimates that between 27 April and 10 May, an average of 148,000 people in England, 0.27 per cent of the population, were infected. Thanks to the utter incompetence of certain people at PHE, the research was much more complicated than it should have been. In an unbelievable blunder, PHE initially produced a survey of blood samples taken purely from blood donors, as opposed to a representative sample from the general population. But to give blood, you have to be healthy in the first place. Since the sample was completely unrepresentative, it was a wasted exercise. The result has been a delay of probably a month in getting a proper high-quality survey. There are only so many times I can put right PHE's basic errors. I despair. They are full of good people, but some are just not up to it.

WHO's health emergencies director Mike Ryan has warned Covid may 'never go away'. I hope this reality check makes it over Hadrian's Wall.

FRIDAY 15 MAY
The Guardian is still harping on about Covid contracts, acting as if this government is fundamentally corrupt and has been gaily dishing out multi-million-pound contracts to ministers' mates. It's complete rubbish and really winds me up. They claim we awarded £1 billion worth of deals without following due process, using illegitimate back-channels. Utter crap. As I've said ad nauseam, we were in a race against time and necessarily fast-tracked the most credible offers of help.

Culture Secretary Oliver Dowden and I are on a mission to reopen competitive sport. It's partly about exercise but also mental health. People are really bored, and televised events might cheer them up. Football and racing are my top targets. I've got Newmarket, the capital of flat racing, in my constituency, so it's close to my heart.

After today's Downing Street press conference, I went back to the Thatcher Room to pick up my stuff and ask the team how they thought it went, then along to the PM's office to download, as I usually do. He wasn't there but the duty clerk said I'd find him in the garden, so we all went through. Gina came too, the first time she'd been in the Downing Street garden. Most of the No. 10 team were sitting around in small groups. The PM came over and asked how it had gone. Like me, he'd just got his results from the antibody test. I had medium to strong antibodies, but his were off the charts. He's so competitive that even winning on the strength of his antibodies cheers him up. He went back to the group he was sitting with on the terrace, grinning all over his face.

SATURDAY 16 MAY

The BMA has come out in support of teaching unions questioning whether it's wise to reopen schools. When the Prof says he's 'slightly irritated', you know that means he's properly cross. He and I are both really annoyed that the BMA are pontificating on this issue, when their members – doctors – are defined as key workers, meaning neither they nor their kids are subjected to home schooling. The Prof pointed out that the BMA didn't kick off when we decided to keep schools open for certain groups. 'It's other people's children they seem to object to,' he observed.

Sadly, so far during the pandemic, the union has behaved in a way that's even lower than my already very low expectations. 'Near the start of this, the Queen said everyone should act in such a way that they can be proud of, when they look back at what they did. I don't think the BMA were watching,' I told the Prof irritably.

Anne Longfield, the children's commissioner, rightly says that we should 'stop squabbling and agree a plan', warning that the education shutdown is having the worst effect on disadvantaged children. I hope the BMA is listening.

In the Mediterranean, they are pushing hard to open up in time for the tourist season. Italy has announced it will reopen shops on 18 May and lift travel restrictions from 3 June. Spain is to reopen some public spaces, including hotels. I'm worried all this may be premature.

SUNDAY 17 MAY

China's top respiratory expert, Zhong Nanshan, has said the country is at high risk of a second wave. India's death toll has reached 85,940, overtaking China. As we now know to our cost, the world is a very small place.

In more positive news, Sarah Gilbert thinks we could have a vaccine by early autumn. If she's right, we could well be the first country in the world to have a mass vaccination programme. Amazing.

MONDAY 18 MAY

I woke up worrying that AstraZeneca are charging ahead doing deals with European countries that give them access to our vaccine without us extracting anything in return. I messaged Cummings first thing, pointing out that we have a potentially world-saving product here, developed with the support of British taxpayers' cash, but as AstraZeneca roll it out around the world, HMG aren't getting anything in return. I joked with JVT that if AZ comes off, in return for saving the world, at the very least, Europe should give us a good EU exit deal.

JVT reminded me that it's no good the UK winning this race if we don't have everything in place to produce the jabs at the speed and scale required. Capacity building won't be time wasted: whichever company/country gets there first, we'll still need to be able to make their vaccine.

I'm also pushing hard for so-called human challenge trials, which involve infecting healthy volunteers with Covid in order to accelerate vaccine development. The ethics are complex, but the potential benefits are huge. JVT described challenge trials as 'risky' but is also keen. My view is that as long as volunteers are fully informed, it's absolutely justifiable.

If we need to legislate, that's fine by me. JVT thinks it may be the only way to get there this side of Christmas.

'Let's make it happen,' I enthused.

In the meantime, President Xi Jinping has said he will make Chinese vaccines a global public good. Nice sentiment, but I'm not sure quite how grateful the world will feel, given where this whole nightmare started.

TUESDAY 19 MAY

I'm worried Cummings is trying to screw over Dido. She's already ensnared in his silly turf wars. While she tries to grip the launch of Test and Trace, he's been busy setting himself up as a kind of alternative expert on testing and is still trying to get her to report 'direct to the PM', by which he means to himself. As she and I discussed when she took the job, the only way her role can work is if she reports to me as Secretary of State and together we report to the PM. It's all so draining.

Meanwhile NHS England are trying to stop her using the NHS logo. Seriously, you couldn't make this stuff up. They want Test and Trace to be presented as a 'Gov.UK' initiative instead. We need it to be an NHS service to ensure we get maximum trust. Since I'm responsible for the NHS brand as Secretary of State, they're not going to win this one, but it's ridiculous that Dido is being tied in knots over such trivia.

The World Bank has announced that all the progress that has been made towards tackling world poverty over the past three years could be wiped out by the pandemic, pushing as many as 60 million people into extreme poverty. How depressing. I keep a copy of Matt Ridley's wonderful book *The Rational Optimist* on my bedside table, a reminder of the many ways the world has improved over the generations. It's a struggle to maintain my natural optimism right now.

WEDNESDAY 20 MAY

There are growing concerns about whether our hospitals have either the technology or the expertise to treat cancer patients in a way that does not increase their risk of dying of Covid.

Chemotherapy makes them more vulnerable, so, where possible, doctors are trying to use radiotherapy instead. The switch has been welcomed by oncologists, who consider it long overdue. The problem is that hospitals don't have the machines to deliver the treatment safely. Publicly, NHS England insists everything is fine. In reality, as I learned today, our equipment is not suited to the type of radiotherapy that's being recommended, not least because it was generally installed ten years ago. There are also concerns about whether staff have the required expertise. I can't quite believe we're having this problem. I worry so much for the cancer patients who can't be treated – and all those who will harbour a cancer undiagnosed for longer thanks to the pandemic – and many more will die. And I really resent the accusations I get sometimes about this, as if I care only about people dying from Covid. I know the impact of cancer. I want to defeat it – and Covid is giving it a boost.

Cummings's interference notwithstanding, the Test and Trace system will be up and running from 1 June. Meanwhile the Queen has approved Boris's recommendation for Captain Tom Moore to be knighted. He's given a fantastic boost to the whole country in dark times.

THURSDAY 21 MAY

Sunetra Gupta, an Oxford epidemiologist who thinks that up to half the population has already had Covid, has been calling for a 'rapid exit' from lockdown. She reckons the virus is 'already on the way out'. Personally I'd like to see her making a rapid exit from this debate: her claims are potentially dangerous. Of course we all want this to be over, but it's not. Annoyingly, the Porton Down data showing only 5 per cent of people have been infected is still not ready for publication. I'm looking forward to countering her nonsense with more facts.

The R number is still very high, and there's not much we can do without Test and Trace in place. However, the summer holidays will effectively reinstate school closures in July, potentially addressing some of the negative effects of reopening.

The total number of cases worldwide has passed 5 million.

FRIDAY 22 MAY

Westminster is abuzz with claims that Cummings broke lockdown rules. The *Mirror* has revealed that he went up to Durham to stay with his parents while he had Covid, which looks like a mega breach. Apparently he was with them five days after he had supposedly gone into isolation at home in London. He seems to have been spotted by several people at various different times. There's some suggestion the family was spoken to by police.

No. 10 claims he didn't break any rules because he and his wife Mary needed his parents to look after their young son while they were sick. They've cited some comments Jenny Harries made about 'exceptional circumstances' in which people could get their families to help out. But it doesn't look good, especially as – just before we closed schools back in March – Boris said, 'Children should not be left with older grandparents ... who may be particularly vulnerable.' My big worry is the impact on public health messaging. Words cost lives in a pandemic. I know Cummings's instinct will be to ride it out – never apologise and never explain – but let's see how long that lasts. Journalists loathe him so they'll go for him hard.

At the Downing Street press conference, Priti Patel finally announced that all travellers entering the UK from 8 June will have to go into quarantine for fourteen days. The Prof's view is that unless other countries are in a worse state than we are, there's no downside to travel, except that planes are not great places during pandemics. Ideally people would take a test before going abroad, but we're a good way off that. I've long been concerned we've been too soft on borders, and at least we're making some progress. Shapps has suggested we create travel corridors with some of the safer countries. Seems a good idea.

SATURDAY 23 MAY

A roller-coaster day on the Cummings story. Boris went out to bat for him after it emerged that the police contact reported yesterday was initiated by his father, who confirmed the family was self-isolating on the property and asked for security advice. It turns out that Cummings and his wife stayed in a separate cottage on his parents' farm, not in the same house. I felt slightly guilty because I was quick to judge him yesterday.

Nonetheless, I wasn't that keen to go out to defend him. Downing Street called asking if I'd do some media, but I'm uneasy. Despite all the reassurances, it feels off. In the end I issued a supportive tweet, saying he was right to find childcare for his toddler when both he and his wife were getting ill. I hoped that was the end of it. Sadly not: the story is still running hard and tomorrow's papers are a shocker. As well as driving to his parents' house in County Durham in March, the *Mirror* says Cummings was seen walking in woods with his wife and son near Barnard Castle on 12 April. Apparently he was spotted there again a week later, five days after he was photographed in Downing Street coming back to work. The witness claims he was commenting on how lovely the bluebells were. Downing Street has dismissed it as 'a stream of false allegations', but nobody is convinced by these denials. No. 10's line is that he 'behaved reasonably and legally', but I am furious. Surely he should resign, if true? When an adviser becomes the story, they've got a problem.

Osborne messaged me this evening warning me not to stick my neck out for him again.

'Lay low' was his advice.

SUNDAY 24 MAY

The media is in full hue and cry over Cummings's jaunts to Barnard Castle and what they consider to be his transparent lying. It looks terrible for the government and for everyone who stuck up for him. Poor Shapps made a valiant attempt to defend the indefensible on the morning media round, but No. 10's line is shot to pieces and it was obvious that even the unflappable Shapps knew it.

All the clinicians on my team are absolutely furious and I spent much of the day fielding angry messages, many of them questioning why the PM is still standing up for him. The answer is that Cummings rules through fear and intimidation, squashing those who dare to challenge him or get in his way. He has already seen off half a Cabinet over Brexit and got Sajid fired as Chancellor just three months ago. A culture of fear is a terrible way to run any organisation, but that's how he operates.

Feeling sickened, I kept my head well down all day and tried to focus on our messaging around Test and Trace. On Wednesday we'll announce that anyone who's contacted by the NHS and told to self-isolate must do so. It's a big ask of people who will probably be feeling perfectly well, so we need to be very careful about how we present the policy.

Jim Bethell took a call from Theo Agnew, who has some concerns about the contract we've signed with the US pharma company Moderna. As a senior Treasury Minister and a minister in the Cabinet Office, he has a duty to safeguard taxpayers' money. He's not at all happy that Moderna is demanding a hefty deposit when we don't even know whether the vaccine they're developing will work.

'He feels it's egregious to hold us to ransom for a pre-payment,' Jim reported. 'I stated the obvious, that we didn't have any options and the sums involved were tiny compared to the benefits and tried to make him feel better about an unpleasant situation.'

The discussion was clearly tricky and was a reminder that plenty of very smart people think the government is being taken for a ride. Jim says some people regard the whole Covid response as a left-wing conspiracy to expand the reach of the state and spend money on useless things. Apparently they suggest that the entire lockdown could have been avoided if only we'd had 3,000 more ventilators. Jim very wisely refuses to rise to the bait, but he is right that we need to be cognisant of the right-wing counter-narrative.

MONDAY 25 MAY

Still under intense pressure, Cummings tried to draw a line under the Barnard Castle affair by holding a press conference in the Downing Street garden. I watched it from the office in between meetings. He sat behind a table, squinting awkwardly in the sun, looking like a sulky teenager who'd been sent outside to do his work for disrupting the class. Doing his best to conceal his loathing for being held to account, he professed himself ready to answer any question, and in so doing only dug himself into an ever bigger hole. He did not regret his actions, he declared (because he is completely incapable of ever admitting he's got anything wrong), though he does regret not making a public statement earlier. He said he and Mary went north because they had been worried that if they stayed in London and became seriously ill they would have 'no reasonable childcare options'. He also said he'd been very worried about staying at home during lockdown because people have been shouting threats outside his house. He said he didn't clear it with the PM as Boris was ill, so he decided off his own bat to stay at a cottage on his parents' farm. The most extraordinary moment came when he claimed that the reason he drove to Barnard Castle (thirty miles from his parents' home) was to test his eyesight, wanting to be sure he had recovered well enough to drive the family back to London. I listened open-mouthed. Did he really say that? What possessed him? Who tests their eyesight by driving a car?

Afterwards, I found myself feeling strangely sorry for Boris. He drafted in Cummings to get Brexit done, which made sense, but the man is completely ill suited to a pandemic, which requires bringing people with you. He only has one setting – divide and destroy – and now the boss is having to say some pretty stupid things as he machetes his way through the resulting mess. The only thing for it was to keep backing Cummings – silence from me would just create an unhelpful story – so this evening I asked Jamie to draft something vaguely collegiate. He was not enthusiastic.

'If we are supportive again and something else comes out, our credibility is totally shot,' he warned, adding that I'll have to defend whatever I say now the next time I'm fronting the Downing Street press conference, 'so it needs to be watertight'. This is the problem when ministers are sent out to defend lies. It becomes impossible to govern.

In the end Jamie suggested that I welcome the fact that Cummings 'has provided substantive answers to all the questions put to him' and that we can all now move on etc., so this was the thrust of my tweet. Apparently it got me some credit in No. 10, but I can't say I felt good about it.

Away from the Cummings saga, we had a Cabinet meeting to discuss plans for easing restrictions. I want people to grasp that opening up is only possible because we got this thing under control. They must understand the need for caution as we slowly ease off the brakes. It was a bizarre Cabinet, held on Zoom without a single mention of the Cummings-shaped elephant in the room. In fact, an absurd amount of bandwidth was occupied by a discussion about whether – when we allow two households to get together outside – people should be allowed to walk through a house to get to a friend's garden. The Prof is in favour, pointing out that in cities it will often be the only way to get into someone's garden, and people will probably do it anyway. I told him that if he thinks it's workable, it's fine by me, but are people going to ask whether they will also be able to go inside to use the loo?

'If they're quick and disinfect the handle?' he replied helpfully.

With charming naivety, he seemed to think that settled the matter, whereas I could see red lights flashing all over it. At the next press conference, I just know I'm going to be asked what being 'quick' in the loo means. I can already see it: the media will try to draw us into pronouncing on whether people can read on the toilet and precisely how long we'll give them on the pan. Do they get to sit there and sing 'happy birthday' or is that just for when they're washing their hands? Who could believe that under a Conservative government the long arm of the state would find its way into people's loos?

TUESDAY 26 MAY

For the first day since 18 March, no new deaths have been reported in Northern Ireland. I sent Robin Swann my congratulations. He called it 'a clear sign of progress'. But the WHO has warned of a second peak as countries start to ease lockdown.

Ecuador's largest cities have seen widespread disturbances in protest at the government's response to the pandemic. This worries me. We're not exactly Ecuador, but how long will public patience last?

Meanwhile the BBC reports that Cummings has edited his blog to give the impression he predicted a coronavirus pandemic. Unreal. Here we are battling hard against a real pandemic, while Dom is spending his time fiddling around with his blog to try to pretend he saw it coming. I tried to imagine the thought process that leads to someone sitting in their bedroom altering obscure old musings in the vain hope of conjuring an image as a seer, while most of us are working eighteen-hour days trying to save lives. What kind of mind must you have to do that?

It's recess, so I was home in time to see all the children before bed – sadly, a novelty these days. I'm really missing them.

WEDNESDAY 27 MAY

Dido spent most of the morning locked in what seems to have been a very stressful meeting ahead of the announcement about Test and Trace. I say 'seems' because to my annoyance I wasn't invited – yet Rishi, who isn't directly involved in this one, was there. This is no way to run things. Afterwards, Dido described the meeting as 'weird' and said they all got super stressed that they didn't understand what contact tracing was. She said most of the discussion was about whether it should be a legal requirement to self-isolate if asked by the NHS to do so. Apparently they went round and round in circles on this question, with Cummings 'quite exercised' (in Dido's words) that for now we are only describing it as a 'civic duty'. The plan is to see how seriously people take the moral obligation. If they routinely ignore the request, we'll have to make it mandatory. Dido and I explained all this at this evening's press conference. Our biggest problem is managing expectations. So many people from the Prime Minister down are desperate to get out of lockdown and are investing huge hope in Test and Trace. Dido did her best not to set us up for a fall, stressing that it won't be perfect at first. In fact, it won't even be fully operational until the end of June. The truth is that this is a heroically fast timetable for creating a system of this scale, but in the context of a pandemic, it still seems an age away. I felt slightly sick as she said it, because while setting realistic expectations is the right thing to do, it gives the press a massive target.

Back in the department, I finally received the results of the study into how many people have had Covid, this time based on a proper representative sample. I was oddly nervous as we sat down with Dido, the Prof, Nadine Dorries and Jim Bethell for a readout of the findings. Unfortunately, they're not good. It finally and comprehensively confirms that only 5 per cent of the population have antibodies, though it's three times that figure in London.

The implications are crystal clear: we're not going to get out of this without a vaccine. I left the meeting feeling more determined than ever to support the necessary research.

THURSDAY 28 MAY

Oliver Dowden has done great work and the Premier League has announced it will restart matches from 17 June behind closed doors. Later Tom Goff, one of my constituents, who's a big figure in the racing world, messaged asking if racing will definitely restart on 1 June as planned. When I confirmed, he replied with just two words – 'happy days' – and a bunch of champagne cork emojis.

Tomorrow's papers claim Cummings is set to leave Downing Street within six months. I don't buy it. 'It's what you brief when you want some breathing room,' Jamie said. 'Like Theresa last year. Or Blair.' Sounds about right.

SAGE reports that one in three people hospitalised specifically for Covid die. Very sobering.

FRIDAY 29 MAY

Cummings messaged early to say that the PM has asked Simon Stevens for a drink on Monday. I guess this is about negotiating an amicable exit. At least Boris is handling this directly himself now.

Jamie alerted me to a figure in *The Guardian* that only 50 per cent of people are self-isolating when they have symptoms. Unsurprisingly, No. 10 is concerned. David Halpern says 80 per cent of people claim they would self-isolate if asked to do so by NHS Test and Trace, but we don't have any actual data yet.

Today we've started a new system for formal decision making. Mark Sedwill has put in the same model we use for Brexit subcommittees, with a 'Covid Operations', or Covid-O, meeting chaired by Michael Gove whenever we need it, and a 'Covid Strategy', or Covid-S, meeting chaired by the Prime Minister for the big calls. Now Michael's onside for the pandemic response this should work well – and make it easier to get cross-government decisions taken.

SATURDAY 30 MAY

Finally my work with Oliver Dowden to get competitive sport up and running has come to fruition. It means Formula One, cricket, racing, golf, rugby, snooker and football will return to TV screens. I'm thrilled. We've pulled it off despite PHE scepticism and without a 'one rule for professional athletes, another for everyone else' public backlash. Just a shame it's too late for Wimbledon.

We aren't yet ready for grassroots sport to reopen as it's too early for the mass relaxation of lockdown rules this would entail. The Prof is actually more worried about supporters on the sidelines than players on the pitch.

At the press conference, journalists tried to trick JVT into wading into the Cummings row by asking him if people in authority should lead and obey the rules. It was a classic 'When did you stop beating your wife?' question, designed to generate a story whatever the response. To his credit, JVT, who isn't supposed to comment on political issues, answered that the rules are clear and have always been for the benefit of all. 'In my opinion, they apply to all,' he said. Deft handling!

He also said the UK was 'at a very dangerous moment' and that infections could rebound 'like a coiled spring … if we don't stay on top of it'. He's right. Japan's Covid cases have risen for the fourth day since its state of emergency was lifted.

SUNDAY 31 MAY

No. 10 is furious about JVT's response to the Cummings question and wants him off the airwaves. There was me thinking he'd preserved his integrity without mentioning Cummings by name, but no humble pie from our antihero, who clearly kicked off. Bluntly, JVT is our best communicator on the clinical side, so we can't take him off the pitch. This is what happens when you try to defend the indefensible.

JUNE 2020

MONDAY 1 JUNE

Abad start to the day as No. 10 omitted to invite me to a high-level meeting with the PM about coming out of lockdown. The Prof, Simon Case, Dido and Simon Stevens were all on the cast list, so I'm not sure why I didn't feature. Probably Cummings's doing. In the end I attended by Zoom, which seemed a base-level requirement, given that I was fronting this evening's Downing Street press conference.

Things took a further turn for the worse when Piers Morgan started laying into me on Twitter. I'm used to his crazed rants, but being publicly accused of deliberately covering up the number of Covid deaths because I 'don't give a shit about people losing their lives' was a whole new level. Morgan thought he'd caught me lying, when in reality several hundred deaths were reclassified as being non-Covid-related because it turned out that the disease was not relevant in those cases. If anything, we have consistently *overstated* the number of Covid deaths precisely to avoid such accusations, so this really got my goat. Normally I try not to get drawn into Twitter altercations, but in this instance I told the team we *had* to hit back, because the accusation was outrageous. There's always a tricky balance when shrill shouters like Morgan attack you on social media. Their whole business model is to create a fight, which I'd rather avoid, but to allow accusations not to be answered implies they contain some truth. What's odd is that these media tormentors tend to be perfectly friendly in person. In my view they contribute very little to political debate other than making it harder for voters to understand what's really going on.

What has cheered me up is tomorrow's fantastic *Daily Express* front page, which rightly declares we're winning the battle against this disease. We are indeed, with no thanks to Piers Morgan & co. At this evening's press conference I was able to say that Covid deaths and cases are now at their lowest since lockdown started. As schools begin phased reopening, this feels like a real turning point.

TUESDAY 2 JUNE

I am so sick of having to endlessly make the same arguments to lockdown sceptics who either don't understand or won't accept why we had to do what we did, and why we're not suddenly abandoning all restrictions in one dramatic fell swoop. It is wearying explaining it over and over again to people who just don't want to listen and would rather act as if the whole episode has been some kind of power trip. It's not just certain backbenchers: some Cabinet colleagues are giving off-the-record briefings to journalists about why we should be unlocking further and faster, and generally winding up the anti-lockdown brigade. There are honourable exceptions – when Rees-Mogg has reservations, he says what he thinks but doesn't go out and brief the media and continues to support the PM – but for some this is all about positioning themselves in the party. It is all incredibly negative and I hate it.

After yet another exasperating meeting with colleagues who don't like our approach, during which I had to explain the reason for everything we are doing for the umpteenth time, I felt like exploding.

'I can't believe we had to have that very basic conversation again,' I told the Prof despairingly.

He doesn't really do emojis, or I suspect his 'Groundhog Day' reply to my WhatsApp would have been accompanied by several eye rolls.

WEDNESDAY 3 JUNE

The scientific consensus that the virus came from wild animals like bats or pangolins is starting to crack, and it does not look good for the Chinese.

Angus Dalgleish, a British professor based at St George's Hospital in London, and the Norwegian virologist Birger Sørensen have identified 'inserted sections placed on the SARS-CoV-2 spike surface' that explain 'how the virus binds itself to human cells'. According to Sørensen, this may indicate that the virus is not natural but man-made. The suspicion among some is that it escaped from a microbiology lab in Wuhan, where scientists regularly work on coronavirus projects and have previously deliberately engineered a hybrid of SARS and bat coronavirus. If true, the implications for international relations are massive. Sir Richard Dearlove, the former MI6 chief, has been ramping things up, describing the findings as compelling evidence that the virus accidentally escaped from the lab. To me, this explanation could be credible. The plausible alternative is that the virus was brought to Wuhan to be studied and then escaped.

THURSDAY 4 JUNE

Boris messaged me at 6.43 a.m. saying he was 'going quietly crackers' about testing. He told me he sees it as our 'Achilles heel'. He's complaining that we can't deliver a sensible border policy or adequate Test and Trace because we aren't testing enough people. He was in a proper flap, asking whether we had followed up on an offer from Angela Merkel to send us more kits, and claiming we've had 'months and months' to sort it out.

'What is wrong with our country that we can't fix this?' he complained.

I tried to calm him down, pointing out that we are doing pretty well on this front relative to other countries.

'Don't go crackers,' I said. 'We now have the biggest testing capacity in Europe.' Tempting as it was, I refrained from saying we did this against the obstruction of his own No. 10 operation.

He thinks people should be able to get out of quarantine early if they test negative. Well, of course! That would be great. The problem is that the virus incubates for ages, and the medics are all against going down this route because of the risk of false negatives.

SAGE has discovered that between a third and a half of hospital admissions 'for Covid' are actually either re-admissions or not acute Covid at all. We need to understand better how the NHS is recording people. Our many critics have no idea how complicated all this is. As I keep saying, far from deliberately playing down the scale of death and illness, we have been as transparent as possible – even though we look worse for it.

Meanwhile Nadine is worrying about how people will behave when we relax restrictions. She thinks we need to sharpen our messaging.

'It should be a three-point policy combined as one. Masks. Hand-washing. Social distancing,' she suggested.

'Four: isolation,' I replied.

I thought about it a bit more and suggested we sum it up as follows: Masks, Hygiene, Social Distancing, Test, Isolate. Not exactly catchy.

'Maybe we could turn it into an acronym?' I suggested.

'SHITM,' Nadine replied, with a clown emoji. Here's hoping Lee Cain can come up with something better.

FRIDAY 5 JUNE

Dom has been looking at TV footage of hospitals and is annoyed that some staff are not wearing masks. He messaged me saying he was 'truly astonished' and asking what we were doing about it. As it happens, I am all over this. I was able to tell him that we're announcing a policy of masks for all staff and all patients at all times.

'When?' he asked.

'5 p.m.,' I replied, astonished he clearly hadn't read any of the huge amounts of paperwork that have been going back and forth on this over the past two weeks.

The truth is that this has been quite a saga: NHS management and the unions were implacably opposed, and I couldn't have done it without chief nurse Ruth May, who went above and beyond to make the case.

Less helpfully, Nadhim Zahawi, a minister at BEIS, opened up a can of worms today by announcing that the Test and Trace app will be ready this month. Cue sharp intakes of breath in the department. Obviously that's what we're hoping, but I've not been advertising that fact because we need to be 100 per cent sure it actually works. Now we're getting a barrage of follow-up questions from journalists, which we can't answer without risking digging an even bigger hole. I messaged him a bit grumpily and he was apologetic. The UK's Covid death toll has now passed 40,000. Test and Trace can't come soon enough.

The NHS are calling for people to donate their plasma if they've had Covid, to help with trials, so this morning I did my bit. I felt dreadful afterwards and had to take an hour out to lie down on the sofa to try to get it together ahead of the press conference. Suffice to say it wasn't my finest performance.

SATURDAY 6 JUNE

Boris is mulling what other restrictions we can ease on 15 June. 'How are we doing? How are the numbers? Seem very hard to squeeze,' he mused. He thinks we might be able to open up non-essential shops and do something more for families, perhaps even allow a bit of outdoor hospitality. However, his media advisers James Slack and Lee Cain have told him that it's too soon. I'm inclined to agree.

'I think Slack and Lee have a point,' I replied. 'All in all, with R just below 1, if we go ahead with non-essential retail on 15 June, we are sailing very close to the wind. My view is that the public are right and we need to hold our nerve,' I told him, adding that if R goes above 1, 'then we are in all kinds of trouble'.

SUNDAY 7 JUNE

One of the SAGE scientists, John Edmunds, has been sounding off on *Marr*, saying we should have gone into lockdown earlier to save more lives.

Boris is furious. 'These SAGE geezers now saying we should have gone into lockdown earlier ... Can we gently ask them why they did not make their anxieties public at the time???' he demanded, not sounding as if he wanted me to ask it gently at all.

Diplomatic as ever, Vallance promised to have a word. In any case all the SAGE minutes are published, so anyone who wants to can see the hypocrisy for themselves. I was also fuming: it's exceptionally unhelpful having individual members of SAGE making comments like this. It undermines us all. There was a very broad range of scientific opinion advising against lockdown in early March, including SAGE, which has more than 100 scientists feeding into it.

Tragically, the worldwide Covid death toll has now passed 400,000. Jim has been banging on about something called 'rockpools'. 'Epidemiologists say when the tide goes out it leaves rockpools of infection,' he told me. 'Homeless. BAME. Sex workers etc.' He wondered if we need a 'rockpools tsar'. If he wants to call it that, I'll happily let him own the idea.

MONDAY 8 JUNE

There's a dramatic spike in the number of cases in Leicester. The Prof says it's exactly the kind of place where we may have problems: some very deprived areas and a lot of casual employment on production lines where workers are cheek by jowl. One of Jim's rockpools.

I'd love to be able to report that PHE is all over it, but, true to form, they don't seem to have any idea what's going on. I met them this afternoon expecting a full update on the local data and more detail about the exact location of the hotspots and they had... nothing. Trying to bullshit their way through the meeting, they told me that their efforts to monitor what's going on are 'progressing well', a claim that collapsed the minute I asked for any numbers or other evidence to back up what they were saying. I gave them a rocket, telling them it was no use coming to me with nothing, and instructed them to return with some proper analysis. The pandemic has exposed the woeful shortcomings of this quango and it is increasingly clear to me that the whole institution will have to go. It just isn't working.

WEDNESDAY 10 JUNE

The PM has announced that from this Saturday single people living in England will be able to form so-called support bubbles with another household to give them some company. They will be allowed to visit the people in their bubble and even stay overnight. I've insisted that the rule also applies to single parents with children under eighteen. I know lockdown was especially hard for them. Hopefully it will make life much easier for a lot of people, especially couples who don't live together. We've also confirmed that from 15 June we're opening shops and outdoor attractions like zoos, safari parks and drive-through cinemas. We are getting there...

THURSDAY 11 JUNE

The Cabinet Office have had a little taster of what it's like dealing with PHE and are deeply underwhelmed. Yesterday they were forced to scrap a meeting with the PM because between them, PHE, NHS England and the Test and Trace team failed to come up with the facts and figures the attendees needed for the planned discussion about what the data tells us so far. Apparently the papers produced were so hopeless that the discussion would have been a complete waste of everybody's time.

I asked what information they needed. It was all relatively simple stuff – breakdown of incidence by community, NHS settings and care homes. They got absolute flannel in return.

I suggested that in future they direct all data questions to the Joint Biosecurity Centre, which I specifically set up to pull together this kind of information. 'They are our intelligence function,' I explained.

Unfortunately, that's where they started with this whole exercise – only to get the 'sad answer' that it would take them 'many weeks'. So frustrating. Sometimes I feel as if we're continually trying to shove water uphill.

In better news, Moderna has said it will begin the final stage of trials for its vaccine in July with 30,000 participants. Progress towards the vaccine is moving faster than I ever dared hope.

My son's seventh birthday. Home in time for celebratory tea!

SUNDAY 14 JUNE

Buoyed by the fact that deaths are now down to the lowest figure since March, I felt confident enough to tweet that we're winning the battle against this disease. Slightly surprisingly, Boris, who sometimes describes his own attitude as 'too boosterish', is wary of getting overexcited. He rang me this evening to talk through the numbers and is worried that more than 1,500 people are still testing positive every day. I shared the PM's concern with Case. I think Boris's caution is actually quite helpful: it keeps him focused on the numbers.

'Yes, but he's got to focus on what we need for winter now too!' I said.

Our backbenchers are increasingly mutinous about the two-metre rule. They're all getting grief from business owners in their constituencies. Pubs, cafes and restaurants are due to reopen on 4 July, but many say they won't bother if we don't ditch or at least amend the rule. We're looking at it.

Now my days aren't quite such a mad, hurtling rush as they were at the peak, I've been thinking about how things are likely to play out over the next few months. I foresee three moments of danger: One: 4 July. Two: early September when schools go back (assuming they do). Three: December when it gets really cold.

We need to prepare.

MONDAY 15 JUNE

PHE finally delivered a proper update on the situation in Leicester, which showed that the only thing 'progressing well', as they described it, is the virus. PHE are clearly not gripping this – I need to act, and fast. I demanded all the data we have, and a full-blown analysis for Wednesday. We cannot leave rockpools of the virus to fester.

Non-essential shops reopened today, though it will be another three weeks before restaurants, pubs, cinemas, theatres, museums and hairdressers reopen. Masks on public transport have also become compulsory.

Then, this afternoon, much more important – and exciting – news.

JVT called practically breathless with excitement. Our much-vaunted Recovery Trial has a tentative, clinically valid result. It seems that a drug that's been around for sixty years can make a huge different to the most poorly Covid patients. It's called dexamethasone, a common steroid, and can reduce the chances of a patient on a ventilator dying by about a third. For patients like Boris who needed oxygen but weren't intubated, it can reduce mortality by a fifth. Bingo! We know this because we organised the biggest and fastest pharmaceutical trial in UK history, to identify whether any existing medicines could be used to treat Covid patients. The data is tentative – at least until tomorrow. Pulling this off involved recruiting masses of volunteers in record time and was a huge effort. I think it's one of the proudest days of JVT's professional life. It's cheap, readily available and life-saving!

TUESDAY 16 JUNE
JVT called first thing to confirm we can go public about dexamethasone.

Around the same time, Cummings messaged demanding to know why we aren't stockpiling it before the announcement. He reckons Steve Oldfield told him that we can't do that because it wouldn't be fair. Dom described this as 'insane' and told me to order him to buy as much as he can, immediately. His implacable, strident attitude is absurd: he's obviously got crossed wires, as we've been hoarding the stuff for months and already have a stockpile of 200,000 courses, which we will double. The NHS is going to start using it as standard from 4 p.m. today. When I told him this, he calmed down a bit but still seemed weirdly twitchy, sending me various garbled WhatsApps about not screwing this up.

'This shd be mega good news, I'm just v nervy there are no cockup that turn it to cockup story, the media is partic deranged right now,' he said. We've been calmly sorting the substance, and he's causing all sorts of tyre-spinning worrying about the comms.

He was clearly in no mood for small talk, so I didn't regale him with my efforts to pronounce the bloody thing. My dyslexic brain finds new words very hard to learn, and I was beginning to panic about fluffing 'dexamethasone' when we made the announcement. JVT was sweetly patient and encouraging while I paced around my study, saying it again and again. Eventually I felt I'd mastered it – only to learn that Boris had decided at the last minute to take the press conference and make the announcement himself. I'm not going to pretend I wasn't annoyed to be stripped of my moment to shine as the word 'dexamethasone' slipped seamlessly off my tongue, but these things happen to ministers. I consoled myself that the PM's eagerness to lead on this one underlines that it's a really big deal. JVT was also obviously upset – it's been his baby – but the Prof will do the press conference with the PM. My job was to make the same announcement to the Commons.

Afterwards, I had my photo taken at a pharmacy in Ebury Street near the office, triumphantly holding up a pack of dexamethasone. Behind my mask, I was grinning, perhaps a bit inanely.

Tedros sent his congratulations to everyone involved in what he described as a 'life-saving scientific breakthrough'. Days like this make it all worth it.

WEDNESDAY 17 JUNE

In an embarrassingly crude power grab, Ursula von der Leyen is trying to wrest control of vaccine research and procurement from EU member states. Never mind that health is a matter for individual countries: the woman who, as Defence Minister, once sent German Army units on manoeuvres with broomsticks because they didn't have any rifles wants to take responsibility for scientific development and manufacture away from nation states and move it into the sticky paws of Brussels bureaucrats. I may have voted to remain, but sometimes I'm genuinely thankful to be out of the EU, and this is one such moment. I simply cannot imagine this turning into anything other than a fiasco. Her justification for the brazen takeover bid is entirely political: she claims there's no point to the EU if it can't play a central role in a crisis like this. Her idea is that the European Commission will set vaccine development policy and bulk buy on behalf of member states. Under the plans, individual countries will have to hand over everything they've done so far on their vaccine programmes to the Commission. What, really? Five months into the crisis? Even if you buy the political argument – and I don't – she's hopelessly late to the game. Now she risks dangerously undermining everyone's efforts. I foresee a complete mess, not least since Germany, Italy and others have already placed a load of orders with pharma companies. So many questions! What does Ursula's initiative mean for our talks with Germany and other EU members? How do we protect the negotiations we've been having with Pfizer for months about buying their vaccines, which are made in the EU? Only last week, France, Germany, Italy and the Netherlands got together to place a joint order for Oxford vaccines. What happens to this now? It's enough to make a Brexiteer out of anyone.

In other news, we've finally abandoned the in-house version of the contact tracing app. 'Dido is putting it to sleep. And moving on. Probably quite right,' Jim told me gruffly. He's worried about how we explain it. The app developers have built a perfectly good system that works – but Apple won't let us deploy it because they don't want us using the data in the NHS to identify contacts and save lives. Their behaviour is outrageous, but despite all our efforts they won't budge. If Google and Apple can come up with something better, then great. Jim thinks it's important it doesn't look as if we're 'jumping into bed' with the tech giants and suggests we tell people that it's all been very diffi-cult and so we're doing a 'strategic review', with Google and Apple as the frontrunner, but also looking at some type of fob that's being used in Singapore, and QR codes, which are being used in New Zealand. He spent the morning talking to other countries about what they're doing, including a very funny exchange with an Australian govern-ment minister who admitted they're on their fifth version of a test and trace app. Apparently they're very proud of it, though there's so little Covid in Australia that it doesn't have to do much: so far, it has only referred thirty people to the health authorities. The Singaporeans ad-mitted they want more than health outcomes from their app – they're looking for data on how to redesign their city.

On my way into the Commons today, I slapped Alex Burghart, the Essex MP, on the back as I greeted him. It was on camera, and shortly afterwards Jamie started receiving calls about me breaking social distancing rules. It was a momentary lapse, so I've apologised for a 'human mistake'. The media seem to think that's reasonable and a large fuss has been avoided.

English Premier League football has resumed behind closed doors. Fantastic! I'm looking forward to the Newcastle game in a couple of days.

THURSDAY 18 JUNE

A day dominated by debate about overseas travel. There's huge political pressure to make some sort of summer holidays abroad possible, so we're trying to figure out what we can do. SAGE still wants to quarantine anyone coming in from countries with higher case rates than ours. They are also pushing for testing ahead of travel to the UK and on days five and eight after arrival. They acknowledge that this stuff needs international agreement and some kind of common standard.

Shapps has drawn up a list of thirteen countries with which we'd most like some kind of arrangement, based on the number of Brits who normally go there and other considerations, like trade. It includes the main tourist destinations in Europe – Spain, France, Italy and Greece – as well as Australia. The US and Canada aren't on the list because we're worried about their case numbers. The idea is that PHE will advise on the health risks of each country and then we'll try to reach a decision. The Prof thinks Shapps's paper is a good starting point, but he pointed out that most Covid imports in March were from Spain, France and Italy – so allowing people to gallivant to and from these countries now might not be the smartest move.

I asked Jens Spahn how successful the German Covid app has been. He says it had 9 million downloads in two days, which sounds very impressive but doesn't mean it works. At the heart of the problem is the difficulty associated with measuring the distance between phones.

We cracked this on the home-grown version and have offered that technology to Apple for theirs.

I'm increasingly worried about Leicester and have sent a mobile testing unit to get a better picture. Cases have rocketed in the past two weeks. At this rate, they'll be stuck with restrictions considerably longer than anyone else.

There's also a significant outbreak at a meat processing plant in West Yorkshire. We're keeping an eye on it.

FRIDAY 19 JUNE

Alok, Steve Barclay and I formally signed off on plans to buy 100 million doses of the Oxford vaccine – though not without a dramatic blow-up with Kate Bingham. Kate simply doesn't see the need to order as many and can't seem to grasp that if the vaccine works, almost everyone may want or need it. Time and again, I've asked her and her team how we go further, faster, and time and again I've been fobbed off. She seems to think that any problems that would arise if we under-order are just a 'comms issue' and kept pushing back during the meeting, prompting me to warn her that if we don't get our act together on this one, we risk a complete car crash.

At the start of the meeting Alok set out the proposal in the paper to buy her suggested number. I couldn't quite believe he was making that case and knew it was a make-or-break moment. If I didn't go in hard and win the argument, the country would not be left with enough vaccine for everyone. Worse still, if everyone needs two doses, that's only 15 million people. Fairly vulnerable people – like those in their fifties – would be left behind. I absolutely had to convince everyone, and took no prisoners.

After my first blast, Alok immediately swung in behind. He was very gracious, having just set out the paper from Kate's team. Next up, Steve Barclay. He holds the purse strings. He said there is no better insurance in the world than spending money on potential vaccines. Bingo. Kate pushed back hard and insisted we won't need all these doses, and when I asked her how we could do more, she just argued it was the wrong approach. But with the other elected ministers on my side, I won the argument. I sat back in my chair, exhausted by what was an extraordinarily stressful but pivotal moment. In the end I secured all the terms I've fought for: 100 million doses, domestic manufacture and an exclusivity agreement.

It shouldn't have been this difficult.

'You can't just tell me I'm wrong when I'm asking HOW something can be done. The question I've been asking for months has been what do we need to do IF we want to go faster,' I told her afterwards.

'I'm not happy with that meeting,' she snapped back.

'Nor me,' I replied, bashing at my phone a little harder than usual.

'We will create a guide for you to explain what we are doing – there are enormous risks with this,' she said, as if I don't spend all my time thinking about how to save lives.

Kate pressed on, claiming that while the global flu jab is 'proven and scales', the adenovirus technology that underpins the vaccine Oxford is working on 'is neither proven nor scaled'.

'We have an expert team who are working round the clock pushing hard. And I don't appreciate being told this is a car crash,' she declared.

'I didn't say it's a car crash,' I replied angrily. In fact – as I told her yesterday – things are in better shape than they were. 'BUT I am acutely aware of the enormous pressures that will come to bear when a vaccine comes good. That is when there is a risk of a car crash if we do not have all our ducks in a row. Simply saying that the unavailability of product for large swathes of the population is a comms issue isn't going to work. We need to have tried everything feasibly possible to accelerate delivery. I've been asking the same question over and over again and not yet had a satisfactory answer – hence my frustration,' I said, horribly mangling my metaphors.

This only seemed to wind her up further, prompting a patronising mini-lecture about the dangers of trying to go too far too fast.

'We will give you a written answer. Sadly human biology is more complex than medical equipment. And a lot more risky. The worse case is we kill people with an unsafe vaccine. We need to tone the comms to register the fact this is risky and unproven – and not raise everyone's expectations of a magical silver bullet,' she said.

If there's one thing I can't stand, it's being patronised.

I walked out on my balcony overlooking Westminster Cathedral to try to get some calm. It's taken a huge effort, but we should now have enough vaccines for the entire population – not just the elderly and most vulnerable. For the first time, I am starting to see how this ends.

SATURDAY 20 JUNE

Delightful as it would be never to talk about the app again, Dido can't get Test and Trace off the ground until it's sorted. Jim is doing a magnificent job managing all the many egos. He met the development team again today and reports that he banged the table 'only once'. Noses are clearly out of joint about the decision to ditch the in-house version and he says the atmosphere in the meeting was 'pretty weird'.

'They were very hostile to alternative suggestions,' he says.

Meanwhile Jim's contact at Apple says they're a bit antsy about our various criticisms. It's a bit rich given they took an active decision to ensure our app won't work on Apple phones, but I told him we absolutely have to turn this into a positive collaboration.

SUNDAY 21 JUNE

JVT messaged this morning to say that the first clinical meeting to design the human challenge trials is meeting this week. The whole thing feels as if it's taking ages, but the machine won't let me move it along any faster, largely because of the ethical assessments needed for a study which involves directly infecting people with the virus to see if the Oxford vaccine works. But the ethics of meaningful consent need to be offset against the ethics of 40,000 deaths and months in lockdown.

During the morning media round I came under a bit of pressure over the app and had to go in quite hard on Apple. Our app worked on Android, and Apple simply wouldn't make the changes required for it to work on iPhones. I pointed out that the company has a history of being intransigent in the face of perfectly reasonable requests from democratically elected governments to work with them on solving particular problems, whether it's solutions to terrorism or other technical challenges.

Trump has hosted a big indoor re-election rally in Tulsa, Oklahoma, where he called the coronavirus 'kung flu'. What a plonker.

MONDAY 22 JUNE

I asked the Prof if he is worried about what's happening in Germany, where the R rate is shooting up. Today it's said to have hit 2.88. He said he's not too fussed for now, because the overall numbers are very low there, so the measured rate can bounce all over the place. Part of the problem is a huge outbreak at a slaughterhouse in Gütersloh in north-western Germany. These meat processing plants seem to be real super-spreaders. Why?!

JVT messaged again to update me on vaccine development and procurement. He promised to give me a 'plain and straight' summary of where things stand, which was his way of preparing me to hear something I might not entirely like. It turned out to be about the size of our order for the Oxford vaccine. Apparently the 'machine' is trying to undo Friday's agreement to buy 100 million doses, reverting to the 30 million cap Kate has been pushing for. Unbelievable!

'I think they probably can't increase production in the timelines allowed if you take into account needing to back multiple horses for manufacturers beyond Oxford, who in my view may be first (they are well ahead now even beyond Moderna) but the vaccine may not best in class and may only be disease-modifying,' he explained.

He says he's happy to 'bank' 30 million doses for a first tranche but, like me, would not stop there. He thinks the next tranche we secure might be a different type of vaccine that takes longer to develop but prevents the disease altogether, if that can be achieved.

I told him that an initial 30 million is fine – especially if the first iteration is only disease-modifying – but if the vaccine requires two doses, that's only enough for 15 million people. He told me not to worry and that he has been 'most explicit' with Kate's team on my behalf that the initial tranche means 30 million people, not doses: 'absolutely no less'. The continual pushback from the Vaccine Taskforce (VTF), which Kate chairs, is so frustrating. Don't they, of all people, understand that this is a global race for a vaccine? Oxford looks well ahead of the field. JVT is pretty sure we will be first in the world to go into mass production, beating Moderna, though their version is coming along well. Global demand will be stratospheric: we can't be left behind.

TUESDAY 23 JUNE

The PM did his great 'independence day' announcement ahead of 4 July, though we're certainly not billing it that way.

'Our long national hibernation is beginning to come to an end' is how he put it in his Commons statement, which didn't sound massively liberating, but we don't want people to get carried away. Cabinet colleagues are divided over how just how prescriptive we should be. When I looked at the final draft of the new guidelines this morning, I noticed that someone had sneakily watered down the new Test and Trace rules for pubs and restaurants. The original (and best) plan was to mandate business owners to keep customer logs to help NHS Test and Trace, but the language had been changed from saying that they 'should' do this to '*could*' do this.

On enquiry, it turned out that Alok was blocking 'should'.

'Well, I'm blocking "could"', I said briskly, pointing out that the PM agreed with me. I was told it would have to be resolved in Cabinet, which I was fine about, because I knew I'd win. What I can't understand is why Alok is against controlling the virus.

Apparently Rishi is also going bonkers about 'should'. The more I thought about this, the more annoyed I got. We must keep R below 1 or we will get a huge second wave, and a second lockdown. This one is not a big ask. This, plus proper funding for the NHS this winter, is the necessary price of liberation. These kinds of negotiations just make everything harder. I told Case that BEIS has gone off the reservation, and whatever is agreed must be in writing. At least Ben Wallace is being helpful. He'd heard about the spate of Covid outbreaks in meat processing plants and asked if I wanted to use military assets 'to target them (not blow them up!)'. He pointed out that the Germans used their army to test the entire workforce in some factories. I told him that military testing units have been mission critical to dealing with local outbreaks so far and that I'm grateful for their support.

I went to bed mulling over how on earth a significant number of people in the UK still don't have any basic understanding of Covid. According to SAGE, only 65 per cent of people realise that a cough or fever are possible symptoms. Where have they been for the past three months – Pluto?

WEDNESDAY 24 JUNE

A truly awful shock: Rose Paterson has died. Rose is an old friend, and as far as I knew she was in excellent health. Later I heard that it was probably suicide. This won't be announced immediately. I am absolutely reeling and am so sorry for the family. I simply can't believe she's gone. It will take a long time to sink in and Owen and the family will be absolutely devastated.

THURSDAY 25 JUNE

The weather is amazing and people have been flocking to the beach and the countryside, triggering a 'major incident' alert in Bournemouth. Dorset Police reported traffic gridlock, fights and a load of people camping. I just hope it doesn't lead to a huge uptick in cases. Dido and I have been trying to draw up some protocols setting out the circumstances in which we might go back into local restrictions, like in Leicester. The PM is taking a close interest. The presidents of the Royal Colleges of Surgeons, Nursing, Physicians and GPs, as well as the head of the BMA, have signed an open letter to the *British Medical Journal* warning that local flare-ups of the virus are increasingly likely.

They think a second wave is a real risk and are demanding that we do more to prepare – as if we're just sitting back with our feet up!

I spent some of the day talking to EU contacts about whether there is any merit in joining their vaccine-buying scheme (as we're entitled to do so under the terms of our Brexit transition). It's against all my instincts at this point, but there's heavy political pressure from some quarters. We've got to do the due diligence. Now I've stress tested it, I'm more convinced than ever that it won't work.

Just one fact says it all: if we joined the EU scheme, we'd have to hand all our existing contracts to Brussels. I spoke to Jens and he also has major reservations. However, he has very limited room for manoeuvre because Merkel is super keen. She is desperate to do whatever she can to bolster Von der Leyen, who is her creation, even though, by law, health is nothing to do with the EU.

In other gloomy news, efforts to get a grip on the virus in Leicester just haven't worked. The whole city is going to be stuck with heavy restrictions when everywhere else is opening up further on 4 July. I foresee a load of problems with the tricksy Labour mayor. At least we're in much better shape than America, where cases are skyrocketing and the official data is all over the place. The CDC thinks the number of people who've had the virus could be ten times the official figure. More than half the states are seeing record increases.

FRIDAY 26 JUNE

Boris is watching what's going on in the US and getting very twitchy about our plans to unlock. 'News from America is horrific,' he declared gloomily. 'What is the difference in the relaxation measures in the badly hit US states (Texas, Arizona etc.) and what we are doing on 4 July? In what way have they gone further than we will?'

Vallance explained that the situation varies significantly from state to state, but a lot of people in the US are just going about their normal business – as a result of which cases are multiplying. He told the boss that if people behave like that here too, we will be in the same boat.

'We need some tough messaging. And we need the protocols for going back into local and national lockdown. And the public needs to understand exactly how they are going to be enforced,' Boris replied grimly. I told him that we are working on exactly that and can accelerate.

He is especially wound up about the scenes in Liverpool last night, when crowds poured onto the streets to celebrate the team's first Premier League title win in thirty years, for the second night in a row. He's reprimanded people for 'taking liberties' and said these mass gatherings have got to stop.

SUNDAY 28 JUNE

PHE claims to have Leicester under control with its mobile testing units, but I'm calling out this non-scientific bullshit. The truth is that they're terrified of upsetting the mayor, Sir Peter Soulsby, who thinks his city is being unfairly targeted and is determined to make life difficult for the government. I'm not taking any lessons on how to handle this pandemic from Soulsby, so we're pressing ahead with plans for a local lockdown. Priti Patel confirmed it on *Marr*, and the Sunday papers are full of it. I'm resolute, but it's going to be a rocky ride.

Meanwhile Cummings is still obsessing about masks. He messaged me this evening saying he doesn't think we are being 'aggressive' enough and that they should be compulsory in shops and for restaurant staff. Boris apparently agrees. The Prof said there was 'no science/medical reason not to', describing the evidence for mask wearing as 'moderate but positive in enclosed spaces where distancing is difficult'. I said I could see no reason not to use the power of the state to enforce it and that the importance of masks should be in all our messaging. Next week the Treasury is launching a new campaign to encourage people to go back to pubs, but in the adverts nobody's wearing a mask, and the tone isn't at all cautious. We'll need to talk to them.

MONDAY 29 JUNE

We're at crunch point with Leicester. This morning I asked JVT for his latest advice and his firm recommendation is that not only should the planned reopening not happen but the recent easing of lockdown should be reversed across the city. Soulsby can jump up and down, but case numbers are spiralling out of control.

We met in my office to make the decision. The Prof, Dido and JVT were all agreed: we need to close all non-essential retail and shut schools early for summer. We're going to tell people to stay at home as much as possible again and we're advising against all but essential travel to, from and within Leicester. This was a tricky call: when other rules are obligatory, why should travel restrictions just be advisory? Priti and Grant were on the Zoom call, and they agreed. Policing a mandatory travel ban in just one city would be nigh-on impossible. My view was informed by what's been going on in Wales, where travel rules are obligatory and the police are manning roadblocks on county boundaries, including on the tiny lanes near my parents' home in Cheshire. It's a very poor use of their time, so travel rules will be advisory.

After the decision was rubber-stamped, I announced it in the Commons.

I asked JVT to brief Jonathan Ashworth, who I am confident will understand the imperative. Liz Kendall, another of the Leicester Labour MPs, is also onside.

By contrast, Soulsby is in complete denial. When I spoke to him myself, he literally claimed there was no problem and despite being given all the data and an explanatory briefing, he dismissed the official figures as 'rubbish'. I tried to be diplomatic, because a huge public bust-up is not helpful, but it looks as if he's just playing politics.

Feeling grateful for everyone who is backing me up right now, I messaged JVT to tell him what a legend he is. I trust him completely and he always gives me such clear advice. His grandfather, Nguyễn Văn Tâm, was a notoriously tough Prime Minister of Vietnam in the French colonial days. After he fell from power, his son, JVT's dad, escaped to England and settled in Boston, Lincolnshire, as a good place to lie low. He met an English girl and started a family. When my Auntie Sandra first saw JVT on TV, she asked me if he was from Lincolnshire, as that's where she's from and she recognised the accent.

TUESDAY 30 JUNE

While Ashworth has been super supportive over the Leicester lock-down, the Labour Party leadership is kicking off, accusing me of being too slow to respond to the outbreak and demanding I give an immediate press conference. By mid-morning I was the target of a mass political pile-on, with everyone from the BBC's Jeremy Vine to my old colleague Anna Soubry laying in. Soubry was particularly aggressive, getting all worked up after Vine encouraged punters to ring him about the local lockdown on his radio phone-in.

Once upon a time she and I used to sit next to each other in Cabinet, when she knew me as 'Matt'. Now she's in the political wilderness, having flounced off to a new political party that collapsed after about five minutes, and I'm 'hashtag Hancock'. Heigh-ho. Given how much work we've put into containing the Leicester outbreak these past two weeks, I don't feel remotely nervous about the political pressure, though dealing with the onslaught is a poor use of my time.

Meanwhile we were subjected to embarrassing levels of incompetence from Leicester Council. Deciding the perimeter of the lockdown is very difficult, so I asked them to do it, given that they know their area best. The result is a total dog's breakfast. I'd made it clear that the whole city should be covered, but parts of the urban area are technically in Leicestershire, so the definition of the city boundary is ambiguous. It was all too much for local officials, whose response was to send over an image of the city with a fat red line round it which looks as if it has been drawn by a child. To make matters worse they added a grey area, which is quite literally that. I looked at it and had no idea what was in or out. Considering what a massive impact this is going to have on people's lives, this kind of confusion isn't an option. It needs to go right down to street level, with a definitive list of which houses are and aren't affected.

There are multiple other complications, including an issue with textile factories. Karamjit Singh, the chair of University Hospitals of Leicester, told Dido that young men working in illegal factories are scared of mobile testing units because they are manned by the military, so we need to get civilians to lead on testing in those places. He's going to connect us with the right local leaders. Priti is going to take away the issue of enforcing regulation of the Leicester garment industry. It's an extremely important issue, but sadly not one we can tackle today. I'll be sure to raise it with the boss once this is all over – we can't let this sort of thing continue in plain sight. It's a clear example of modern-day slavery.

JULY 2020

WEDNESDAY 1 JULY

Helen Whately sent me an alarming message about possible neglect in care homes after regular inspections were suspended during the first three months of the pandemic. Apparently the independent regulator, the CQC, has raised various concerns with local authorities. Initially, they seem to have kept her out of the loop, though she says they have 'at last' shared what they know. She says there is a 'material risk' now they are restarting inspections that they will uncover cases of neglect.

'The processes put in place in March were meant to prevent that, but Kate Terroni [chief inspector of adult social care at the CQC] is not confident,' she told me.

This is very worrying indeed. Helen has asked the CQC to keep us updated. She sounds upset and anxious. 'I really pushed CQC to have a system in place that would pick up and stop neglect/poor care. It's frustrating that Kate could not assure me on this in my meeting with her today,' she added.

'Better to know and better to get it sorted,' I replied. I asked the team to ensure we get on top of this.

Boris was nervous about getting beaten up at PMQs over Leicester and asked me to help him prep in No. 10. I was very happy to oblige as we have nothing to hide. Afterwards, we headed over to the Commons together, and I sat next to him on the front bench in case he needed any prompts, but in the event Starmer was very lame. I had been worried that he would wallop us over the recall of a batch of masks that went out to care homes and turned out to be seven years past their expiry date, but he didn't even mention it.

PHE can't identify any specific source for the Leicester outbreak, despite much speculation in the media about the role of some of the fast fashion factories that supply the likes of Boohoo, but there's disturbing evidence that some of these businesses appear persistently to flout lockdown rules. I talked to Priti again about what to do with these places. Dido thinks we need to take action against illegal sweatshops, and she's right, but Step 1 is to stop them infecting everybody. I confided in her that I don't think PHE is up to dealing with the local response. Happily, she's already on it and is bringing in one of Ben Wallace's military men. Meantime I need to watch her back. Rumours have reached me that some inside No. 10 have her card marked. Any slip-up will be used as an excuse to get rid of her.

Trump has announced what he's calling 'an amazing deal' to snaffle almost the entire global supply of the Covid treatment remdesivir for the next three months. Amazing for Americans, maybe, but what about the rest of the world? Nadhim Zahawi's been on Sky News trying to react in a way that doesn't cause a diplomatic spat. I checked in with Steve Oldfield, who reassured me that we've got solid contracts for UK supply, but it shows what we're up against.

In the past two days alone, 12,000 people have lost their jobs in retail and aviation. Everything we are doing is about buying time.

THURSDAY 2 JULY

Jim has had a very positive conversation with Sir John Bell, who says progress on the vaccine is faster and more encouraging than he expected. 'He's moved his central case from mid/early next year to before Xmas,' Jim reported. Great!

Less great is progress on the forty hospitals, which is glacial. I have pushed and pushed and pushed on this, and the Treasury just won't engage. I'm up against constant low-level resistance and muttering that HMT never signed up to the pledge in the first place etc. etc. Boris staked his reputation on delivering the hospitals, and my department has slaved over the policy for months, but I'm banging my head against a brick wall. I told Simon Case what had been going on and he sounded almost as exasperated as I am.

'Oh FFS,' he said, promising to do what he can to help break through the roadblock.

FRIDAY 3 JULY

Leaning into his role as my long-range radar system, Jim is worrying about anti-vaxxers. These fringe groups are already spreading misinformation and could seriously undermine public confidence. He shared worrying research suggesting that as many as half of Americans and a fifth of people living in the UK will decline the jab. A load of nutters are putting it about that it is part of some great global conspiracy, and we need to limit their influence.

We've pulled together a team from the Cabinet Office that was involved in tackling Daesh propaganda during the existence of the Caliphate. The online campaign they led was based on providing an overwhelming counter-narrative. Instead of focusing on responding directly to false claims, the main effort is to provide clear, objective positive material. The way it works is a bit like an election campaign. For the purposes of the jab, they'll divide everyone into five groups: enthusiastic adopters (a small proportion); early adopters; the mass ranks; the hesitant; and finally the anti-vaxxers. There's no point getting in a tangle trying to win over hardcore anti-vaxxers – it only gives them the oxygen of publicity, so they're best ignored. What we want to do is harness the enthusiasts, reassure the mass ranks and stop the anti-vaxxers persuading the hesitants not to have the jab.

It's clear we're going to have to rope in social media companies. Here we have a major asset in the shape of Nick Clegg – David Cameron's Deputy PM in the 2010 coalition government and now effectively number two at Facebook. I still have his number and messaged him right away, flagging up the potential problem with Facebook being used as a platform for spreading medical misinformation. He sounded concerned and said he was happy to help, so we've scheduled a more detailed discussion. Not so long ago Clegg was mooching around in the political wilderness after leading his party to electoral oblivion. Now he's Zuckerberg's right-hand man, earning millions, and more powerful than he ever was as leader of the Lib Dems. Evidently the world is full of possibilities.

The rest of the day was about rolling the pitch for tomorrow's big easing of restrictions. At this evening's press conference, Boris called it 'the biggest step yet on the road to recovery'. As part of our plans for the summer, Shapps announced a list of seventy-three countries and territories where people can travel without having to quarantine for two weeks on return. Safe places include Spain, France, Italy and Germany, but not the US or Portugal. The Portuguese are indignant, but we can't let diplomatic pressure skew clinical judgement.

SATURDAY 4 JULY

People have been calling today 'Super Saturday', an expression that makes me wince. I'm terrified of all the hard work and sacrifice going to waste. I just pray people are sensible and don't blow it. I marked my own liberation with a trip to my hairdresser, an experience I have been eagerly anticipating.

To my surprise, he was nervous, not only because he wasn't sure whether we should both be wearing masks and aprons (we did) but because he hadn't wielded his scissors for over three months – the longest break of his career. Roger is the only person who's ever been able to tame my thatch and has proper political pedigree, having cut Harold Wilson's hair back in the 1970s. Sitting there while he snipped away felt ridiculously good, as did meeting up with my brother afterwards. We had a beer in Notting Hill, and it was glorious.

SUNDAY 5 JULY

Andy Burnham, former Labour Health Secretary turned Mayor of

Manchester, is whinging about not being given enough data on cases in his area. On ITV today he performed his usual oh-so-reasonable routine, acting as if he's all cross-party-collegiate and thinks of nothing but the greater good, when in truth he's all about Andy Burnham, wannabe Labour leader. I see right through it and it really pisses me off, especially as I'm assured his complaint about lack of facts and figures is rubbish.

Challenged about it on *Marr* this morning, I adopted an air of weary patience and graciously offered to provide Andy with more help in understanding the figures that are readily available. If he's struggling to interpret the data, I said, we'd be more than happy to give him some additional support. I'm sure my tone was incredibly patronising, but he deserved it: he knows exactly what he's doing.

To top off an already annoying day, someone has been briefing against me and the department to *The Spectator*. In an article speculating about who will succeed Sir Mark Sedwill as Cabinet Secretary, the magazine's well-informed political editor James Forsyth says it won't be my brilliant Permanent Secretary Chris Wormald, because No. 10 thinks the 'institutional response' of the Department of Health to the pandemic has been 'deeply flawed'. What?! Wormald is the best Perm Sec I've ever had, and he's working incredibly hard. Though he's both professional and thick skinned, I don't need him getting demotivated. Friends in No. 10 say the piece is the result of 'extremely cock-eyed briefing' by Cummings & co. and that it has annoyed a lot of people. I messaged Boris asking him to tell whoever is briefing this stuff to Forsyth and others to cease and desist. The PM replied that he hadn't read it.

'I love Wormald,' he added.

Why oh why does No. 10 create this awful, destructive atmosphere when the rest of us are working every hour to save lives? It's horrific.

MONDAY 6 JULY

JVT and I have finally persuaded the Treasury to go full throttle on the full 100 million vaccine orders. As well as the argument about how many Oxford doses to pre-order, there's also the question of how many international companies to back. The Vaccine Taskforce has argued that we only need to back three brands. My view is we need to hedge our bets. Any one of the vaccines could fail in clinical trials. What if we back the wrong horse? Fortunately, Rishi and Steve Barclay at the Treasury are totally onside. When the cost of lockdown is approximately £4 billion a day, anything that gets us out of restrictions sooner rather than later is a complete no-brainer – or, as Steve put it, the cheapest insurance policy in the world. If several of our contenders come good and we end up with far too many doses, I doubt they'll go to waste. We can sell them on or donate them to developing countries. 'I know which problem I'd rather have!' I told JVT.

A setback with the Oxford vaccine today underlined the wisdom of covering all bases. JVT texted to say clinical trials are being paused because someone has symptoms that could suggest an adverse reaction. An investigation is under way. JVT assured me that these things happen all the time with trials, but it could turn out to be something serious, derailing the whole Oxford vaccine programme. A very, very tense moment that left me feeling physically shaky. So much is at stake.

Perhaps unsettled by the news, the PM wasn't on top form on a visit to Yorkshire. He was supposed to be bigging up our plans to reform social care funding, but for reasons best known to himself he launched into a totally unscripted attack on the way the sector has responded to the pandemic. Naturally the providers have gone crazy, and he's now being accused of trying to shift the blame for the government's failures, insulting hard-working carers etc. etc. We spent half the day trying to 'clarify' his remarks, but unfortunately there was no mistaking what he'd said.

More positively, I've been drafting a letter to everyone who's been shielding, to say that it is finally safe to come out. Given how much people have sacrificed, and how frightened many still are, these communications demand real sensitivity. I hope I get it right.

Dido's been on a fact-finding mission to Leicester, where she reports that 'even the chicken shops' on Evington Road are closed. Apparently the place is a ghost town. Her main worry is that some communities still aren't getting enough information. She thinks we need more ethnic language videos and posters and fewer military uniforms at testing centres to make them more welcoming. It's funny: I think of the military uniforms as reassuring, but for many they are an intimidating presence.

TUESDAY 7 JULY

Labour MPs are frothing at the mouth over the PM's 'clumsy and cowardly' words yesterday, so I went out to bat for him, stressing that care homes had done 'amazing work' during the crisis. I tried to get him out of it on the basis that care homes could not have known what procedures to follow before asymptomatic transmission was known to be a thing. The *Telegraph* described my performance as 'a dazzling masterclass of spin', which I took as a compliment. I forwarded the article to Jack Doyle at No. 10 accompanied by the message 'Objective achieved.' I may have sounded a bit self-satisfied, but since I've gone out of my way to get the boss out of trouble, I want them to know they owe me one.

There are reports of pubs in Yorkshire, Hampshire and Somerset closing after customers tested positive and landlords were alerted. They're getting staff tested before they reopen. 'The system works!' I said excitedly. Even accounting for all our efforts, it was never a given.

Friends have been getting in touch saying how relieved they are that shielding is over. Some people were even hiding away from their own families in their own homes. What a relief it must be.

Yesterday there were only 352 new cases, the lowest since lockdown began. Fantastic progress. Let's hope it holds.

WEDNESDAY 8 JULY

Rishi's announced a new 'Eat Out to Help Out' initiative, so diners will be able to get a tenner off meals and non-alcoholic drinks on Mondays, Tuesdays and Wednesdays in August. I did my best to sound supportive and refrained from expressing disapproval at his photo op, which saw him serving food to customers at a branch of Wagamama near the Royal Festival Hall on the Southbank, but in truth I'm worried that it might backfire and lead to a spike in cases. I am torn: I get on really well with Rishi and think he has done a brilliant job supporting people through the crisis, but I'm not at all sure about this scheme.

It's part of a much wider £30 billion package of economic measures designed to stave off mass unemployment, including a £1,000 bounty for businesses for every employee they keep on and cuts to VAT on food, accommodation and attractions for the hospitality sector to 5 per cent until January. I told Rishi truthfully that I was 'really thrilled' about a part of the package relating to traineeships. The first policy I ever took from idea to reality was on this subject, back when I was Skills Minister. When we launched the programme, the headline was about how the new scheme would help people 'get to work on time'. Then I overslept and missed the morning TV slot to talk about my pride and joy. Total humiliation. 'I've never overslept since,' I told Rishi.

THURSDAY 9 JULY

A mad scramble to sort out the 'safe travel corridor' scheme. When the FCO is involved, there's usually some farce, and so it was that a ridiculous situation arose whereby one part of the government was saying that people will be able to travel to Serbia without having to quarantine on return to the UK, while another part of government was saying the exact opposite. While we were all scrabbling around trying to coordinate, with Grant Shapps becoming increasingly irate at this latest demonstration of Whitehall incompetence, we discovered that two flights were due to take off for Serbia before 9 a.m. tomorrow, giving us a matter of hours to get our act together.

Earlier I'd found myself with a rare bit of breathing space and sat down to do some big-picture thinking. I want to give a speech about the future of the NHS, but Cummings hates the idea, basically because he wants to 'own' any new thinking. I also want to talk about the importance of reducing red tape – something the pandemic has really hammered home – but he's blocking that too. I messaged him asking what his problem is and he denied all knowledge. Typical.

This evening I returned to my constituency for the first time since March. For the best part of six months, Elizabeth Hitchcock, who normally runs my parliamentary office, has essentially been MP for West Suffolk in all but name. She's kept the show on the road, handling an avalanche of correspondence and spotting when my work as Health Secretary links up with what happens on the ground in West Suffolk. She's a bright, super-charming American and everyone in Suffolk loves her. She can be direct and is not remotely afraid to challenge me, frequently taking the time on her journeys to and from Suffolk to tell me she's not really sure lockdowns are a great idea. Sometimes I think my constituents would prefer her to me.

I was glad to get away from dealing with Sir Peter Soulsby, who is like a stone in my shoe. He keeps complaining that we don't give him enough data about case numbers in Leicester. He's now issued an 'open letter' repeating his claims. Nadine is even angrier than I am. 'Odious' is how she describes him, saying that while I have to be civil, everyone else should be 'taking him down'. She suspects Starmer's office is pulling his strings. 'We need to be a bit more ruthless' is her view.

Is this what he was given his knighthood for? His continual attacks are particularly uncalled-for as case numbers are finally improving in Leicester, proving that what we're doing is right. Unfortunately, other hotspots are starting to crop up, mainly in the north of England and the Midlands, and particularly in deprived, densely populated areas with high populations of Asian descent. The ethnic dimension requires great sensitivity and is going to need pitch-perfect comms.

Despite all my fears, the numbers are still going in the right direction, with cases down a quarter on last week. The next stage of reopening is competitive grassroots sport, starting with cricket from this Saturday. On Monday, it'll be spas and tanning salons. Indoor sports like gyms, swimming pools and climbing walls will follow on 25 July, and there will be some careful pilots for theatres and concert halls with socially distanced audiences.

FRIDAY 10 JULY

We've formally decided we're definitely not joining the EU vaccination scheme. As I always feared, they were adamant that we would have to hand over all the contracts we've already signed and, what's more, we would have no say over how the doses we've bought are distributed. I was worried that the machine would try to resist this decision too, but in fact it was easy and everyone agreed. Once we announced it, though, the usual suspects went bananas, trying to paint me as some kind of mad, ideologically driven Brexiteer, which is something of a stretch, given how I voted. Actually, it's very simple: we're way ahead of the rest of the EU countries on vaccine procurement. If we clamber on board the Brussels bandwagon, we'll be forced to mosey along a scenic route, with frequent stops in laybys, when we're currently in the fast lane of the motorway.

In the constituency, I dropped into the market in Mildenhall and visited Newmarket Community Hospital to open the new GP surgery which has been added to one wing of the building. The hospital tripled its bed numbers during coronavirus – a complete turnaround on the threats to close it when I became the MP in 2010. I finished off with a beer on Haverhill High Street. It was oh-so-sweet a day. I've been away so long, going home to Suffolk felt like an adventure.

The PM was out and about in a mask today, an uncomfortable look that was only slightly improved by a very evident recent trip to the barber, but it did set an example. In Scotland, face coverings are now mandatory in shops and on public transport. We'll go the same way, but Sturgeon was desperate to get in there first.

The Sunday papers have been told that I'm unhappy about Rishi's Eat Out to Help Out scheme. They think I'm worried about the impact on the anti-obesity strategy. I hadn't even thought of that angle, which allowed me to issue a completely truthful denial. I've no desire to fall out with Rishi. We may not agree on everything, but I admire how he's risen to the challenge.

SATURDAY 11 JULY

Catherine West, Labour's shadow Europe Minister, has called our EU vaccine decision 'dumber and dumber'. Pure ideology. Time will tell who is dumber on that front. Meanwhile the Belgians have put Leicester on their red list. I hoped that this might encourage Soulsby to turn his fire on Brussels, but no such luck.

MONDAY 13 JULY

I'm getting really stressed about the NHS winter budget. Several vital funding issues have been repeatedly kicked into the long grass.

I sent Simon Case a memo warning that these decisions cannot continually be deferred.

I've got to the point where I don't care if I sound desperate, because the situation is now dire. Rattling off a list of urgent issues, I said, 'We need to sign off the Nightingales by Friday or we lose them. We need to sign off on the independent sector contracts this week or else we lose the capacity to roll over again – at much worse cost to the Exchequer. We have already lost a month on this at great cost due to HMT foot dragging.'

Continuing my rant, I told him we absolutely have to sign off extra money for social care or people who should be getting care at home will be taking up hospital beds over the winter. We also need to sign off the flu vaccination programme and tell the NHS system its financial plans for the rest of the year, because right now they have no financial arrangements beyond the end of this month. This is all before we discuss actual capacity for this winter and, of course, funding the forty hospitals.

I literally can't believe we are still in this position, having been debating it for two months now. I distracted myself over the weekend by building a zip wire for the kids in the garden, but it absolutely cannot wait. When I raised my concerns, I was told that the PM wants to announce all this on Friday and that the issue will have to be resolved before then. Simon Case suggested I write him a simple note setting out where Rishi and I have agreed and where we differ. He also wanted to double check that I'm still in favour of mandating masks, telling me that when it was discussed in No. 10 yesterday the PM 'leant into it', whereas Gove was trying to row back. He thinks Boris will want to go firm on the policy tomorrow. I told him I'm in favour.

'I have no idea why Gove was so remiss,' I said.

Helen has received a very unsatisfactory update from PHE on the latest Covid outbreaks in care homes. Some cases were not previously reported; some have emerged as a result of blanket testing; and some are suspected but not confirmed. 'I find their report frustratingly vague and dismissive about new outbreaks. I have asked for a proper breakdown on how many fit into each of the new categories, going down to named individual care homes,' she said.

She told me she wants to adopt a 'zero tolerance' approach to the virus in these settings. 'Every single outbreak should be treated as a problem requiring immediate action and investigation,' she said.

'Totally agree. We should have zero tolerance for both Covid and crap data,' I replied.

PHE is simply exasperating. Four days before the latest lockdown, they told me that Leicester was 'progressing well' – the exact opposite of what the city was doing.

'It was only because I blew up at that imprecision that they acted,' I told Helen.

As an aside, my appearances in official Zoom meetings today were not impressive. Clearly my son had been fiddling around with my laptop, and instead of appearing as the Secretary of State for Health and Social Care, I kept popping up under his name. I couldn't figure out how to change the settings and was stuck with it until I was able to summon him. It has got to the stage when my twelve-year-old son is better at these things than I am – and I was the Digital Secretary! Humbling.

TUESDAY 14 JULY
Gove is behaving very strangely regarding masks. This morning he and Liz Truss were photographed coming out of the same branch

of Pret A Manger in Westminster, just eight minutes apart. She was wearing a mask; he wasn't. Cue a very unhelpful front-page story in the *Standard*. I was up in the Commons two hours later and knew I'd have to field hostile questions.

The scientific advice is still pretty mixed, but I told Parliament that we have decided to make masks compulsory in shops from next Friday, as they may have some preventative effects. Masks also give some people more confidence to get out and about. Ashworth was uncharacteristically petulant, and I can't say I blame him. We've given the opposition an open goal on this one.

Alastair Campbell, who's presenting *Good Morning Britain* this week, is trying to suggest that my ministerial team is ducking the media. This morning he was mouthing off about Nadine, asking when was the last time anyone heard or saw her talking about mental health. She is already extremely sensitive about not being on TV/radio as often as she would like and it clearly touched a nerve. She thinks No. 10 prefers to wheel out younger ministers who went to Oxford University and made it clear she wants to do more. I told her we'll keep pushing.

The best moment of the day was a message from JVT saying the MHRA have told the Oxford team their trial is safe and can be restarted. 'Thank Christ for that,' I replied.

I am beyond frustrated about the situation with NHS finances/winter planning, so this evening I called the boss direct. He didn't pick up, so I sent him a blunt message.

'We've gone fast on releasing lockdown. New cases entering Test and Trace starting to rise. And I'm getting no traction on doing what's needed to protect the NHS this winter,' I said. 'We can either take a risk on releasing lockdown OR we can take a risk on not building up the NHS this winter. We can't do both. The second option – 10,000 extra beds – is far cheaper. But if we decide against that then I can't see how we can take any more steps out of lockdown.'

No reply so far.

WEDNESDAY 15 JULY

Boris messaged at 6.42 a.m., concerned about my reference to case numbers ticking up. It was sabre rattling because the figures are still very low, but it got his attention. I asked him when we could have a proper discussion about making sure the NHS can cope this winter and he replied that he was 'v keen to talk', though he pointed out, somewhat grumpily, that the NHS is 'already about a third of government spending'.

'I know – all I want is to ensure we can keep saying "We protected the NHS,"' I replied evenly. This is all about risk judgement. 'If we are taking a risk on opening up, it's unwise to take a risk on NHS capacity at the same time.'

Anxious not to overplay my hand, I didn't mention the forty hospitals saga, but he's clearly going to have to get involved, because the Treasury has put the brakes on yet again. If the PM wants to honour the pledge, he is going to have to kick some backsides.

I used the morning media round to try to end the confusion over masks. The position is actually very simple: face coverings are already required on public transport and in NHS settings; now they will also be mandatory in shops, supermarkets and takeaways. I am not sure what is so hard to grasp. Gove did his bit by going back to Pret, this time very ostentatiously sporting a face covering, while Rishi also tweeted a masked-up Pret photo of himself. As far as I'm concerned, that should have been the end of the matter, but certain colleagues who are 'too busy' to master the detail keep making matters worse. I told the *Today* programme I was 'not frankly interested' in why Gove had got it wrong and set out the position once again, only for No. 10 to screw it up again at the lunchtime lobby briefing by suggesting masks in places like Pret are 'voluntary'. Cue another set of 'Hancock says one thing; Downing Street says another' headlines that make me look an idiot. It's just an unnecessary own goal. Lately No. 10 has been literally *begging* ministers to do the morning media round. Is it any wonder nobody volunteers, if they just get dumped on afterwards? As I told Simon Case, this may not seem like a mega issue, but the principle is very important, and the look is terrible. He promised to investigate and ensure that the poor sod doing the rounds tomorrow is properly briefed so we can move on to more important matters than 'PretGate'.

I was still feeling annoyed about being hung out to dry when No. 10 had the brass neck to suggest I give an oral statement in the Commons tomorrow.

'Tell them no chance', I instructed my private office. 'They've just completely fucked me over on masks!'

In no mood to mince my words, I fired off an email to No. 10 making it clear that a) the policy I set out is the policy that will be implemented, b) if I set out a policy in a morning media round in future, they need to follow it at the midday lobby, not freelance and c) because the science isn't clear on masks, to date I've not taken a strong position one way or another, but our collective approach has led to total chaos. Maybe I should have adopted a clear stance, because the vacuum has been part of the cause of the problem, but I've taken one now, and it needs to be followed across the board.

When I eventually calmed down, I relented on the Commons statement because there were other important updates for MPs, on the Leicester lockdown and an issue that has cropped up with the quality of some Randox tests.

My punchy email to Boris on winter planning seems to have paid off, resulting in a crunch meeting in No. 10 with Munira Mirza, the director of the Downing Street Policy Unit, and Simon Stevens. I emerged semi-triumphant, with money for extra A&E capacity, a commitment on measuring waiting times and an agreement to promote NHS 111 to take the pressure off hospitals. It's a start. Today we also looked at the business case for the Pfizer BioNTech vaccine, which is based on mRNA technology. It's less advanced than either the Oxford or the Moderna vaccine and wasn't one put forward at first by the VTF, but to their credit they're now moving fast. We need more data to evaluate it properly, but on the principle of backing all horses, I was insistent that we should do the deal.

THURSDAY 16 JULY

I woke up looking forward to a Pret-free day, which turned out to be a hopelessly optimistic. Last night, Simon Case and I agreed the definitive government position, only for Alok Sharma to reignite the whole thing this morning. When I heard that he was due to go on Sky, I wanted to make sure there could be no scope whatsoever for any further confusion, so I texted him the precise situation. Alok is a very fine man, but, somehow, he'd still been given the wrong line, which he said instead of what I'd texted him. He even messaged me afterwards saying that he'd stuck to the lines to take. Cue more chaos.

By this point I was so worn down I didn't have the heart to break it to him that he'd just ruined my day and prolonged PretGate for another twenty-four hours. Next time, I might as well act as a human autocue, holding up the script in big black letters behind the TV camera. In my Commons statement, I announced that most of Leicester will come out of lockdown in ten days, though some restrictions will remain in certain hotspots. Neil O'Brien, the normally level-headed Tory MP for Harborough, Oadby & Wigston, went tonto, telling Nadine we've handled it badly and that he should have been invited to take part in discussions ahead of the decision. While he went off on one that his constituents are being unfairly targeted, we had Soulsby sounding off that we're releasing all the Tory areas from lockdown while targeting Labour wards. You just can't win.

Meanwhile the debate about measurement of deaths has come back with a vengeance. Two professors, Yoon Loke and Carl Heneghan, have highlighted the fundamental flaw. Under the system we've used, if a person tested positive in April, recovered in May and died in a car crash in July, they are counted as a Covid death. While this was fine at first, now that it's four months since the first peak, we've got to fix it. Otherwise the problem will grow and grow. I have ordered an urgent review with no blame attached.

Better news on my NHS funding efforts. The PM is about to announce an extra £3 billion to get us through the winter. Not a moment too soon.

In my box tonight was one particularly startling note relating to the way Covid has been getting into care homes. The main takeaway is that the virus is primarily being brought in by staff, not by elderly people who've been discharged from hospital. This explains a lot, including why the rise in care home deaths came so much later than would have been the case if hospital discharges were the primary cause. The policy consequence is clear too: we must ban staff movement between care homes, fast.

FRIDAY 17 JULY

True to his word, Nick Clegg made time to talk to me about how Facebook can help tackle anti-vax misinformation. When he popped up on Zoom, I was genuinely alarmed by his appearance: sitting in front of a bright yellow screen he looked dirty and dishevelled and bore the air of a man who had not slept for days. His face was covered in stubble and his flowing locks were all greasy. I know the pandemic has been stressful and we've all aged, but this was next level. He was such a mess that pretending nothing was wrong wasn't an option, so I just came right out with it.

'What the hell's happened to you?' I asked. Surely life in California isn't that bad?

'I'm in my tent in Yellowstone National Park,' he replied breezily. 'I've been out of communication and haven't washed for three days, but you said you wanted to speak to me, so here I am.'

I was pretty impressed that he'd interrupted a family trek through the wilderness – that in itself showing commitment to the cause. He was right on it and very helpful, saying Facebook will do what they can to direct searches about vaccine safety to credible sources of information – and that they were keen to have access to the objective truth from the NHS to promote globally. Soft power in action.

Re. the possible cock-up over the way we've been counting deaths, it turns out that if like Scotland and Northern Ireland we only counted deaths within twenty-eight days of a positive test, our death toll would be measured at around 4,000 lower. I am going to have to work out how to handle this. My instinct is full transparency – especially as the truth is better news than what we've been saying so far. Why not align our approach across the UK? Normally getting Scotland on board for any change is extremely painful, because the SNP want to be different just for the sake of it, but if we align our measurement with theirs, how can they complain?

In his first No. 10 press conference for a fortnight, the PM announced the extra £3 billion for the NHS to prepare for a possible winter wave and testing capacity to rise to at least 500,000 a day by the end of October. Playing hostage to fortune, he also said we are aiming for a 'more significant return to normality from November, possibly in time for Christmas'. The Prof and I tried very hard to persuade him not to say anything of the sort, because it will probably come back to haunt us, but he was not in listening mode.

The brilliant Captain Tom Moore has been knighted by the Queen at Windsor Castle, standing on the grass with his walking frame. Her Majesty did the honours in her first official engagement in person since lockdown. I cannot think of a more deserving case. He's raised £33 million for NHS charities, a magnificent achievement, and is a symbol of stoicism.

Israel is the latest place to reimpose some lockdown measures because of a spike in cases. They fear they're heading for a full-blown second wave. They've been criticised for being too gung-ho with opening up – a warning to the rest of us.

SATURDAY 18 JULY

The PM called about the vaccine rollout. He was at his most bullish and scrawled 'Project Speed' next to the timing options on a note on where we're up to. He's adamant that the programme needs to be UK-wide, with no silly differentiation policies from the devolveds.

Councils have started taking advantage of new powers to introduce local restrictions if cases are rising in the area. This is how we want the system to work going forward. Rochdale has put extra social distancing rules in place and Blackburn and Pendle are doing something similar.

JVT told me today that a group of Boston Utd fans are petitioning to have a stand at their new ground called the JVT Stand. Both of our forebears were season ticket holders, and now he is something of a local celebrity. 'Where do I sign?' I replied.

SUNDAY 19 JULY

I've been discussing the US with Jens Spahn. The situation there is shocking, with new cases climbing over 60,000 a day. Meanwhile the White House is exerting massive pressure on industry to hoard medication and testing kits to reduce the scope for negative publicity about Trump in the run-up to the election. They're once again threatening to invoke the Defense Production Act to keep stuff in the country. This is precisely why I've been so determined to have exclusivity clauses in our contracts with vaccine companies – not to spite the EU, or any other country for that matter, but to safeguard the UK from such protectionism.

As if to make the point, just after I heard this news I finally received formal sign-off from the Prime Minister to spend £469 million to buy the full 100 million doses of the Oxford AstraZeneca – and to pay for 80 million of them to be bottled in Wrexham. Hooray! What a battle it's been getting all the terms right – exclusivity, onshore manufacture and enough doses for the whole UK adult population – but it's finally formally signed off. Then, even better, JVT called to tell me the first results of the Oxford vaccine human trials should be public tomorrow. It's safe and triggers the immune response we need. They're fact-checking the exact figures overnight, so I'll have to wait until tomorrow to get the actual numbers.

MONDAY 20 JULY

Today was undoubtedly the best day since this whole awful thing started. The vaccine programme is on a roll!

The Oxford results were published first thing by *The Lancet* – one of the world's most respected medical journals – having been through the normally months-long publication schedule in just forty-eight hours. They show not only that the vaccine is safe but that it stimulates antibody and T-cell response. It's a major breakthrough, meaning we can now trial it in large numbers of people to see how strong the protection is in practice. In short: we know it triggers the right biological response, but to be effective, that biological response has to stop you getting Covid in practice – and we need to know there are no major side effects when it's injected into many thousands of people.

Finally we are starting to win this race. We might even have a vaccine by Christmas.

On top of this great news, the VTF have worked wonders with Pfizer and landed a binding agreement for 90 million early doses of the BioNTech vaccine they're developing, plus an agreement in principle for 60 million from the French company Valneva. This last deal is particularly good, as we're funding its expansion in Livingston and contributing to its clinical trials here in the UK.

I've been urging people to sign up to the NHS vaccine research registry as potential volunteers for these trials. It's usually a real slog to find people to take part in this kind of research, but the response so far has been overwhelming. People really want to do their bit.

So, in the space of a few days we've gone from angst over the EU scheme and battles over how much to buy to securing 250 million doses of three different vaccines and discovering that our home-grown one probably works.

It's not just the size of the portfolio but the diversity in the science that's maximising our chances of success. Oxford's uses adenoviral technology – which basically means you inject a chimp virus that doesn't affect humans to get the vaccine into the body. Pfizer BioNTech and Imperial use mRNA and Valneva uses an inactivated whole virus.

At lunchtime we all trooped over to No. 10 to go through it with the boss. He'd already heard the news and walked into the Cabinet Room fists aloft. His team were oddly subdued: they kept saying that we can't be sure, explaining that we might never get a vaccine, and nothing is certain etc. etc. Sure – but this really is a huge step forward.

To cap it all off, there was a note in my box this evening saying we've got agreement in principle with AZ for 1 million doses of a treatment containing Covid-neutralising antibodies for those who can't have vaccines, mainly cancer patients or others with compromised immune systems. I punched the air – and, for once, let myself enjoy the moment.

What a day!

TUESDAY 21 JULY

We're finally easing restrictions in care homes.

These restrictions have been some of the hardest for people to bear. Throughout lockdown the sight of very old people stoically waving at their relatives through windows has affected me more than almost any other part of lockdown. The stereotypes are usually of younger relatives visiting parents and grandparents, but the ones I feel for most are separated husbands and wives, especially those close to the end. I've felt the duty to protect them very keenly, so I've been very cautious about lifting restrictions until the clinical advice is clear.

We've been working on it for a couple of weeks, and residents will now be able to nominate two 'constant visitors' who will be able to call in one at a time. It's not a legal requirement as such, just a strong recommendation, which gives managers scope for discretion according to local circumstances. I'm worried that not every care home will make it happen – but we've got to move carefully, as we're caught between the desperate sadness of the separation and the huge vulnerability of frail, old people to the disease. If we have to, I'm up for making allowing visitors a legal requirement, but better to try to make it work with sensitivity to what's going on locally in the first instance.

Managing what's happening in care homes is one of the hardest parts of the job. We don't have clear policy levers, because social care is formally the responsibility of local councils, but we get all the scrutiny.

The balance of policy is very difficult and the people in care are so vulnerable. The sector generally does a wonderful job, but it's not easy.

WEDNESDAY 22 JULY

Sir John Bell has discovered that the White House is plotting to give the Moderna vaccine FDA approval before full clinical trials are complete, in an effort to boost Trump's flagging re-election campaign. The scientists who know about it are all horrified. By all means accelerate other aspects of regulatory approval for inoculations, but compromising safety is madness. Any short-term political gain would come at huge societal and public health cost, undermining public confidence in vaccines generally. I understand Trump's impatience – I feel exactly the same – but we would never go there.

Conveying Sir John's concerns, Jim also told me that the White House has called in Roche and demanded the company's entire global supply of PCR tests, many of which are made in New Jersey. We may need to get the Foreign Office involved. I imagine Europe would want to retaliate too. Ominous.

This evening Cummings shared a Bloomberg piece describing the British response to the pandemic as 'world-class'. It highlights our work on dexamethasone and the Oxford and Imperial vaccine trials. Nice to get some recognition, rather than the usual agenda-driven, click-bait bashing.

THURSDAY 23 JULY

SAGE has confirmed a case of a cat with Covid. It's the first known case of an animal being infected with this particular strain of coronavirus in the UK. I immediately had a flashback to the beginning of the year, when there were real fears over the possibility that the virus might be spread by pets. We are waiting for more info from the chief vet, but I'm told the cat caught it from its owners, who are also unwell, rather than the other way round, so thankfully still no need for a cat cull.

The mask mandate comes into force tomorrow. Tongue in cheek, I suggested to the team a symbolic trip to Pret. My SpAds didn't find this funny. They suggested I should go to Greggs instead, but Emma thought that would look too try-hard. Jamie suggested a quick trip to the House of Fraser store a few minutes' walk from Parliament, but then someone reminded him that chief executive Mike Ashley tried to keep his Sports Direct stores open when other non-essential shops were closed, so that was the end of that. In the end Natasha went out to buy me a sandwich.

My brilliant SpAd Ed Taylor is leaving the department. His contribution has been phenomenal, helping with media and leading on all things data. As a small token of our collective appreciation for his work, we got him a face mask with the data dashboard on. Surely he will treasure it.

FRIDAY 24 JULY

Tony Blair messaged asking why the UAE is still on the quarantine list (he does a lot of business over there). I told him I'd questioned it too but the expert advice is very clear. 'Spain isn't looking too pretty either,' I told him gloomily.

Blair protested that the reason the UAE is still reporting over 200 cases a day is 'because they do so much testing'. I resisted the urge to ping back an eye-roll emoji at that old chestnut as he went on to argue that the disease is well under control there. He says virtually all the cases are in the migrant worker community and are asymptomatic. Hmm.

It's Boris's first anniversary as Prime Minister. I can't believe it's only been a year.

I tweeted my congratulations this morning, saying that since the boss came into office 'we've delivered Brexit, defeated Corbyn & protected the NHS in the face of this unprecedented coronavirus'. In honour of the occasion, the PM subjected himself to a grilling on the BBC, during which he acknowledged that in retrospect we could have locked down earlier. This is a question I've spent lot of time considering, as I'm frequently hit with the accusation that we were 'too slow'. That suggestion fails to recognise how little we knew. I was of course in favour of a lockdown, but we had to balance the huge cost of such a move against its necessity – based on scant information. No doubt people will be debating it for years to come.

More prosaically for the future, the latest ONS figures were published this afternoon, showing that the decline in cases in England is now levelling off. I got the first cut of the data on Wednesday morning and it was then polished over Wednesday and Thursday before publication today. I've been worrying about it ever since I saw it.

A packaging factory in West Bromwich has shut after forty-nine out of 117 workers tested positive. Straws in the wind? I look at Spain, where there have been 1,000 new cases, the highest figure since early May, and at what's going on in France and Germany, and I am nervous.

We're in a very odd phase, where the vaccines are going far better than expected but I am certain that a second wave is building.

SATURDAY 25 JULY

I called the PM first thing about the situation in Spain and he gave the go-ahead to remove it from the corridors list. It means anyone coming back from Spain from midnight tonight will have to self-quarantine for fourteen days. This is very bad news for a lot of British holidaymakers, so no surprise that both the Foreign Office and the Department for Transport had strong views. Cue a lot of frustrating to-ing and fro-ing as we debated the precise timing and whether Gibraltar and the Canary Islands should be included. DfT officials kept pushing for twenty-four hours' notice for the Spain decision, which I thought was curious – Grant is normally an 'action this day' minister – until I discovered that Grant and his family had just flown there on holiday. They were trying, perhaps too hard, to protect their minister. When I called Grant himself, he was typically phlegmatic and saw the funny side.

'It's good – it shows the rules apply to everyone,' I told the team.

'Including Members of the House of Lords who were rather hoping to go to Mallorca and instead are summering in the Wiltshire Riviera,' Jim replied ruefully. Well, yes.

The other reason to crack on with these travel restrictions is Sturgeon. Her political games are incredibly debilitating and significantly limit scope for open discussion in COBRA. She sits like a statue, lips pursed like the top of a drawstring bag, only jolting into life when there's an opportunity to say something to further the separatist cause. The minute someone presses 'End Meeting' you can almost hear her running for a lectern so she can rush out an announcement before we make ours. We now chew over big decisions elsewhere and relegate formal meetings to rubber-stamping exercises. Otherwise, we might as well invite *The Herald* and *The National* along too.

Boris asked me what we should be doing. I said we need to shift the emphasis towards more caution and delay the planned opening up of beauty salons and other 'close contact' businesses on 1 August. Even though numbers are still low, once they start rising there's only one thing that can happen.

MONDAY 27 JULY

Downing Street is in a semi-panic about a second wave.

'Folks, looking at Spain and France and remembering March, it is completely obvious we are about to be hit by a second wave. We have to get out there in front of it and explain what we are doing to prevent it,' Boris declared to me and the Prof this evening.

I told him that we're all over it and are organising a big package for this week.

'Much stronger comms, tightening the isolation rules and providing support for those isolating,' I said briskly. I am under no illusion about what's at stake, which is why I've been so tough on the Spanish quarantine policy. I told Simon Case that dealing with the FCO on this has been a complete nightmare and the process needs to be seamless next time. We can't have the FCO pulling in one direction and the rest of government in another, especially if it results in contradictory travel advice.

TUESDAY 28 JULY

Sturgeon is on manoeuvres again, trying to persuade us all to sign up to her impossible and anti-scientific zero-Covid plan. Sure, we'd all love zero Covid, but that's about as realistic as a bagpipe-playing unicorn. As always, this is all about her: she knows we won't sign up to zero Covid because all credible scientists say it won't work. She can't be in any doubt about this, because she gets the same scientific advice we do. This isn't a game and she shouldn't view it as one. She just wants to look and sound tough, then blame us when her policies don't work. It is all so cynical that I can hardly bear to watch her on TV any more.

WEDNESDAY 29 JULY

'Achtung achtung,' Boris boomed over my WhatsApp. It was just after 9 p.m., but he was unusually worked up, lashing out at what he sees as 'total complacency' on the part of the public about the spike in cases. Today's first cut of ONS data, unveiled to us this morning in the Cabinet Room, shows that Friday's publication will reveal cases have soared from 2,800 last week to 4,200 this week. The boss has obviously been chewing it over all day and now he's on the warpath, sending a blizzard of garbled messages to me, Case, the Prof and Vallance this evening instructing us to get 'absolutely militant'.

'If correct the R above 1. Or at least that is what I assume. We need a really strong message tomo and some tightening.' Simon agreed, saying the figures in parts of the capital were particularly worrying.

'I'm not remotely surprised about London,' the PM replied. He said it tallied with his own observation of the streets in outer London boroughs and blames 'the general collapse' in social distancing at home and in social settings.

'We need to tell people that if they want to save the economy and protect the NHS then they need to follow the rules. And we may need to tighten the rules. You can now have six people from different households indoors. Do people really understand that and are they observing it?' he demanded.

Case and I did our best to calm him down, assuring him that we have a plan. When people see the figures on Friday, they'll know we're not bullshitting.

Meanwhile long-range prep continues. We signed a deal with GSK/

Sanofi today for up to 60 million vaccines, the fourth in our portfolio. We also have a huge reserve of people willing to participate in trials. In the first week alone, an amazing 72,000 people signed up to the NHS Covid-19 vaccine research registry. Normally, finding a single volunteer for vaccine trials is a nightmare.

Ben Wallace messaged asking what more the military can do in the event of a second wave. He also wanted to know whether we're going to give people more warning before changing travel quarantine rules next time. Dodging that question, I told him I thought the armed forces have been brilliant so far, especially on logistics, though we could fine-tune the process for civilian authorities requesting military aid. When pushed on travel, I pointed out that there are downsides to giving too much warning, as people then move in droves before the ban comes into force.

'I think people have now got the message that travel during a pandemic is not a risk-free option,' I said, which he seemed to accept.

Capacity for testing is a continuing concern. We still haven't sorted procurement for what Boris calls 'Operation Moonshot'. The idea is to carry out not thousands, not hundreds of thousands, but literally *millions* of Covid tests a day to keep the economy going. Getting to the millions point will obviously take time, but we've got to get the basics in place.

After the research last week showing the best way to protect care homes is to stop staff movement, I found an extremely weak and disappointing submission in my box. Officials say we mustn't eliminate staff movement across care homes because it might lead to a shortage of carers. Yet the research shows the risk of outbreaks in care homes doubles if workers are coming and going. I'm pushing to ban staff movement fully. Now we know how to stop the virus getting into care homes, I'm not allowing it to happen again.

THURSDAY 30 JULY

Weird new advice from the behavioural scientists, who have suddenly taken against the word 'lockdown' and want everyone to start talking about 'areas of intervention' instead. Setting aside the fact that this phrase sounds somewhat medical, I just don't think it will fly.

The behavioural lot think the word 'lockdown' sounds like a punishment, and they're right, but this genius observation has come almost six months too late. In any case, how would that expression work if the whole country is an 'area of intervention', as I very much fear will sooner or later be the case?

In any case, we have started toughening up. We met in the Cabinet Room to discuss what we need to do in response to yesterday's ONS data. SAGE now advises that R is probably above 1 in much of England. If it stays at that level, we're back into exponential growth, and we all know where that leads. The PM knows action is the only way to stop this spiralling. On clinical advice we decided to increase self-isolation from seven to ten days, and from midnight tonight much of the north-west will be in lockdown. In Greater Manchester, West Yorkshire and parts of East Lancashire, socialising in other people's homes will be banned. Dealing with Labour leadership wannabe Andy Burnham proved a lot less painful than dealing with Soulsby, and I was able to square him off in advance. In fact, he went out of his way to be helpful, suggesting we announce that we're doing this in partnership, which made my life much easier.

Amid the maelstrom, at the suggestion of Tony Blair I had a Zoom with Larry Ellison, founder of the American tech giant Oracle, a business that helped make him one of the richest men in the world. He's pushing various data-driven solutions to the pandemic. Jim has been looking into it and is excited. He thinks the UK could become some kind of global hub for Larry's innovations and wonders whether it might be possible to add tests for other conditions into Covid tests. The question is whether Ellison's data solutions can help drag the NHS into the twenty-first century.

FRIDAY 31 JULY

A day of dark warnings. Boris's afternoon press conference, coming shortly after the ONS data dropped, had an air of urgency. He didn't ladle it on too thick but said it was 'time to squeeze the brake pedal'. After the discussion yesterday, we have decided to postpone the 1 August reopening of indoor sports, beauty salons and the rest for at least two weeks – and put back the opening of wedding receptions of up to thirty people. Face covering rules will be extended to all indoor venues like churches, museums and cinemas. Sounding quite stern, the PM warned we might have to go further if people don't follow the rules.

For now, people are still able to go abroad on holiday, though it involves a lot of form filling. Jamie has been struggling with the paperwork required to get into Greece and asked if any of us could help. I told him that my one contact with the Greek authorities involved telling their Culture Minister that we wouldn't give them back the Elgin Marbles, so I'm probably not best placed to put in a call.

Good news on banning staff movement in care homes. After I blew my top at the weak advice, officials have got the message. However, Helen thinks the number of outbreaks in these settings may have been higher than PHE's data suggested. 'Oh Christ,' I replied, head in hands. I'm worried that we're still not doing enough testing to keep residents safe. I will talk to Dido to see if Test and Trace can divert more capacity.

In the parallel universe that is Westminster, I'm under some pressure to undergo a 'Valuing Everyone' course to learn how to be a good boss. All MPs have to do it. Allan Nixon messaged from his sunlounger to say that Vice News has submitted a freedom of information request to the House of Commons authorities to find out who has (and hasn't) turned up. Jacob Rees-Mogg's SpAd, who is handling the enquiry, wanted to give us the heads-up that my name isn't on the list of MPs who have already attended, nor on a list of MPs who have booked.

Allan asked if I was bothered, to which I replied that I was rather too busy right now managing the pandemic. Jim chirped up that he'd already done the course.

'Was it any use?' I asked.

'Yes,' he replied cheerfully. He says that even though he's 'quite modern' (his words), he still found it helpful. Apparently the dinosaurs – of which there are many in the House of Lords – found it 'life changing'.

Today a whole posse of my 'One Nation' liberal Conservative friends received peerages: Ken Clarke, Jo Johnson, Philip Hammond, Ed Vaizey, Ruth Davidson and Patrick McLoughlin. They are mostly Remainers who have been somewhat in the political wilderness since David Cameron stepped down. Old wounds are healing.

AUGUST 2020

SATURDAY 1 AUGUST

Yesterday was the third hottest day ever recorded in the UK – 37.8C at Heathrow. Beaches are packed and social distancing has disintegrated.

Boris is worried and sent an SOS this evening demanding a rethink about what we're telling people. 'Folks, my private focus groups telling me our messaging now so mangled as to be totally incomprehensible,' he announced.

He wants 'a big reset' involving simple themes pumped over the airwaves, especially on social distancing and how many people you can have in your house.

Lee Cain agreed. He thinks we give too many updates and have confused people by continually shifting policy. Instead he thinks we need to 'drill the basics hard'. We agreed to discuss on Monday.

Jens has been dealing with a huge public protest against Covid restrictions in Berlin. His vaccine procurement programme is also being crippled by the EU. It looks to me as if they've lost about a month of progress. It's the same story with other member states that pre-ordered vaccines and now have to wait for the Brussels machine to splutter back into life in September when they put away their flip-flops and Factor 15 and get back to work.

SUNDAY 2 AUGUST

I took advantage of a quiet moment to update the Cabinet Office on a bunch of things that are stuck in the No. 10 paper jam. Downing Street has now been sitting on my proposal for the future of PHE for ages. Much worse is the situation with the forty hospitals. I've got the PM pushing us to go faster, and the Treasury saying we need to delay for eight weeks. As a senior Cabinet Office official said to me, the mess over hospitals is a classic of the Johnson era: 'Go fast – no, go slower – listen to me – no, agree it with Rishi...' The official got onto it immediately, coming back to me less than an hour later. As if to confirm the 'go faster – no, go slower' point, he discovered that the PM himself agreed to the eight-week delay! Unbelievable. So while Boris has been pushing me to go further and faster, he's also let the Treasury press pause. The official thinks he's almost certainly forgotten he did so. Swallowing hard, I said that we can work with this new timeframe as long as there is no further procrastination. Otherwise the whole policy will fall apart.

We've rightly been getting flak over delays in publishing the PHE review of the methodology for recording deaths. I'm actually embarrassed by this and agree we need to sort this ASAP.

MONDAY 3 AUGUST

Boris is delighted that he was able to correctly recite the rules for indoor socialising during the morning meeting. To ram home his point about how complicated the measures have got, he went round the table asking everyone to set them out simply. We had endless different answers, and he got them all right.

'I hope colleagues feel I have justified my general reputation for mastery of detail by being RIGHT this morning about the rules. It's two households inside and six outside and always has been,' he said triumphantly.

'Bravo,' I replied obligingly, adding that the collective confusion among colleagues had confirmed that we need to sort out our messaging.

TUESDAY 4 AUGUST

Tony Blair is backing Operation Moonshot, writing an article calling for a mass testing system for people who are asymptomatic, which is what the goal is all about. As controversial as he is, his views still carry a lot of weight, so this is a plus, even if he can't resist presenting it as his own idea. Dido wants to have a background chat with him about Test and Trace, which I encouraged. Former PMs are a valuable source of advice.

WEDNESDAY 5 AUGUST

Clegg may have looked a mess when he Zoomed me from Yellowstone, but he got straight onto it re. combatting fake news. Facebook has taken down a wild-eyed Trump post declaring that children are 'almost immune' to coronavirus. Twitter followed suit. I'm delighted he's been sanctioned for this nonsense. It's irresponsible.

We've moved fast on the Valneva vaccine. Less than a week after officials submitted the business case, we've signed off £620.5 million to develop this one all the way down the supply chain, from science to trials to manufacturing to fill-and-finish to distribution. If trials are successful, we'll get 60 million doses, with options to go up to 100 million in 2022. It's a French company, but the vaccine will be made in Britain, with a UK supply chain centred on the company's plant at Livingston near Edinburgh.

The Prof has been banging heads together with the CMOs of the devolved governments about agreeing a consistent way to report death numbers. We can't have different parts of the country calculating the figures in different ways. Whether the agreement is that we count deaths within twenty-eight days of a positive test or sixty days of a positive test is less important than that we all do it the same way. In the end the four CMOs went for twenty-eight days as the headline measure, publishing sixty days too – though they're not quite ready for a formal recommendation.

Back in London, the PM held a long meeting on population testing. The idea is that if you test everyone, and everyone who tests positive isolates, then you can massively hit the pandemic without social distancing. I think it's worth a shot – though we haven't nearly got enough tests yet. Maybe we should try it in one city first? Some of the No. 10 crowd are very excited by the idea. I can see the logic – but I can see the cost too.

THURSDAY 6 AUGUST

For the first time since February, there were no Covid stories on the 7 a.m. news bulletin on the *Today* programme. Long may it continue.

Obviously we keep working away. Finally we reached agreement on how to measure deaths. We will all publish deaths within twenty-eight days of a positive test. England and Wales will also publish deaths within sixty days, but not as a headline measure. Scotland and NI refused to add this measure – but it doesn't matter, because now we have a standard, reasonable measure that we can stick with. It really shouldn't have taken all this time to sort out. Afterwards, I told the Prof we had agreement. He sighed heavily.

'The only real measure is afterwards, when you see how many people died compared to a normal year. It's impossible to measure accurately why someone died, especially frail elderly people. But what we do measure very accurately is how many people actually died,' he said.

What a palaver, and a huge amount of effort, to reach an interim measure that isn't itself accurate anyway. Still, at least it's done now.

FRIDAY 7 AUGUST

Boris is having a sugar rush about DIY Covid testing, which he believes could lead us to what's he's dubbed – in emphatic capital letters – 'COVID FREEDOM DAY'. I have no idea who he's been talking to, but he's very fired up.

He thinks rapid home tests are the way to 'get Whitehall and the whole British army of bludgers and skivers' back to the office and 'douse all remaining embers of the disease'.

'If we can get this project going well in the next few weeks, we should be in a position to promote our methods to the rest of the world,' he enthused. 'I know that I am sometimes accused of over-optimism/boosterism etc. but I truly think [this] could be a turning point. The prize is immense. If we can offer the British public a simple and rapid turnaround test to show whether or not – to a high degree of probability – they have the disease then we have the glimmerings of a route out of the nightmare.'

He thinks the new lateral flow tests have 'the makings of a freedom pass – a green light that flashes figuratively over your head and tells your family and your co-workers that you are v unlikely to give them the disease ... People will be able to take a test in the morning and, as Matt says, go to Hamilton the musical in the evening.'

The *Hamilton* reference followed a comment I'd made in Cabinet when we were discussing how lateral flow tests could liberate people. He'd looked at me quizzically when I'd mentioned the show and it was immediately obvious he'd never heard of it, which surprised me, given his interest in American history and the fact that there are adverts for it plastered all over central London.

I think he must have been WhatsApping from a laptop, because the message arrived in one big chunk, with various bits in ALL CAPS to underline his excitement.

Scrolling down, I became increasingly alarmed. I didn't mind the bit about 'throwing absolutely everything at it' – I couldn't agree more – or the idea that Dido and her team should be given everything they need. Of course I also agree with his observation that this is a national emergency and the faster we can get going, the less damage we will continue to do to the UK economy. His sudden determination was actually quite marvellous to behold: a breathless outpouring of hope, energy and enthusiasm culminating in a call to arms. He has instructed us all to 'work flat out' in the next few weeks to get it done.

What worried me was that he put a date on it. He wants 'COVID FREEDOM DAY' to be 7 October, i.e. just two months today. Why then? Is it achievable? Maybe, maybe not – but I'd rather not be set up for a fall.

Re. the debate over how we record Covid deaths, I received a note from the eminent Cambridge statistician Sir David Spiegelhalter criticising the way PHE explains the numbers. He described their communication as 'consistently poor' and said it had led to 'deeply misleading media coverage'. He's right, of course – but he knows as well as the Prof does that the only true data will be available in a year's time, which isn't much use now.

I dealt with all this while on a short family break in Hay-on-Wye. I love the Wye Valley. For two hours I paddled down the river with no mobile phone reception at all. Bliss.

When we got to the pub at the far end, there was great excitement. I'm not used to people spotting me, except in Suffolk, where I've been on the leaflets for years, so the universal recognition is a bit of a shock. Something I'll have to get used to, I suppose.

SUNDAY 9 AUGUST

An unwelcome landmark today, with UK case numbers going back over 1,000 for the first time since late June. Preston Council is using a new slogan: 'Don't Kill Granny'. It's punchy but quite distressing at the same time. If it helps hammer the message home, I'm all for it.

A disturbing poll in *The Observer* suggests that only half the population would definitely have a jab. We've got to hit anti-vaxxers hard.

MONDAY 10 AUGUST

The *Mail* has run a piece about our trip down the Wye. They had a friendly chat with the owner of the canoe hire company. Fortunately, he said I'd been 'very careful with everything', washing my hands with antibacterial gel and elbow bumping instead of shaking his hand. The only thing they could find to pick on were my crocs. I'm now being dubbed 'Matt Hancroc'. I can't quite believe me going down a river then having a pint in a pub is news. I've had worse.

A boost from Tedros, who's publicly described local lockdowns in northern England as an example of a 'strong and precise' approach to suppressing spikes in the virus.

Then late in the evening, I took a really worrying call from Pascal Soriot at AZ. He says they can't manufacture based on the terms of the indemnity we are giving them, and they may have to press pause on manufacturing the Oxford vaccine. This would obviously be a disaster. I called JVT, who says they're in endgame on the commercial negotiations on the indemnity, so this is Pascal trying to play me into it. 'Fine,' I replied. 'By all means protect our interests, but don't let manufacturing stop, and take AZ's concerns seriously. They're doing all this for no profit, so we can hardly expect them to carry commercial levels of liability too.'

TUESDAY 11 AUGUST

Boris finally announced £300 million for A&E upgrades at 117 trusts – the culmination of a lot of pushing on my part. We went on the 'getting the NHS ready for winter' angle, but it's also about making sure these departments are less crowded in future. Plans for the announcement were very carefully choreographed. Unfortunately, one of our backbenchers had one too many beers last night and pre-announced half of it in a drunken group WhatsApp. The first rule of social media: only message when sober.

We're looking into what to do about the AZ indemnity issue. We absolutely can't afford for the deal to collapse.

WEDNESDAY 12 AUGUST

The Cabinet Office is doing my head in. The procurement team takes for ever to sign things off, even when contracts are patently urgent. I messaged Cummings saying they need to turn around clearances much faster or, even better, be removed from the process.

We've finally formally announced how we're going to define coronavirus deaths. Now that the numbers only include people who died within twenty-eight days of a positive test, the official death toll for England has immediately fallen by 5,377, to 41,329. I wanted the Prof to clear my quote before we issued a press release, but the team couldn't get hold of him. It turned out he was on a hospital ward. Typical Prof: no fuss, no publicity – just serving his patients and the public. He never lets up. What a star.

THURSDAY 13 AUGUST

Media coverage of Test and Trace is dire. Our press releases and briefings have been hopeless. We need to drive the narrative. 'No flabbiness. Tight messaging. Not spraying figures around,' I told the team, knowing I didn't sound very chilled for someone who was supposed to be on holiday.

The truth is I wasn't in the best of moods, partly because it's not remotely relaxing being away at a time like this and partly because I discovered there's been another blunder over the way we record figures which is distorting Test and Trace records. Apparently when Test and Trace teams call a house with multiple occupants and ask everyone in the property to isolate, they only count that as contacting one person. So if there are four people in the house and the team speaks to one member of the family, that is recorded as '25 per cent contacted'. Thanks to this screw-up, we're reporting that we're missing the targets set by SAGE and we've been getting worse write-ups than we deserve. It's an easy fix, but it's a stupid, unforced error.

Thank goodness we only went as far as Wales for this mini-break: France and the Netherlands are about to come off the safe travel list, as is Malta.

FRIDAY 14 AUGUST

France's Europe Minister, Clément Beaune, who always relishes a swipe at the British, says they will retaliate over our move on travel corridors. Nothing to do with the science, just petty. As a courtesy, I texted my French oppo, Olivier Véran, about the change. No reply.

Dido, who's also on holiday, is as worried as I am about the PM's 'COVID FREEDOM DAY'. She pointed out that if we hadn't described Test and Trace as 'world-class' two months ago (when we weren't), we could actually have been fairly described as 'world-beating' now, instead of which, we are just getting a kicking. We're doing more tests now than anyone else, and once we fix the stupid measurement error, our contact tracing is well ahead of where the scientists say it needs to be. Yet there are constant stories about it not being good enough. In part that's because some people who hate lockdown thought Test and Trace alone could hold the virus down. Self-evidently it can't. But that doesn't make it worthless – just not magical. Dido's frustration is palpable. She thinks that if we introduced some kind of financial support for people who are self-isolating, it would make a huge difference to compliance. Naturally it would also be very popular. The question is whether we'd have any hope of getting it through the Treasury. Right now I can't even get them to sign off my announcement about breaking up PHE – and that doesn't even have a big price tag. Amid the usual foot dragging, the PM is on holiday next week. His team say he's 'not taking any boxes', their way of pretending he won't be making decisions. It's rubbish – he never stops – but I can't imagine he'll particularly want to think about health quangos.

In better news, we've added another couple of arrows to our quiver of vaccines – 60 million from Novavax in the US and 30 million from Johnson & Johnson/Janssen in Belgium. We're now on 340 million doses across six products. Amazing.

SATURDAY 15 AUGUST

The PM announced the next stage of easing from 15 August, with beauty treatments, indoor gigs and wedding receptions of up to thirty allowed as well as bowling alleys, soft-play centres and casinos. This was the measure we delayed before; I'm still nervous.

The Times got wind of my plans for breaking up PHE. Now that Downing Street can't ignore it, they've suddenly become quite helpful and it's good to go. I'm looking at Tuesday for the long-over-due announcement.

SUNDAY 16 AUGUST

The *Sunday Telegraph* has gone big on the PHE story, running it under the headline 'Farewell to Public Health England, and good riddance'. Certain officials and health policy types are going nuts, including Chris Hopson, chief executive of NHS Providers, who never misses an opportunity to opine about how difficult things are for his 'members', aka NHS trust managers. After listening to him rubbishing the announcement, I was ready to lose my rag. I asked Jamie whether we had a problem or whether he's devalued his own currency with his constant low-level attacks.

'He's totally rogue,' Jamie replied wearily.

Unfortunately, we can't just ignore him, not least because he still has enough currency to get his hatchet jobs onto BBC bulletins. It sticks in the craw, but maybe I'm going to have to show him some love.

MONDAY 17 AUGUST

The Prof couldn't make the senior team meeting today because he's on his ward rounds again. This is what he's doing instead of going on holiday – what a legend. The Treasury finally signed off my PHE speech. The organisation will be split in two. Fighting pandemics and other communicable diseases and external threats will rightly be the preserve of one organisation – which must focus on this not just in the middle of a pandemic but when there's no threat on the horizon. Non-communicable public health – fat-busting, pollution, healthy eating etc. – will come back to the department and be led by the CMO.

I've looked round the world to design the best system for the future. It's no good just spotting that PHE was too much of an amalgam, which had diluted its pandemic-fighting preparation and leadership – it's also that promoting non-communicable public health is largely done through other departments, and PHE got no purchase on that as a quango.

TUESDAY 18 AUGUST

My PHE speech seemed to go well. On reflection, I should have been more brutal earlier. It wasn't fit for purpose, and I should have cleared out senior figures who blocked the expansion of testing, basically because they didn't want the private sector involved. In relation to one individual, I did try, but I wobbled when Duncan Selbie heard about it and threatened to walk too. 'If they go, I go' was his response. At that time, I wasn't ready to blow the whole thing up. In retrospect I should probably have taken him at his word.

I told Jens about my plans and said I want the new body to be more like Germany's Robert Koch Institute, their main agency for disease control and prevention. I promised to send him a draft copy of some work we are doing on wider population testing. I'd also like to see a complete change in culture over diagnostics. No longer can it be OK for people to struggle into work with a dripping nose. Go home and get a test! Same for cancer/flu/heart disease/other infectious diseases. 'If in doubt, get a test' is not just a Covid instruction but a way to keep the population healthy. I told Dido that we need to signal to the market that diagnostics are the place to bet their investment.

In response, Labour's deputy leader Angela Rayner has been tweeting the usual tripe about Tories wanting to privatise the NHS by stealth. Does anyone seriously listen to this nonsense any more? It's what Labour always parrot when they can't think of anything else to say. Why don't they just do a recorded message and press play every time a journalist phones? Do they really want no private sector support for testing, pharmaceuticals etc? The truth is, we wouldn't stand a chance of winning this fight against Covid if it wasn't for support from business. From manufacturing tests to developing the vaccine, the private sector – alongside the NHS and academia – has been critical to the fight.

WEDNESDAY 19 AUGUST

Boris is on staycation somewhere in Scotland but is bombarding colleagues with calls and messages. Another person who never stops is

Dido. We need to find several more senior people for her team, but civil servants are increasingly nervous of applying for any role involving Covid. They just don't want to touch it.

Tedros has been warning against 'vaccine nationalism'. I'm caught between two opposite facts. First, it's not nationalism to look after your own people first – it's the basic duty of any government. But second, we should also help others, and I'm proud we were one of the first countries to commit to providing vaccines to developing countries. The whole debate seems to be about pledging doses – but our AstraZeneca contract does much better than that, allowing anywhere else to make their own at cost. We need to get this message across, before the smears start to stick.

THURSDAY 20 AUGUST

Cases are rocketing in areas with a high concentration of ethnic minorities, especially in parts of the north where there are big Asian communities. I'm told the reason is quite simple: many families in these communities live in bigger households, often with grandparents living under the same roof as grandchildren. We can see the patterns of infection right down to ward level.

We have to explain this, but I also have to choose my words carefully. The question is how to protect these communities without being seen to single them out. I don't want to impose local lockdowns on nearby areas with very low Covid rates just so that nobody can complain that Asians are being targeted. It is very tricky indeed. Nadine reminded me about the Burnley race riots, back in 2001, when simmering racial tensions in Lancashire exploded into violence. She reckons the town ward of Colne, which has more than a dozen pubs and is a predominantly white working-class community, would be 'like a tinderbox' if its pubs closed because of high infection rates among people in the neighbouring, predominantly Asian, area. The solution is to get the right messengers: clinical voices, preferably from the affected communities. It's going to be a huge challenge if this gets worse.

Meanwhile Sturgeon has delayed reopening in Scotland because of various local flare-ups, including forty-three cases at a chicken plant in Coupar Angus. The army has put in a mobile testing unit. NB – that's the British Army, though Wee Jimmy Krankie (as Boris once called her) won't be giving the union any credit.

FRIDAY 21 AUGUST

Border enforcement is a mess. Everyone who flies into the UK has to fill out a passenger locator form, which they're supposed to hand to officials on arrival at the airport, but half the time the documents go straight in the bin.

One of our MPs says her son has just returned from Malta with a bunch of other lads and they all brought their forms home with them. He had a bit of a cough on his return, so they got him tested and the result came back positive. One of his mates also has it – and who knows how many more? Test and Trace is none the wiser. She tried to do the right thing by contacting them, but there's no way of ringing them. So now we know that Brits are pouring back into the UK having picked up Covid on holiday and our borders system hasn't got a clue.

This is an epic fail. I got straight onto Simon Case and told him we need a mass focus on enforcement. HMT and BEIS continually argued that we should ease off on enforcement when numbers were falling. Now we have massive gaps. It risks undermining everything we've been trying to achieve. Luckily the PM agrees and wants to know what more we can do.

Still a lot of to-ing and fro-ing about the outbreak in the north. We announced what we called 'targeted intervention' (i.e. local lockdowns) in eight council wards in Blackburn but took nine other wards out of restrictions at the same time. Nadine's been doing a great job of keeping the local MPs on board, though our outreach work to Burnham was less successful. This evening he tweeted that our policy had 'taken him by surprise', sniffing that it's 'problematic'.

That's code for him not finding a way of disagreeing with it but wanting to be against for political reasons. So wearying.

Separately, Jeremy Farrar of SAGE is going to have to be reined in.

He took to social media a couple of days ago to lay into my PHE announcement, posting a blizzard of hostile tweets. Raging about 'arbitrary sackings' and 'passing of blame', he labelled my reforms 'ill thought through', 'short-term' and 'reactive'. He didn't address the fundamental problem at all – which is that having one organisation with two objectives meant no one focused purely on preparing to fight pandemics – and suggested it is only being abolished to pre-empt the 'inevitable public inquiry' into the handling of Covid. What total rubbish. A week ago, he busied himself writing an article for *The Guardian* in which he opined on the perils of vaccine nationalism. But he didn't mention that the vaccine we're developing is available to the whole world. Jim has volunteered to have a word and – as he put it – 'nicely explain' that we don't need trusted advisers behaving this way. Apparently Vallance and the Prof have also spoken to him. Such a pity he can't be a team player.

Later we officially signed off the decision to spend £469.44 million buying 100 million doses of the Oxford vaccine, plus £80 million to Wockhardt to fill and finish – to put it in the vials and label it all up. Having shepherded this amazing project since January, signing the metaphorical cheque was an amazing moment.

The day didn't end on a great note after so-called 'Whitehall sources' briefed the *Telegraph* that I've 'lost the plot' over plans for a £360 million new headquarters for the successor body to PHE (the National Institute for Health Protection). According to the article, I 'spend money like water' and 'don't know what I'm getting' for the cash. Treasury officials have barely bothered to hide their fingerprints. Actually, we've junked the £360 million HQ plan, and I have no problem with people knowing it's been killed off, but I don't appreciate the suggestion that I'm profligate.

Jamie says he knows for a fact the Treasury briefed it and has rung his counterparts to give them hell.

SUNDAY 23 AUGUST

Rishi messaged first thing apologising about the *Telegraph* story. He says he has no idea where it came from and that all his media SpAds are on holiday. 'Hand on heart, I personally have never heard of this HQ project,' he added. He seems genuinely upset and is going to deliver appropriate bollockings. He has always been honourable and we have a very good working relationship, despite our differences of opinion on certain policies, so I trust him.

Trump has announced emergency authorisation for the new Covid treatment which involves giving patients blood plasma containing antibodies from patients who have recovered from the virus. Efficacy data is patchy, but there's no evidence it's dangerous and the FDA decided that the benefits outweigh the risks. According to Jim, UK teams are working on something similar and are actually closer to finalising a trial than the Americans. He thinks we can beat them to it.

Overnight, police broke up more than seventy house and street parties in Birmingham. Greater Manchester Police said they dispersed 126 illegal gatherings, including a child's tenth birthday party. Chief Constable Ian Hopkins said it wasn't a 'jelly and ice cream' type event but 'mostly adults celebrating'. These people are playing with fire.

MONDAY 24 AUGUST

Perhaps the Gods think I am becoming too self-important, because they have delivered a new humiliation: I am having to work from the kids' treehouse.

When we moved into our rented constituency house in Suffolk, I happened to be the minister responsible for broadband rollout. By happy coincidence, soon after, Openreach upgraded the whole village to full fibre. Annoyingly, it crashed today, and despite the best efforts of the department's IT team it proved impossible to reconnect me. As a stopgap, the team wearily suggested that I use an iPhone hotspot instead. Unfortunately, I only get 4G in the garden, and even there, it's patchy. Ridiculously, the best spot is twelve feet up an old ash tree in the treehouse I painstakingly built with the kids last year. Behold the temporary new offices of the Secretary of State for Health.

TUESDAY 25 AUGUST

My heart sank when I woke up to see the rain hammering down and remembered that the broadband was still on the blink. It was so wet I knew I wouldn't be able to take calls while wandering around the garden and would have no choice but to crawl back into the treehouse, which in any case has a leaky roof. Blame the builder! After a certain amount of silent swearing about the deficiencies of the 'Rolls-Royce government machine', I did my best to crack on from my humble new headquarters. Eventually, to my immeasurable relief, the connection miraculously leapt back into life, though I still don't have a secure phone line.

Sadly, that wasn't the end of my travails. Just as I was attempting to sign off the latest local lockdown regulations, the printer packed up. No amount of opening and shutting the paper tray and switching the thing on and off would revive it. In despair, I sent an SOS to Jim asking him to complete the formalities.

While I was enmeshed in this techno farce, Nicola Sturgeon blind-sided us by suddenly announcing that when schools in Scotland reopen, all secondary school pupils will have to wear masks in class-rooms. In one of her most egregious attempts at one-upmanship to date, she didn't consult us or give us any notice, leaving us scrabbling around to formulate a response.

The problem is that our original guidance on face coverings specif-ically excluded schools. As she knows full well, unless Vallance or the Prof are willing to go out and say the Scots are wrong, we now have to do a U-turn.

Cue much tortured debate between myself, Education Secretary Gavin Williamson and No. 10 about how to respond. Much as Stur-geon would relish it, nobody here wants a big spat with the Scots. Meanwhile there's only so long we can get away with a holding po-sition about our policy. So, U-turn it is. There's a general view that if we're going to shift, we might as well get on with it. Masks are ex-tremely divisive, and Simon Case messaged me privately saying we need to keep everyone calm. 'If we did start a fight, all that happens is we spook parents,' he warned. The Cabinet Office view is that if we are going to change tack, it has to be in an ordered fashion, not chaotic lurching around. Amen to that.

WEDNESDAY 26 AUGUST

For all our best efforts to avoid chaotic lurching, the PM has veered off the reservation, suddenly going off on one about how the virus isn't really killing many people any more so 'how can we possibly justify the continuing paralysis?'

I was minding my own business, making the most of that golden half-hour between 6 a.m. and 6.30 a.m. when hardly anyone messages me, when suddenly, ping! Ping! He sprang into life. It was 6.29 a.m., and he wanted to know about mortality rates for Covid.

'I have just read somewhere that it has fallen to 0.04 per cent from 0.1 per cent. So by my maths that is down from one in 1,000 to about one in 2,000. (And I seem to remember that when this plague began we thought the fatality rate was one in 100),' he observed.

Either he's extremely speedy at mental arithmetic or he was sitting there punching numbers into a calculator, because he was throwing figures around like Archimedes, musing that if all 66 million people in the UK were to be infected, 'we could expect 33,000 deaths'. Yet 'we have already had 41,000'.

His new theory is that Covid may be 'starting to run out of potential victims' and he doesn't think we can justify restrictions for a disease that's only killing one in 2,000 people.

I stared at the messages, hoping someone else in the WhatsApp group would reply but… nothing. By 6.55 a.m., neither the Prof nor Vallance nor Case nor Cummings had replied to him and I was beginning to get nervous. The figures he was wheeling out – recited from a badly written article that appeared a couple of days ago in the *FT* – are hopelessly misleading and should have no bearing on our response. Firstly, measured mortality rates are dependent on testing rates, so as the world produces more tests, death rates obviously fall. Secondly, the death rate is much higher for old people, though it may be declining overall because of better treatment and shielding of these groups. I thought this would come across better from the scientists. To my immense relief, just before 7 a.m. the Prof and Vallance rode to the rescue, putting the flawed *FT* figures into context and emphasising how dangerous the virus remains for old people.

Unfortunately, the PM just wouldn't let it go, continuing to interrogate the figures and fixating on the 'negligible' risk of death for anyone under the age of thirty-five. Studying some charts, he noted that an eighty-year-old now has a 6 per cent chance of dying, which he didn't think was enough to justify what we're doing.

'If I were an eighty-year-old and I was told that the choice was between destroying the economy and risking my exposure to a disease that I had a 94 per cent chance of surviving, I know what I would prefer,' he argued.

This exchange, which continued on WhatsApp pretty much all morning, was more than a little stressful, given that it represented a fundamental challenge to our entire pandemic response. I'm not quite sure what he expected – that the chief medical officer, chief scientific adviser, Cummings and I would all suddenly throw our hands up and say, 'You know what, you're right, this whole thing has been a huge mistake. Let's ditch everything we're doing and pretend none of it ever happened'? Hopefully he was just playing devil's advocate, something he does periodically to stave off groupthink and keep us on our toes. If so, all credit to him for stress testing our approach: that's his job. Nonetheless, it was disconcerting.

Fortunately, after a few hours he ran out of both statistics and steam, and Cummings managed to close the discussion by promising him a briefing note.

All the same, I sense a very definite shift in attitude. Something has unsettled him. Who has he been on holiday with? Someone has got under his skin – at the end of July he was rightly fretting about a second wave. Now he's regurgitating flawed maths from a flaky newspaper article, and not letting it go.

THURSDAY 27 AUGUST

The PM has turned his ire on capacity problems in Test and Trace and is on the warpath. Overnight, his creeping suspicion that everything we're doing has been a catastrophic overreaction has evaporated as quickly as it appeared, to be replaced by annoyance at the discovery that there is a supply/demand gap for testing. MPs are being bombarded with complaints from constituents who are being asked to travel miles for tests, including, in at least one case, from Lewes to Manchester or the Isle of Wight. Buckinghamshire Council has been telling MPs that people in that area may not be able to get tests until the end of next month. I'm particularly worried about what's going on in care homes, after Jim received what he called a 'slightly gruesome update' from the team in charge of testing. He describes the situation as 'rickety', with only around 1,000 staff a day being tested. He says there's no system to speak of, just thousands of private institutions doing their own thing.

Simon Case messaged me just before 7 a.m. warning me that the PM is really frustrated about the situation, which is code for 'going batshit'.

Dido and I had been planning to argue – truthfully – that we are a victim of our own success. Our advertising campaign encouraging more people to come forward for tests has been a bit too effective, and now we're overwhelmed. Simon doesn't think the PM will buy it and told me to expect the next meeting on this issue to be 'bumpy'. Jim rightly says that we need to be open about constraints caused by the increase in demand (a positive story) and about supply problems (which show that this stuff is difficult).

A shrieking headline on the front of tomorrow's *Telegraph* suggests No. 10 wants to sack workers who don't return to the office. Case is fuming. He messaged me in high dudgeon at 11.15 p.m. labelling it bullshit.

In other news, Tedros is sending a team to Wuhan to study the origins of Covid-19. It would be nice to think they'll leave no stone unturned. I'm not holding my breath.

FRIDAY 28 AUGUST

The virus is on the rampage in France, just when tens of thousands of Brits head back across the Channel from holiday. They're supposed to quarantine on return, but if their passenger locator forms head straight for the bin, we are going to have a major problem.

I messaged Simon Case, saying we MUST enforce quarantine rules. He asked who's in charge of making sure people do it, to which the answer, in theory, is the police. In practice, they are not at all committed to the cause. I told Simon that we are going to have to get heavy. He's suggested a meeting with Priti and some chief constables/police commissioners to bang heads together. Last time this was discussed there was a police/border/PHE stand-off over who's responsible. This time there should be no messing about.

In better news, we're lifting local lockdowns in Greater Manchester and Yorkshire from 2 September. We'll review Leicester restrictions in mid-September. These local lockdown measures are working.

SATURDAY 29 AUGUST

Something of a panic on both sides of the Channel about the situation in France, where they recorded 7,379 new cases yesterday. Macron is now openly talking about imposing a national lockdown. Spain is also in trouble.

Boris is galvanised. 'Bound to be us in two weeks unless we have some outlandish luck or really sort out Test and Trace and local lockdowns,' he said grimly, followed swiftly by: 'WE MUST GET THE MOONSHOT.'

He wants mass testing of everyone who's vulnerable, and has started going on about 'freedom passes' again. He envisages some sort of app that would allow anyone who can prove they're negative to get back to normal. I can see the appeal, but I can also see the likely furore over anything resembling 'papers please'.

It's unclear why cases are rocketing in France and Spain, though they've both had big problems with testing. In Spain they reopened nightclubs and pushed a lot of people back to work, but this doesn't really explain it. Anyway, the PM was told we should work on the basis that we're next.

'We need to draw lessons pronto,' Boris replied, asking if the French have tried local lockdowns or whether it is 'a case of the whole frog (ahem) getting slowly boiled?'

I rang Ed Llewellyn and a few other contacts for more intel. Ed told me our local lockdowns are much tougher than theirs. Apparently we also have much greater testing capacity. International comparisons show the British return to normal social activity has been among the most cautious in the world. This may go some way to explaining why we've only seen a gradual increase. I told the boss we should continue well-enforced local lockdowns, increase testing and ensure positive cases isolate, and keep hammering home the 'hands, face, space' message.

In truth I doubt any of this is going to be enough. Kids go back to school next week: a second wave feels all but inevitable. One person who's not scared is Piers Corbyn. Jeremy Corbyn's climate change-denying, conspiracy-theorist-pushing big brother spent today bumbling around Trafalgar Square with a megaphone and a bunch of straggly haired weirdos in anoraks, shouting into the wind about 're-sisting' vaccines and lockdowns. Obviously none of them were social distancing or wearing masks. What a bunch of dangerous losers.

SUNDAY 30 AUGUST

Corbyn the Elder has been fined £10,000 for organising yesterday's rally. Quick work by the cops and strangely pleasing. Of course I respect differing points of view, but his antics yesterday were downright irresponsible.

The leader of Norfolk County Council has alerted me to a problem on chicken farms. He says certain poultry processors are supremely unconcerned about either employment law or Covid restrictions. He wants me to exercise my powers to shut them down. Dido counsels caution. She thinks that if we swoop, more reputable operators will be reluctant to work with us. In the end we decided to do all we can while keeping the farm open: another tricky balancing act.

MONDAY 31 AUGUST

Big jump in infection rates today. Boris asked when we last saw numbers like this.

'Not since the end of May,' I replied grimly. I told him we need a simple plan to end the confusion over social distancing rules. Then we need to enforce the hell out of it. Vallance thinks that if this uptick is sustained, rates will soon be doubling every week to ten days.

'We've seen the wave coming for miles, so should be ready,' Boris replied.

Well yes, as long as the Cabinet Office doesn't drag us backwards. Formally, they're the ones who propose social distancing rules. Their exceptionally unhelpful contribution is suggesting we allow groups of eight to get together 'in all circumstances'. Seriously? This would represent a massive *loosening* of the rules and completely undermine everything else we're doing. I told the team to treat it with the disdain it deserves.

I spent the rest of the bank holiday trying to figure out how we improve the local lockdown system. We need something much clearer, which doesn't involve negotiating a tailored set of rules for each area with local politicians while councils and local health officials add bells and whistles.

I talked to David Halpern, who thinks the answer is a tiered system with clearly defined rules at each level. Areas can move up or down a tier depending on the local situation. If people know what tier they're in, they'll know what rules they have to stick to. Next step is to sell it to the Prof and get Boris to buy in.

Simon Case has been appointed Cabinet Secretary, a fantastic and well-deserved promotion. He and I are almost exactly the same age. I congratulated him and told him I think forty-one is a great age to be in these very big jobs. Encouragingly, he says he doesn't want to move too far from Covid. He's brilliant at making things happen; now he'll have many more levers. I told him that the civil service will now see him in a different light. Every email will have more punch.

SEPTEMBER 2020

TUESDAY 1 SEPTEMBER

Parliament's back. The Speaker asked me to update MPs on the latest figures and make sure everyone understands what we're facing. I told Parliament we've got to go all out to prevent a second wave, but I also said there's a real prospect of a vaccine by the end of the year.

Re. Moonshot, Jim is worried that the mission will be thwarted by vested interests trying to block cheap home testing. He messaged me to say there's 'huge pushback from the system' against lateral flow tests. He put it down to what he called 'typical pathology snobbery' from people who just want fancy stuff from big pharma companies and bridle at anything 'lesser'.

Apparently this snobbery extends to Porton Down, where 'PHE snobs railed against LFTs' and took them off their projections altogether. This is a big mistake. Of course people want gold-standard tests, but we'll never deliver mass testing without home testing. It all comes down to your attitude to people. I think you can basically trust the British public to do the right thing. In stark contrast, the public health system basically thinks you can't. The past six months have supported my view – but we've got to make it happen.

Doug Gurr and Gina Coladangelo have been formally approved by the Cabinet Office to join the DHSC board as non-exec directors. Two brilliant people who will bring so much. The board I inherited was excellent but composed entirely of health specialists, when the whole point is to bring a wide range of expertise to the running of a department. Doug, as head of Amazon UK, understands the modern use of data to serve the public more than anyone. Gina, who I first met at a student radio station, is a marketing and communications specialist and joined my team initially as a volunteer – wanting to do her bit. I'm pleased her hard work and value to the team have been recognised.

A bit of drama with Jamie, who had to rush home in the middle of the day to deal with a 'rogue cleaner refusing to leave my flat'. The police were summoned. Intriguing!

WEDNESDAY 2 SEPTEMBER

Test and Trace is now identifying over half of new cases.

'It's like the system actually works!' I messaged Dido excitedly.

'Who would have guessed!!' she replied.

What is not working is my relationship with Andy Burnham, who's in a state of high dudgeon. Parts of Greater Manchester are coming out of most restrictions at noon today, but neighbouring areas aren't, because the numbers don't justify it. He wants the whole region to move as one, waiting until all areas are ready before lifting restrictions. After taking to the airwaves to label our approach 'completely unsustainable', he sent me a whiny WhatsApp complaining about being out of the loop – despite the fact that I spoke to him yesterday to keep him up to speed.

THURSDAY 3 SEPTEMBER

As expected, Burnham is still stirring. He messaged Dido this afternoon asking if they could speak, and she asked me how to play it. 'Please don't tell him anything you wouldn't say in public. He's absolutely 100 per cent in political mode' was my advice.

The guy is all over the place. Now he wants the whole of Greater

Manchester to be taken out of household mixing restrictions altogether. When she pushed on what action he would take that would drive the virus down, he tried to argue that we should accept a higher level of the virus. Literally the opposite argument to yesterday, except he thinks that the whole of GM must move together – whether the facts justify that or not. I loathe his posturing.

While the PM obsesses over Moonshot, I'm increasingly worried about the number of tests we have for the here and now. This happens so often in government: you're trying to pull off something massive, but the immediate pressures take up too much bandwidth. People say 'just focus on the long term', but in truth you have to handle both.

The latest tale of woe involves someone being told to go more than 100 miles from Devon to Carmarthen in north Wales for a test. On the BBC, Dido did a mea culpa. The problem is that the algorithm that finds the closest testing site measures in a straight line, not via road. No one told the computer about the Bristol Channel.

MONDAY 7 SEPTEMBER

The PM keeps looking at what's happening in France, which is in a bad way. I told him that Belgium has managed to turn the curve via strong messaging to young people and the introduction of a curfew. He didn't comment. We shall see.

Much better news on the vaccine though. We've sorted the indemnity and AZ has started production of 100 million vaccines per our order. I think this is the first time ever that a pharma company has begun manufacturing a vaccine at scale before the drug has been formally approved. They're only willing to do it because we're carrying the risk. It's part of the strategy I've insisted on since February of doing things in parallel, so we cut time without cutting corners. Obviously I've welcomed this in a big way – people need to see there's a way out.

TUESDAY 8 SEPTEMBER

After my bit of optimism yesterday, I got a blast from No. 10 about talking up the vaccine. Other than Boris, nobody there has ever really believed we can make it happen. But what on earth is wrong with talking about it – so long as we're honest about the risks?

In reality their scepticism suits me, because it means they're not meddling. The last thing I need is Cummings interfering or the project going through the Cabinet Office mincer. No. 10's messing with testing is a horrible example of what would happen: bungled attempts to run a parallel operation which only complicate the whole process. The Cabinet Office apparently call Downing Street's cackhanded attempt at controlling things from afar 'the long screwdriver': sporadic interference at too low a level at too far a distance. I've issued an edict that absolutely nothing about the vaccine rollout goes to No. 10 except through me. Nothing. I've got to protect my rollout team from the whole saga over there. Simon Stevens is completely onside for this approach too. We will design the rollout here and take it to the centre when we're ready. I'll keep the PM up to speed directly. It'll be on a need-to-know basis.

JVT has been on a diplomatic tightrope at a global health security conference hosted by Taiwan. I tried to get hold of him first thing to discuss the latest on the vaccine programme, but he was about to give a speech to a gathering of Asia Pacific health officials via Webex so couldn't talk. He told me that some representatives were trying to get him to criticise the WHO's links to the Chinese, a temptation he resisted, given the ranks of hatchet-faced Communist Party apparatchiks eyeballing him on the screen.

'Trying not to start WWIII,' he informed me breezily.

Lee Cain has come up with a new idea for social restrictions, which he's calling a 'rule of six'. For an ex-tabloid reporter who spent the 2010 election campaign dressed as a chicken for the *Daily Mirror*, he's come a long way. (According to my old friend Ken Clarke, who encountered him out on the stump, 'he seemed a decent chicken'.) The thinking is that instead of saying that 'two families' can meet, we put a number on it. I'm in favour. Meanwhile the Cabinet Office proposes that restaurants and bars close from 10 p.m. to 5 a.m. They're desperate not to call it a curfew so are describing it as 'late-night restriction of opening hours'. Not sure it will catch on.

WEDNESDAY 9 SEPTEMBER

Just as production starts, AZ has had to pause clinical trials. Apparently a participant is suffering from a condition known as transverse myelitis, an inflammation of the spinal cord which can be linked to viral illness. Kate Bingham says it 'could be fine or it could be terminal' for the vaccine. We are all on edge. JVT did his best to keep spirits up, reminding everyone that this is the nature of Phase 3 clinical trials and why they are done. With any luck an investigation will rule out any concern that the condition was triggered by the vaccine and the trial will be able to resume. For now, there's nothing any of us can do but wait.

The setback underlines why we have to keep buying time. I just wish the Cabinet Office would stop throwing up obstacles. The Rule of Six is going ahead, but they want to create an exemption for public protests. I've enlisted Gove to kill it off. Demonstrations in places like Parliament Square and Hyde Park just undermine public confidence in social distancing.

'Nothing wrong with protests under six!' I said. Gove agreed and is trying to sort.

THURSDAY 10 SEPTEMBER

God, I loathe the BMA. Doctors: great. Their trade union: awful. Their in-house magazine, the *British Medical Journal*, has done a joint number with *The Guardian* attacking Moonshot, having got hold of some internal document about what we're trying to achieve. They repeated an absurd suggestion by consultants that it could cost 'over £100 billion', which is more than the entire education budget. Ludicrous! My heart sank as I skim-read the piece, complete with depressingly predictable negative quote from BMA chair Dr Chaand Nagpaul. Chaand is utterly charming in person, then signs off these absurd quotes which it is difficult to believe he's written himself. This one sniffed that mass testing won't work because of lab capacity issues and problems with false negatives.

Feeling in need of moral support, I messaged Jeremy Hunt, who holds the BMA in even more contempt than I do. When he was Health Secretary they put him through hell.

'Dealing with the BMA is a path well trodden!' he said sympathetically.

'It's all the same people who were against the 100,000 testing target. What's wrong with these people?!' I replied.

I spent most of the afternoon in the Cabinet Room going through the testing options for Moonshot. In the past few days various companies and inventors have come forward with innovative testing systems. Some of this stuff is amazing, but right now lateral flow tests, which use thirty-year-old technology, look by far the best option. An update on Test and Trace was messier, not helped by a barrage of tough questions from Steve Barclay. Dido looked very uncomfortable throughout.

She messaged me afterwards apologising that it had been 'such a car crash' and admitting she is getting frustrated with her team.

'I am taking action and pushing them hard,' she said ruefully.

FRIDAY 11 SEPTEMBER

Boris has unveiled a plan for local authorities to recruit so-called Covid marshals to help enforce restrictions. Suffice to say there are a lot of raised eyebrows – including mine.

In a classic case of policy making on the hoof, nobody thought about getting the police on board before announcing it; nor have they figured out who is actually going to pay for it. The marshals won't have any powers, so what's the point? This isn't the Olympics.

I hope I don't have to go out and defend the initiative when it inevitably hits the buffers.

Worse news though: Jamie is finally leaving. He has worked so hard for me and the government for so long. He just can't stand the

Whitehall grind – especially when No. 10 undermines you at every turn. I'm gutted to lose such a bright and brilliant linchpin from my team. I'll miss his ability to talk to the lobby – a very specialist skill – but even more I'll miss his political chess skills: being able to see five moves ahead. He's off to UK Music, but he's a loss to politics – and to his country.

SATURDAY 12 SEPTEMBER

The Oxford trial has resumed. JVT says the MHRA did a thorough investigation and the illness was nothing to do with the vaccine. Thank God.

MPs are still inundated with complaints from constituents about testing. Labour's Chris Bryant messaged flagging up what he described as a 'major saga' in his Rhondda constituency, where cases are soaring but people with symptoms are routinely being turned away. Bryant is a skilful self-publicist who is fire-and-brimstone in public but entirely reasonable in private. He has to be on this one: the problem is in Labour-run Wales.

I got the team onto it, but I'm afraid it's not a one-off. Against this backdrop, a nice message from Ben Wallace asking if there's anything more the military can do to help was particularly welcome. He's also been getting feedback about people being offered testing slots hundreds of miles away or – just as bad – not even being able to get on the website. He offered to return to providing mobile testing teams. I told him the issue is lab capacity, not mobile units, but that we could definitely do with more logistical support for the labs and may need some squaddies. I warned him that I will soon be coming to him for help with the vaccine rollout. He replied that he's recently returned from the Middle East and Ukraine, where they are all really hoping Oxford wins the race. He said that if we do get there first, we should put a Union Jack on every packet. He's not wrong – I've been trying to! Since the summer I've been working with Allan on what we can do to underline the point that this is a UK vaccine funded by UK taxpayers. It matters for two reasons: at home, especially in Wales, Scotland and Northern Ireland, where it will be administered locally, we need to ram home the point that we are better off, and physically safer, by being one union. I can't think of a more physical manifestation of the value of the union than actually being injected with life-saving medicine thanks to being part of the UK.

Second, we need to tell the world this is a UK vaccine. We can give all the money we want to the COVAX vaccine-sharing initiative, but the biggest contribution we're making by a long way is providing the Oxford vaccine at cost, anywhere. The left don't get this at all – like so many things given for free, the contribution is less, not more, appreciated. Figures like Gordon Brown are running around saying we need to vaccinate the whole world. Well yes, that's exactly what we're going to do – just not via their favoured approach of a patent waiver. Rather than giving the world a fish, we're teaching them how to catch one.

As Culture Secretary I fought – successfully in the end – for Union Jacks to be displayed at the Edinburgh Festival, given the amount of UK taxpayers' money that goes into it. Under Cameron we also successfully changed the UK Aid symbol to a Union Jack. Both took enormous efforts against a slew of naysayers. This time we don't have as long, and we have medical regulators to keep onside. As a patriotic unionist Scot, Allan is the perfect person to lead the project. I hope we can pull it off.

SUNDAY 13 SEPTEMBER

I spent a stupid amount of time today discussing whether hunting and shooting should be exempt from the Rule of Six. The PM is under a load of pressure from the Tory family – including the Chief Whip, Mark Spencer, and Boris's unofficial personal whip, Nigel Adams. Safe to say he is unusually highly engaged. (He's not personally that sympathetic, telling us he 'hates shooting', which didn't surprise me. Somehow I can't imagine him in the heather in a pair of plus fours or taking aim at a pheasant. He'd be hopelessly unsubtle bumbling around in the

undergrowth and would have endless problems with his unruly hair.)
As with cricket, the main transmission threat with shooting is the
socialising afterwards, or as Boris put it 'the steamy shooting lunches
and the stirrup cups and all that malarkey'. When it comes to hunting,
as the boss pointed out, you're on top of a horse and well over two
metres away from anyone, so Covid isn't much of a risk. He proposes
we allow both to continue minus associated social gatherings.

The PM has agreed to my suggestion that we bring in some heavy
hitters to support Dido at Test and Trace. She's also onside. The question is whether anyone will want to do it or whether they'll see it as a
hospital pass. Continuing my efforts to back her up, I've been in touch
with Cameron, Letwin and Blair, all of whom made supportive noises.
They all think we should publish something setting out our plans for
mass testing and explaining why it's so important.

Over in the US, there's mayhem on college campuses where in-person teaching has resumed, fuelling a huge outbreak among students.
I shared a *New York Times* article with Gavin Williamson, hoping it
might make him feel a little less alone.

'A whole new tidal wave of grief,' he replied gloomily. He's confident
universities here will do everything they can to avoid becoming caul-
drons of infection but isn't convinced it will be enough.

As predicted, the Covid marshals policy is unravelling. Councils are
moaning that they can't afford to hire anyone, and the police aren't
especially eager to deal with a whole additional layer of paperwork
courtesy of jobsworths in high-viz jackets. Rob Buckland did his best
to defend the scheme on the Sunday media round but looked like a
man who'd ordered steak and been served spam. He is a real gent.

The day ended with a farcical rush to rubber-stamp the regulations
for the Rule of Six. The paperwork had to be signed by midnight, or
the new measures wouldn't come into force on time. As far as I was
aware, everything was in place, until I received a message from the
office saying there was an issue with the National Archives. At first
I thought this was some kind of autocorrect malfunction and they

meant No. 10, but it turned out that the issue really was in Kew. It turns out that until *they* receive a new law, it isn't legal – and at the stroke of 4 p.m., the only member of staff on duty went home. Cue a frantic operation to disinter an archivist and order them back to the office. By the time all this was sorted, I was on a train to Newcastle, so I asked Ed Argar to do the physical signing. I was just delivering myself a metaphoric pat on the back for overcoming the absurdities of government in a pandemic, when ding! Ding! Up popped an apologetic message from Ed, who had some family crisis and could not sign the regulation after all. Eventually the office managed to get hold of Priti, who did the honours just before midnight. Is this really the most effective way to run a country?

MONDAY 14 SEPTEMBER

Blair messaged to say that the FCDO, as we must get used to calling the FCO now it has taken over international development, is refusing to provide him with the paperwork he needs to avoid a fourteen-day quarantine on his return from a trip to the US. Apparently the White House has invited him to attend a signing ceremony for a new peace treaty between Israel and the UAE, but Raab's department say they have no authority to grant him an exemption from quarantine when he comes home 'because it's a Department of Health issue'.

Blair says he's literally going in for the ceremony and flying straight out again. He points out that it's an official invitation and that if he were a government minister, he'd have a diplomatic exemption. I cannot believe the FCDO is messing him around in this way. He's not a junior minister: he's a former Prime Minister. I told him that of course he should have an exemption and that I'd sort it right away. He sounded relieved and grateful.

Meanwhile the testing crisis is escalating. Never mind Moonshot: we can't seem to provide a single test in Rochdale, Pendle or Bradford. In Bury, people queued for five hours. In Walsall, a father with a sick child travelled seventy-six miles to Wales only to find there was nothing available when he arrived. More and more children are out of school, and hospitals are starting to cancel operations. At the weekend, there was great excitement in Bolton when they were promised a mobile testing unit. It failed to show. I received a courteous message from David Greenhalgh, who's the first Tory to lead the council there in four decades. He said they're trying their best, but the national booking system is failing and they're getting the blame. 'I have released a statement tonight saying the current situation is unacceptable,' he told me. 'I'm sorry, but we're fighting for our political lives here.' An apologetic way of saying he's going to dump on me. I'm on it with the team, who are trying to sort it out, but I understand where David is coming from.

I spent most of the day visiting hospitals in the north-east in Stockton, Bishop Auckland, Darlington and Shotley Bridge, thanking staff and telling them about plans to protect the NHS, expand A&E, build forty new hospitals and beat the virus. While I was coming home on the train, I had a message to say the Cabinet Office has been talking to the PM, Cummings and Vallance about the state of Test and Trace. They all think that Dido is being asked to do too much. They think Moonshot needs to be separated out from normal testing. She's got enough on her plate trying to get testing to Macclesfield, never mind to the Moon. Up to a point, yes, but Moonshot can't be totally separate as it has to be built on the existing system. I pointed out that any change will have to be handled exceptionally carefully. That includes managing egos. We do not need the whole thing blowing up.

TUESDAY 15 SEPTEMBER

Jim says he misses me, which is curious, as he's seen considerably more of me this year than has my long-suffering family. I think he's getting a bit ground down by life in the Lords, which he says he 'sort of loves' but can be heavy going. He spends an inordinate amount of time dealing with the unintended consequences of basing Covid restrictions on the 1984 Public Health Act, a relic of the pre-devolution era. Suffice to say that the architects of these regulations did not envisage a political landscape featuring characters like Nicola Sturgeon.

The PM is still dithering over tiers, a classic Boris battle between head and heart. I want it to start from 1 October so I have tougher measures I can put high-Covid areas into to stop the spread, but there's endless deliberating and hand-wringing in Nos 10 and 11.

Meanwhile a strange message from Nadine, saying she doesn't think we should ease restrictions in maternity units. Making women give birth without their partners by their side has been one of the painful restrictions we brought in. I hate it and want to reverse it ASAP. Surprisingly, Nadine is pushing back. She worries about exposing frontline workers and midwives to more risk. I thanked her for her comments but won't change course.

WEDNESDAY 16 SEPTEMBER

Boris got hammered on testing at PMQs. Later, appearing in front of the Liaison Committee in the Commons this afternoon, he sounded a lot more hostile to another national lockdown than I would have liked, given how fast things are moving in the wrong direction. I was sufficiently alarmed by his bullish rhetoric to ask the Prof to go to No. 10 this evening to talk him through the numbers. What we absolutely don't need is him ruling it out.

More positively, I called a meeting of the team leading the vaccine deployment effort to talk about timing. I explained that, ironically, our task will be hardest if the scientists hit their best-case scenario for approval and it all happens sooner than later. I set them the task of delivering from 1 December. I got some pretty blank looks, as if no one believed it could possibly happen that fast, so had to go into a little motivating speech about how mission-critical this task is for the country and we must not fail. I've asked for a weekly meeting from now on to go through the plans – all based on the 'reasonable best-case scenario'. Makes a pleasant change from the reasonable worst-case scenario we've been dealing with until now.

THURSDAY 17 SEPTEMBER

R is now well over 1 and cases are growing at 3–7 per cent a day in England. SAGE thinks we need a two-week 'circuit breaker'. Cue another long and circular discussion with the PM. Cummings is in favour, telling the boss we should keep schools open but close bars, restaurants, gyms, nightlife etc. and order people to work from home. He thinks we should go hard and fast now and consider doing something similar at the end of November or beginning of December to 'save Christmas'. He suggested we may need to do it all again in 'Miserable Jan'.

Boris seemed confused, doing that thing he does, emphatically verbalising the arguments for and against out loud – which alarms everyone as they try work out where he's going to land. This time he ended up asking what happens if it doesn't work. Rinse and repeat while praying for the vaccine?

My view of a circuit breaker is that it's nice in theory – if no one infected anyone for two weeks, cases would end – but in practice, it's just a short lockdown. Better to try to avoid a national lockdown with very firm local action. But for that I need tiers, with a very tough top tier.

FRIDAY 18 SEPTEMBER

'We've been fucked over by a rhinovirus,' Dido declared miserably, as we braced ourselves for another day of Test and Trace pressure. She was referring to a nasty common cold doing the rounds that everyone now thinks is Covid, creating massive queues for tests.

We are now at 6,000 new infections a day in England alone, excluding hospitals, care homes and prisons – nearly double the figure last week. Simon Case messaged first thing to say the firebreak idea is gaining traction in No. 10. By 10 p.m. they'd done a complete about-turn. He says they want to double down on our existing strategy, i.e. tougher local lockdowns and more warnings about what happens if people don't follow the rules. Apparently the PM wants to explain that we have to balance Covid with other health and economic factors. Well, yes, but if we end up in a national lockdown, the economy will get smashed, so it's better to act sooner and harder to avoid that. I was in the constituency so was unable to join what sounded like a whole series of rolling discussions about what to do – but what's really infuriating is that the people who want action to control the virus didn't insist on me being there to press the point.

I'm increasingly worried about team morale. Jim is indefatigable but feels marginalised on Moonshot and is tied up with endless work on the 1984 regs in the Lords. He is trying to push workplace testing but feels like a lone voice. To cap it all, he thinks HMT is going to shaft the Office for Life Sciences, one of his responsibilities, in the forthcoming spending review and that he'll become a lame duck.

If ever there was a time to be investing in life sciences, it's now.

Later I visited a care home in West Suffolk. As I arrived the staff were outside kindly whooping and cheering – it was a lovely reception. I waved and smiled at residents through the window. They've had no cases at the home and are doing everything right. When I told the manager she was going to get free PPE, she nearly cried. I understood the emotion she felt and it made me more determined than ever – even if it meant dragging certain people along.

SATURDAY 19 SEPTEMBER

A real 'oh shit' moment. Boris has had Sunetra Gupta and Carl Heneghan in – who both thought the pandemic was over back in the spring. This is very bad news. The two of them are massive lockdown sceptics and claim this whole thing can be managed by letting the virus rip through the general population to achieve herd immunity while protecting the elderly and vulnerable. They've got it wrong at every turn. The last thing we need is them messing with his head. Equally worryingly, Anders Tegnell was also at the meeting. He is also running Sweden's light-touch response to the pandemic and will have been busy telling Boris that we can get through this with hope and hygge. Apparently SAGE's John Edmunds was the only scientist pushing the other side of the argument. No wonder I wasn't invited – I would have given them hell for their alarming and absurd suggestions.

Anyway, we'll soon see whether circuit breakers work, because Ireland is going into lockdown for three weeks. The advantage of national lockdowns over local action is that you don't get people pouring out of areas with restrictions to places they can party. We're learning this the hard way: right now, Blackpool is like Benidorm in August, as half the north-west has figured out that it's more fun taking a day trip to the illuminations than it is sitting around at home where everything's shut.

MONDAY 21 SEPTEMBER
Boris is torn. Everyone's getting heavy with him, from Patrick and the Prof, who did a joint press conference without him this evening, to SAGE, which says there will be 'catastrophic consequences' if we don't act now. They've formally proposed a two-week circuit breaker and warned that some measures will probably have to remain in place 'at least throughout the winter'.

It's so frustrating. The last thing we need is a public row about what is in fact a very difficult judgement.

At least they've got the debate moving. The PM has signed up to a 10 p.m. curfew for hospitality, limits on weddings and working from home again. Sporting events with spectators have been paused again. My view is it's a half measure and if it doesn't get R below 1, it won't stop a national lockdown.

TUESDAY 22 SEPTEMBER
A bizarre rear-guard action from Kate Bingham today to limit the number of people we vaccinate. She's still adamant that we only need to target the clinically vulnerable. I have made it crystal clear that this isn't enough. In any case, it isn't her call. JVT put her right, telling her that it's up to the Joint Committee on Vaccination and Immunisation (JCVI) to recommend who gets the jabs and then we – the government – make a decision. I was grateful to JVT for laying down a marker. 'Thanks for clearing that up,' I messaged him afterwards.

Shadow Education Secretary Kate Green has been caught saying Labour shouldn't 'let a good crisis go to waste'. Very embarrassing.

She's had to grovel, but it exposes the mindset of some in the Labour Party.

WEDNESDAY 23 SEPTEMBER

Businesses seem to be realising they need to be much more proactive in testing employees and want information on how to go about it. Unfortunately, BEIS just doesn't want to know. We tried to get them involved in issuing guidance a while ago and they were actively obstructive. Jim's looked at existing testing guidance and says it's 'gobbledegook'.

I asked him to sort it out, whatever the opposition from officialdom.

THURSDAY 24 SEPTEMBER

Another sobering meeting on the figures, which are awful in the north. Dido thinks we need to take a step back over the next twenty-four hours and work out whether the existing tier system will actually halt the exponential rise.

'The danger is we are fiddling rather than intervening,' she warned. She's right that we need a tough Tier 3, the highest level, or the whole thing will be pointless. She says there's a lot of grumbling from local leaders in the north and thinks we need to work harder to keep them on board or they'll 'rear up in horror' at any further tightening of restrictions.

We've finally released a new version of the Covid app. Every single person who downloads it is helping the battle against the virus. Having downloaded it myself, I'm now slightly fearful every time I open my phone. I wonder how people will react to the chance of being pinged by their own phone.

FRIDAY 25 SEPTEMBER

Depressing message from the Prof this morning saying we're losing the argument on tiers. Apparently the PM and HMT 'aren't quite ready' to put any area in Tier 3. The scientific advice is absolutely clear and I told the Prof we need to be 'stark about the problem' with the PM, but he thinks it could be counterproductive if we push too hard.

Private office sent me an alarming note from the modelling people who advise SAGE. They say the epidemic is 'close to breaching the agreed reasonable worst-case scenario on which NHS, DHSC and HMG contingency plans are based'. Unless we can get R below 1, infection incidence and hospital admissions 'will shortly exceed the planning levels'.

Meanwhile public finances are a horror show. According to official figures released today, the government borrowed £35.9 billion in August, up by £30.5 billion in a year. From April to August, the figure was £173.7 billion, six and a half times the figure for last year. Rishi has clearly been using these figures to freak out the PM, but the fact is there's no trade-off: the only sustainable way to get the economy back on track is to defeat the virus, not pretend it's gone away. We've got to suppress it until the vaccine can do its work.

I asked Dido where we've got to on lateral flow tests and she says we're negotiating with various suppliers. She agrees we need to buy as many as we can. Manufacturing in the UK looks possible but unlikely to bring real volume until January at the earliest.

'Team's instruction is to buy, buy, buy!' she reassured me.

'Excellent – and don't let any Cabinet Office nonsense stop you!' I replied.

SATURDAY 26 SEPTEMBER

We've spent millions promoting the app, including buying wraparound ads in loads of publications. I was thrilled when Jim sent me a picture showing them on the front of every national newspaper. Just as I was allowing myself a moment of satisfaction at a job well done – or at least not ballsed up – there came news of fresh horror. A major glitch has emerged: the app can't take data from NHS Covid tests, only from the Lighthouse Labs. I sat very still, trying to absorb the full implications of the fact that we've just spent tens of millions of pounds of taxpayers' money on an NHS app that… doesn't link to the NHS. Which genius thought it would not need to do this, first and foremost? Which other genius signed it off on this basis? Given the multiple overlapping responsibilities of the various quangos involved, Whitehall's institutional buck passing and the involvement of two mega tech companies (Google and Apple), we just didn't know. What I did know was the buck stopped with me, and it was probably time to adopt the brace position.

Privately, I was absolutely furious, but I did my best to hide it. I told the team that what mattered was not who was to blame but how we could fix it. They looked extremely relieved.

I prayed that word of this hideous blunder would not reach Cummings, but that was of course too much to hope. Naturally he went nuts when he found out, and I can't say I blame him.

'This is absurd and makes the government look like utter clowns,' he fumed.

I tried to calm him down by telling him how many people have downloaded it (10 million!), but I didn't disagree. Annoyingly, the Sunday papers are onto it, and tomorrow's headlines aren't pretty.

I find this sort of screw-up personally mortifying. I'm known for my tech background, so the media delight in killing me over any tech problem. The app caused huge embarrassment when Apple screwed us over in the summer. Should I have asked such a basic and obvious question? With hindsight the obvious answer is 'yes' – but I took it for granted that we would link our own app up to our own tests. Never assume!

SUNDAY 27 SEPTEMBER

Dispiriting update from the office: they say it's very unlikely we'll get tiering over the line for Monday. We don't have the PM's steer yet and we need to agree which place goes in which tier. Not looking like we'll get anything before Wednesday now.

We had a late tussle with No. 10 over funeral regulations. They don't want anyone who's self-isolating to be able to attend these services – even if it's for a spouse or their own child. I am not prepared to tolerate this. Not allowing a parent to say goodbye to their child is grotesque and will cause outrage – I had to clear this up in the spring and I'm not going through it again. New mistakes are forgivable, but we can't repeat old ones. Part of the problem is that there are new recruits in No. 10 who weren't with us in the trenches in the first peak. In the end we reached a compromise which involves encouraging people who are self-isolating, either with symptoms or as close contacts, to attend online if possible. If they go in person, they'll have to maintain social distancing, travel to and from the funeral alone and mask up. The picture of that thirteen-year-old boy being buried alone still haunts me. It was utterly heartbreaking and that desolate image is a permanent reminder that we must never allow such a situation to arise again.

MONDAY 28 SEPTEMBER

The PM is in competitive mode and pushing hard on Moonshot. After he watched Trump giving an update on America's testing strategy, he sent a blizzard of WhatsApps demanding updates on lateral flows, who we are targeting, how it will work etc. 'Trump clearly on it and we can't be beaten to punch,' he said.

Right now, I'd rather he focused on tiers. MPs are in open revolt over the current hotchpotch. If the PM wants more stability in the system and a proper strategic approach then this is the way to do it.

'All this shit in Parliament can be avoided by this policy. We agreed this in principle WEEKS ago. Currently I have to deal with massively stroppy local MPs in a messy way,' I told Simon Case grumpily.

To make matters worse, Simon Stevens is being spectacularly unhelpful over Test and Trace. He doesn't want the NHS brand anywhere near it, basically because he doesn't want to be associated with anything that's not going perfectly. This is not very collegiate, to put it diplomatically, especially since he literally runs the in-house part of it. Jim messaged me this evening saying he thought I was 'amazingly zen' about it. He says that in my position, he'd have 'gone totally ape' and rung Stevens to give him 'the full-on "attitude adjustment"', as the doormen apparently used to call it at the Ministry of Sound, the nightclub Jim used to run.

'It's just pathetic,' I replied. I've put Test and Trace on the agenda at the next meeting with Stevens, to ask how he's delivering his part of it.

TUESDAY 29 SEPTEMBER

Nick Forbes, leader of Newcastle City Council, has been sounding off about the impact of the new restrictions on the local economy, accusing me of imposing them in 'knee-jerk' style and claiming it's 'confusion and chaos'.

Boris was indignant. 'Who is this tosser from Newcastle?' he asked.

I told him Forbes had called for the measures and we worked all weekend with his council to agree them. 'Then he's come out against them. Unreal,' I said.

It's part of a pattern: Soulsby, Burnham and now this guy. All Labour chancers, who cooperate with us privately and then the minute we announce everything we've been talking to them about, they take to the airwaves to bleat about it all being a mess.

We've recorded a new high in the past twenty-four hours – 7,143 positive cases. Deaths recorded within twenty-eight days of a positive test are now rising ominously and hit seventy-one today, the highest since 1 July. This appears to have concentrated the PM's mind: he's finally agreed to tiers. Someone in No. 10 hit on a winning formula: taking him through the multiple ways it's currently legal for people to behave in a pub, depending on where they live in the country, and he's seen sense. We'll be announcing the new system on Thursday 8 October, to come into force the following Tuesday. The end of an unnecessarily long saga.

In a quiet moment during a G7 call, I texted Jens to ask what he thought about Trump's announcement on rolling out mass testing. 'I'm ignoring it, like all his other statements,' he replied dismissively.

WEDNESDAY 30 SEPTEMBER

Simon Case has struck a deal with the PM that will allow him to spend most of his time on Covid. He keeps getting dragged into other things, including endless wrangles with the EU that could be dealt with by David Frost, our chief Brexit negotiator. Our response is suffering as a result.

'Great. I'm sure Frosty can sort Brexit,' I replied.

'Hopefully if things calm down, I can actually focus on the biggest issue of the day!' he said.

I told him that I love Chris Wormald, my Perm Sec. And I think he loves me. At least that's what he tells me.

'He tells me the same,' Simon replied. All peace and love over here at the Department of Health.

OCTOBER 2020

THURSDAY 1 OCTOBER

I congratulated Gavin Williamson on his announcement that children self-isolating at home will be entitled to the same education online as they'd get at school. Well of course they should! Needless to say, the teaching unions are kicking off. I thought they were all 'passionate' about their vocation and put the best interests of pupils first? Evidently not.

A bouncy JVT messaged to say the JCVI have been scouring the Ambush data (codename for Pfizer's vaccine), and it works well for the elderly. Great news: whether it would protect the oldest and most vulnerable was one of the biggest questions.

On the Oxford front, I called Adar Poonawalla, chief exec of the Serum Institute of India. They're one of a number of places making the Oxford vaccine, thanks to the deal we signed with AstraZeneca. In fact, if all goes well, they'll be the biggest manufacturer in the world. Given we're allowing them to do it at cost to supply to India and Africa, he said it would be 'an honour' to sell us some. I accepted with delight and asked the team to get onto it.

FRIDAY 2 OCTOBER

I've turned forty-two. Allan Nixon, who reminds me about every birthday from the Queen to *Pulse* magazine, didn't mention it till seven this evening. Presumably mine is the only birthday he doesn't have in his diary. There wasn't much scope for celebration, for obvious reasons, but I did receive a work-related gift: lift-off for the forty hospitals. The PM finally announced the sites and – crucially – the money to go with it. The budget is £3.7 billion – clearly less than we need for all forty, but at least we can get going. Given this was a manifesto pledge and these things take years to construct, I cannot believe No. 10's general torpor or the level of obstruction from No. 11. Challenging, to put it diplomatically.

Donald and Melania Trump have got Covid. The President's disciples, many of whom still think the pandemic is a global conspiracy to microchip the human race, have gone quiet. Tempting as it was to take to social media and suggest he try treating himself with a blast of UV light or drinking bleach, I left it.

Kay Burley from Sky News suggested I tweet good wishes. 'What's there to say?' I replied languidly. The 45th President of the United States has not been a positive presence in this pandemic.

I rang Grandie, my step-grandfather, in his retirement village near Liverpool to warn him about a new round of restrictions coming in at midnight for the north-west and north-east. I haven't been able to see him once since all this began, and now his visits from family will be heavily restricted. He was laid-back, said he'd got everything he needed and that I had to do what I had to do. I appreciated his support. What a star.

SATURDAY 3 OCTOBER
A day dominated by the discovery of a hideous blunder involving a week's worth of Covid data. Somehow or other we have failed to log around 16,000 cases, which all had to be piled into today's figures. We might as well just hang a giant neon sign above the Prof's 'next slide please' screen, saying 'See here: Spectacular Screw-Up.'

PHE, which staggers on for another few months before being replaced by the new body, knew about it last night but failed to tell Dido's

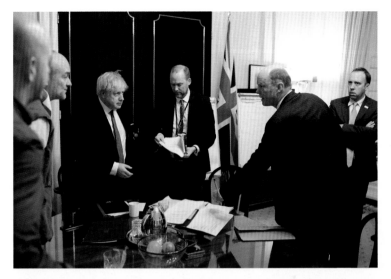

With Boris and his advisers as he's given the latest on the novel coronavirus in February 2020. The total number of UK cases was nineteen at this stage. *Left to right: Lee Cain, Dominic Cummings, Boris Johnson, Jack Doyle, Chris Whitty and me.*

© Andrew Parsons / No. 10 Downing Street

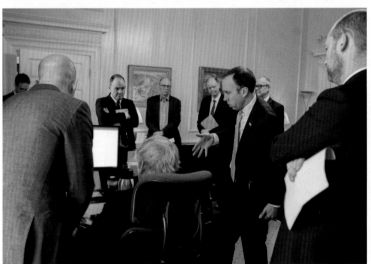

Helping Boris refine his lines before addressing the nation. *Left to right: Lee Cain, James Slack, Boris Johnson, Stephen Powis, Chris Whitty, me, Patrick Vallance and Jack Doyle.*

© Andrew Parsons / No. 10 Downing Street

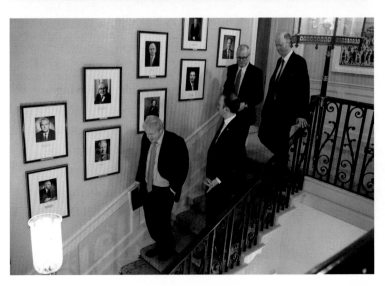

On the famous No. 10 staircase, on our way out from an early coronavirus press conference. Boris had just told the public to stay at home for seven days if they had Covid symptoms, having confirmed we were in a global pandemic.

© Andrew Parsons / No. 10 Downing Street

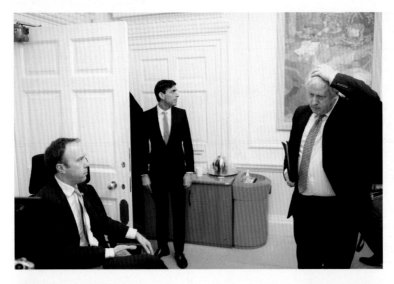

Rishi Sunak and I join Boris after another Covid press conference inside No. 10. The boss had just told everyone to avoid all unnecessary social contact. We were discussing the market reaction, which was not pretty.

© Andrew Parsons / No. 10 Downing Street

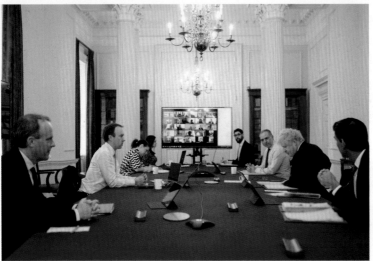

Boris holding one of many digital Cabinet meetings in No. 10. I spent many hours sitting opposite the boss at the Cabinet table as we struggled through tough decisions, often with very little information.

© Andrew Parsons / No. 10 Downing Street

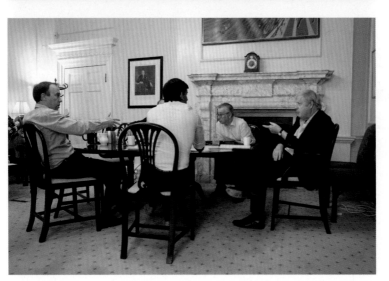

Talking to the boss in his study in No. 10, with Rishi, Dominic Raab and Michael Gove, about when we should reopen schools during the height of the pandemic. These judgements were very difficult, with huge pressures on all sides.

© Andrew Parsons / No. 10 Downing Street

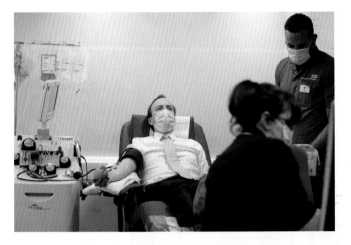

Two months after testing positive for coronavirus, I donated Covid-19 antibodies as part of a trial to see if the antibodies in the plasma could be used to treat those battling to recover from the virus. Big thanks to the nurse from the NHS Blood and Transplant service, Kevin, for looking after me.

© Andrew Parsons / No. 10 Downing Street

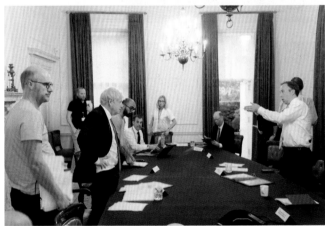

Talking the boss through our plans for locking down Greater Manchester, following an emergency meeting in the Cabinet Room.

© Andrew Parsons / No. 10 Downing Street

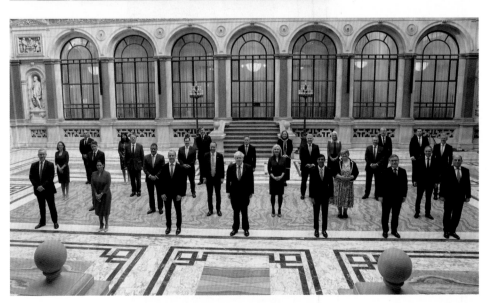

The Cabinet often met in the Foreign Office during the pandemic. Here we line up in the Durbar Court on 1 September 2020 for a socially distanced group photo after the summer recess.

© Andrew Parsons / No. 10 Downing Street

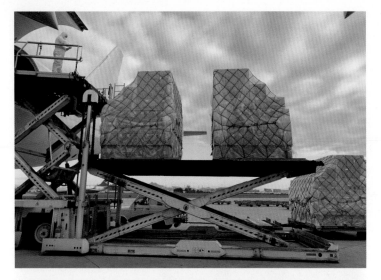

The first big batch of millions of lateral flow tests being loaded onto a plane in China in October 2020. Mass testing helped us keep more things open than would otherwise have been possible.

© Tanner Pharma UK Ltd

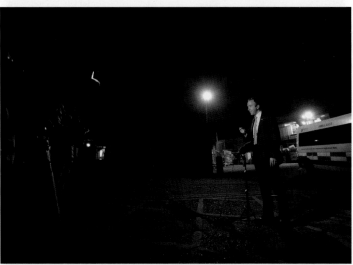

The night before the big advance: visiting King's College Hospital hours before the vaccine drive starts, to check everything was ready. It was on this day that I saw the vaccine in person for the first time – albeit in −60° freezers. It was an extraordinary day and one I will never forget.

© Pippa Fowles / No. 10 Downing Street

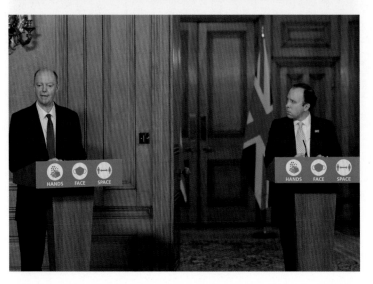

Listening to Professor Chris Whitty delivering the data as we announce that the UK has seen a 14 per cent increase in Covid cases in the past week. Life had quickly veered from the elation of the vaccine rollout to the depressing reality of a sharply growing second wave, driven by the Kent variant.

© Andrew Parsons / No. 10 Downing Street

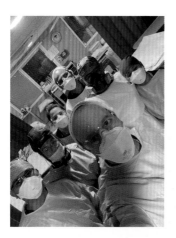

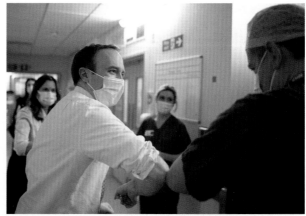

ABOVE LEFT With intensive care staff during a night shift at Basildon University Hospital in January 2021. The team were like so many across the NHS: brave, determined and compassionate. The night shift experience was harrowing and humbling in equal measure.

ABOVE RIGHT With handshaking out of the question, I took up the elbow bump. Here I am greeting staff at the Royal Marsden on World Cancer Day. They worked wonders to keep treatment going as much as possible.
© Simon Dawson / No. 10 Downing Street

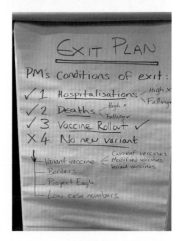

RIGHT In February 2021, I wrote down our early ideas for what became the roadmap that guided us out of lockdown.

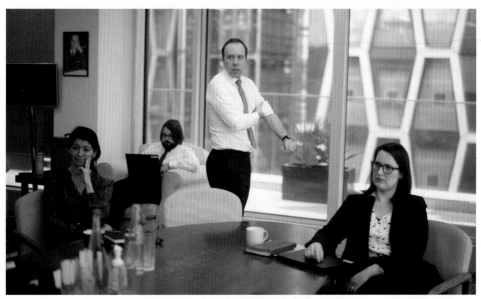

In my office working through and writing the February 2021 Commons statement in which I announced the hotel quarantine scheme. *Left to right: Gina Coladangelo, Joe Reddington and Emma Dean.*
© Simon Dawson / No. 10 Downing Street

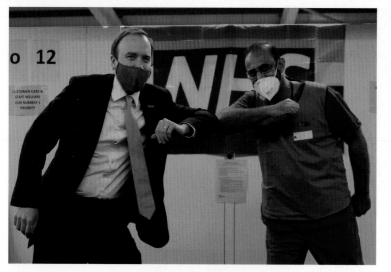

Another day and another elbow bump – this time with one of the wonderful medics at the Covid-19 vaccination centre at Stoke Mandeville Stadium in Aylesbury. We owe so much to the many thousands and thousands of volunteers who helped to administer the jabs. Thank you each and every one of you.

© Pippa Fowles / No. 10 Downing Street

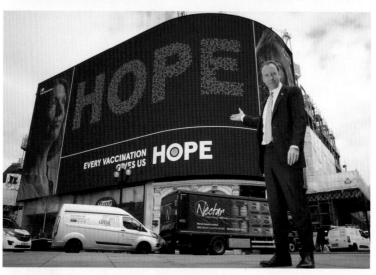

Launching our new push on vaccines in Piccadilly Circus in April 2021 – opening up access to people in their early forties… including me!

© Tim Hammond / No. 10 Downing Street

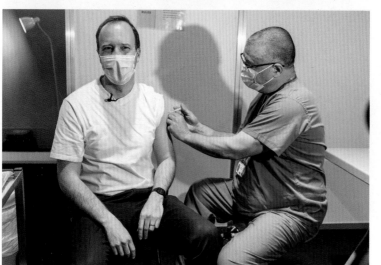

An incredible moment as deputy chief medical officer Jonathan Van-Tam gives me my very first vaccine shot at the Science Museum on 29 April 2021. We are both smiling broadly behind the masks. What a moment! A truly incredible feeling.

© Tim Hammond / No. 10 Downing Street

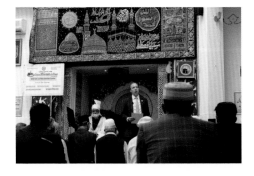

Speaking to worshippers at the Central Mosque of Brent. Many mosques and other places of worship did so much to reach people with the message of the importance of vaccination.

© Simon Dawson / No. 10 Downing Street

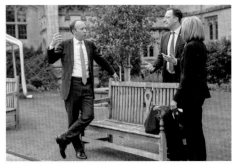

Chatting in the garden of Mansfield College, Oxford, during the G7 health summit with Jens Spahn, German Health Minister, and Stella Kyriakides, EU health commissioner. Jens was a true friend to Britain and a real support to me.

© No. 10 Downing Street

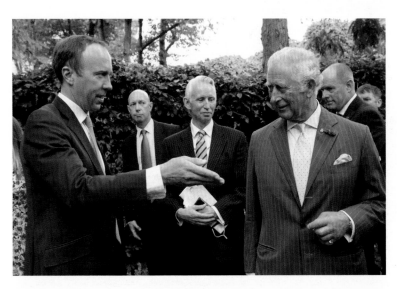

With the former Prince of Wales – now King Charles III – during a visit to the Chelsea and Westminster Hospital as part of the Prince's Trust NHS and Social Care scheme. I've always thoroughly enjoyed Charles's company and find him both interesting and charming.

© Tim Hammond / No. 10 Downing Street

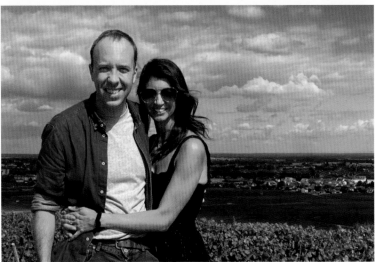

With Gina in the summer of 2021. Our relationship began unexpectedly, taking us both by surprise. It was publicly exposed after only a few weeks, causing huge pain to our families. We are now slowly rebuilding our lives, together.

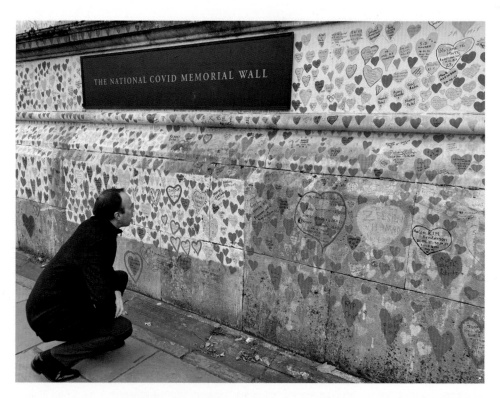

The National Covid Memorial Wall – a remarkable memorial to all those who lost their lives to Covid-19. Not a single day goes by that I don't think about those who either died or lost loved ones during this unprecedented global pandemic. Every heart symbolises a life. It's beautiful, powerful and truly touching.

team until two hours before the data went public at 4 p.m. While I was absorbing the full implications of this latest disaster – after all, case numbers shape our entire response to the pandemic – the PM sent me an ominous 'uh, oh… can we have a call later', which at least gave me some time to figure out what to do. By the time he and I eventually spoke, the Prof and I had worked out that the correct figures wouldn't have changed our response.

Chris did such a good job on the phone to the PM that he quickly agreed that the real data actually bears out all our arguments and that while the mistake is a very bad look, it doesn't change anything. It was some comfort to reflect that it would probably have been much worse to have dramatically *overstated* the figures, prompting unnecessary interventions.

SUNDAY 4 OCTOBER

I just don't understand what Kate Bingham is up to. She's been telling the *FT* we should only vaccinate the vulnerable. 'People keep talking about "time to vaccinate the whole population", but that is misguided,' she told them. Except she has nothing to do with the deployment – only the buying. And what she's criticising is the government's agreed policy.

Kate has done fantastic work on the contracts but has no place setting herself up as some kind of clinical expert on deployment when she's not.

'We absolutely need No. 10 to sit on her hard,' I told the SpAds, adding that I consider her 'totally unreliable'.

I've got Wormald on the case to try to explain the limits of her remit. It's a very peculiar fight to pick. Given she's so respected for the job she's so good at, why keep undermining the team and upsetting everyone?

The Tory Party conference is taking place online. Instead of the usual gig addressing the party faithful from a floodlit stage in a Birmingham or Manchester convention centre, I delivered my set piece to a Zoom screen, sitting in a glass tower in Canary Wharf with my friend Nimco Ali, the campaigner I got to know when I set up NHS clinics for women who've been subject to the horrendous and despicable practice of female genital mutilation. We were live-streamed from our empty room. It was really weird, and apart from the fun of doing a joint gig with Nimco, I hated it. I normally love the gregariousness of conference. The smallest of travails, of course, but I can't wait for the buzz of live audiences again.

MONDAY 5 OCTOBER

Plumbing new depths, PHE is trying to frame Dido for the data fiasco.

I messaged Damon Poole, who's replaced Jamie on my team, venting my frustration. 'Even more infuriating than their original fuck-up is them trying to shift the blame,' I said. It's yet another reason to drive through the reforms I've announced. We should have just one organisation responsible for pandemic response – and only pandemic response.

Meanwhile, for reasons best known to themselves, No. 10 is rowing back on tiers and has pulled the planned announcement from this week's grid. We need to act – preferably this week – with serious interventions in the north-east and north-west. 'How then are we going to control the virus given it's going tonto in about a quarter of the country?' I asked Cummings, genuinely bewildered. If we don't act now, it will be much worse later.

They want tough action; then they don't want tough action; then someone gets to the PM and he changes his mind all over again.

TUESDAY 6 OCTOBER

Lockdown-sceptic scientists have presented a grand plan for conquering Covid. Their genius idea? Protect the vulnerable and let everyone else crack on. It's another version of the old herd immunity argument. Led by Sunetra Gupta, a Stanford University professor called Jay Bhattacharya and a Harvard-based Swedish biostatistician named Martin Kulldorff, they've packaged this up as a 'declaration' signed at the American Institute for Economic Research in Great Barrington,

Massachusetts, and got a bunch of other academics on board. It's going to take a lot of effort to rebut. The number of professors from impressive universities who've signed up make it sound respectable enough to be a rallying point for sceptics. I looked through the names. No public health experts – mostly professors in random other subjects.

Having lobbied Boris the other day, Gupta is finding a ready audience in the White House. Yesterday she went with a couple of American professors to see my counterpart Alex Azar along with Scott Atlas, Trump's Covid adviser. I'm only relieved she didn't have any direct access to the President, who made a great song and dance about getting back from hospital today, whipping off his mask on the White House balcony and issuing bullish messages on social media about 'learning to live with Covid'. Just one problem: a lot of people don't learn to live with it; they die.

I saw myself in the new *Spitting Image* today. Hard to believe I'm featuring on the show I loved watching when I was growing up in the 1980s. My favourite puppet was John Gummer, Thatcher's Agriculture Minister. Surveying my puppet with a critical eye, I wasn't entirely unhappy. Though it doesn't sound anything like me, I was pleased to see it has plenty of hair.

The Economist has got wind of an old vaccine deployment plan. I instinctively asked my SpAds if Kate might be behind it.

'Well, I don't know that for sure, but I have some evidence to suggest it might have been, i.e. the fact she had a meeting yesterday with the journalist who has the story', came the reply. Who knows, but I wouldn't be surprised.

WEDNESDAY 7 OCTOBER

Daily infections are twice what they were a week ago and we've hit the miserable milestone of 100 new cases per 100,000 people in England. Just when we need unity, we've got more division and dither. Mayors, council leaders and MPs in the north are furious about local restrictions and clamouring for more Treasury money. Boris seems scared of them. He messaged me this morning asking how we can prove the NHS will be overwhelmed in the north-west and about space in the Nightingales. I replied that everything we're doing and saying is backed up by the data and the public is onside. He seemed unconvinced. 'We've chosen this plan. It's the right one, and the alternatives are catastrophic,' I told him firmly.

The surge is spreading into the over-sixties, and care home infections are rocketing again, mainly brought in by staff. Nadine had a meeting with Boris about care homes last night and says he now wants us to 'follow the approach in the Netherlands', which is more visitor-friendly. God knows who he's been talking to this time, but Helen Whately agrees: she fears our restrictions now mean too many care homes are allowing little to no visiting. She has asked her private office to ascertain whether that really is the PM's position and is checking with Jenny Harries. Meanwhile she suggests we refrain from publishing any more restrictive visiting guidance based on No. 10's previous 'ban visiting' steer.

'Well done. And 100 per cent agree with you,' I replied.

Let's hope we get a clear steer from Downing Street, because in the past they've been in favour of banning visitors. They're all over the place.

THURSDAY 8 OCTOBER

Boris has belatedly woken up to the fact that it's now going to take ages to build the forty new hospitals – including the one in his constituency.

'Aaaargh now I am being told that Hillingdon won't be done until 2030!!' he said. I stared at the message, suppressing the urge to scream.

Taking a deep breath, I calmly pointed out that the reason the new hospital earmarked for his constituency won't be built for the best part of another decade is that a) we didn't get going on this earlier, and b) HMT have only funded the first phase of the scheme.

'That's the official position because we only got £3.7 billion out of the Treasury,' I explained calmly. I told him I could find another way to do it for Hillingdon – but this would involve delaying other projects. He didn't reply.

More pressingly, the second peak is here. SAGE is waving every red flag it can find. ICU and hospital admissions are soaring close to early March levels. Case numbers are double the worst-case scenario from the summer and the increase is exponential. The scientists have demanded 'decisive interventions', especially in relation to restaurants and bars.

Nadine is utterly militant, urging me to be 'brutal'. She asked me why we aren't closing hospitality 'from midnight'.

'It'll be the Wild West over the weekend, not the north-west,' she fears.

FRIDAY 9 OCTOBER
JVT is worried that unless HMT gets its act together on clearing the funding for vaccines, we won't be able to hire the 25,000 vaccinators in time. He isn't sure if the block is Rishi or his officials, but either way, lives are at stake and it's us who'll get the blame if we don't hurry up. I promised to chase, saying I didn't think the issue was ministerial. JVT says similar bids into HMT have been taking three months to process.

'Three months?' I replied, shocked.

'No typo. Three months,' he confirmed. 'That is officials making work for themselves!'

'We've barely got three weeks, IMO,' he added.

Rishi and Steve Barclay have been brilliant on the buying of the actual vaccines – they get the importance of moving fast – but this is for the nuts and bolts of deployment. Unless they push the whole time, the machine goes through its normal grind for assessing a business case. The reason is to protect public money, which is vital, but business as usual doesn't work in a pandemic.

Later JVT sent me an alarming warning that we're on the verge of running out of the antiviral drug remdesivir because so many people are being hospitalised. Apparently we've got enough for the next ten days, after which we'll probably be short all winter. He says it's nobody's fault: we just can't get enough to meet hospital demand. Perhaps the thought of 'hospitals running out of drugs' headlines may concentrate the PM's mind on the need for stronger measures.

SATURDAY 10 OCTOBER

Boris has finally agreed to announce tiers on Monday.

Starmer's been at his most sanctimonious, puffing about it being 'grossly irresponsible' for details to come out via media briefings etc. It's Labour at their worst, focusing on the comms when they don't have anything of substance to say – and when the briefings are almost certainly coming from the Labour mayors anyway.

I texted Steve Barclay about the vaccine rollout money, doing my best to highlight the importance of pushing it through fast. He was constructive and said senior officials are meeting soon to sort it.

We gave the Sunday papers some interesting polling numbers. Only 15 per cent think current restrictions are too strict and 45 per cent say they should be stricter, while 75 per cent support local lockdowns. 'The people are with us,' I told Damon.

One of the papers is running a rubbish – and untrue – story tomorrow that I broke the rules by having a glass of white wine after 10 p.m. on Monday night in the smoking room at the Commons. Bollocks. I left before the vote at 9.40 p.m. and didn't go back. The Deputy Speaker is my witness! An irritating distraction.

SUNDAY 11 OCTOBER

Nadine is feeling undervalued and wants more airtime. I received a plaintive message from her this morning saying that every time there's a media request for her it gets blocked by the SpAds, even on mental health, which is her patch. She's especially aggrieved that Sky went to Alastair Campbell after someone this end stopped her going on and says there's always 'some spurious excuse'.

'I'm done with it now,' she concluded darkly. I resolved to be more appreciative.

Nadhim Zahawi passed on some exciting intel from Kate, who expects Pfizer to be the first vaccine approved. I'd love Oxford to get there first, but the key thing is we get the public jabbed as soon as possible with a safe, effective vaccine.

A really alarming Covid-O this afternoon. 'Never been on a meeting like it... I do not think we are doing enough, and we know it,' I told Damon afterwards. Too many in government are running scared of further measures, even though the Prof believes Tier 3's too weak and the public want more.

'A conversation among people who don't want to act, clutching at straws,' I told the team wearily.

But if we don't take the tough action we need now, we will end up in national lockdown. The numbers are clear as day and they're exponential. At least I've got Gove onside – and Boris has squared Rishi – so the weak policy proposed got through unscathed.

MONDAY 12 OCTOBER

A carefully orchestrated day announcing the tiers, which come in on Wednesday.

At the morning COBRA we signed it all off, after some late haggling. The final package has made concessions to the mayors by – infuriatingly – softening Tier 3 even more while giving them the option of bringing in tougher measures locally, which of course sacrifices the clarity that's meant to be the main selling point.

Then a press conference like no other, with the PM saying that a national lockdown will do 'a lot of immediate harm', so 'we don't want to go down that extreme route right now', while the Prof warned that Tier 3 won't work on its own and local areas will have to do more than the minimum required by law if we're going to suppress it.

I've never seen a performance like it. There's the PM announcing a policy to the nation, and the government's top expert beside him basically saying it won't work. In the six weeks since I proposed the tiers system there's been delay and watering down at every stage – while the virus has grown faster than the worst-case scenario. What's most frustrating is that I'm being portrayed as the one who's pushing for lockdown, whereas actually it's those with their heads in the sand who will lead us to a full-blown national lockdown unless they agree to action now.

TUESDAY 13 OCTOBER

The debate and vote in the Commons on tiers were pretty straight-forward, which gave me a chance to lay into the so-called Barrington Declaration from Gupta et al. I did my best to demolish the argument, explaining that you can't *just* shield the vulnerable. Of course we're doing that, but it's not enough. What about everyone who looks after them? In turn, what about those who come in contact with carers? And so on and so on.

MPs didn't seem to need much persuading, and the measures whistled through.

We've had our first big delivery of the new lateral flow tests. Four million. I sent Boris a picture of them being loaded onto the plane. Hooray – testing and vaccinating the whole population is our route to normality.

WEDNESDAY 14 OCTOBER

Shades of PretGate. Tiers came in today and we ran straight into a ridiculous row over pub snacks.

One of the concessions on Tier 3 was that pubs can open if they serve 'substantial meals'. Cue a barrage of entirely predictable questions about whether salted peanuts and pickled onions are meals if you buy enough of them. It's a stupid bureaucratic phrase, put in because the Cabinet Office assured us it's got an existing definition in licensing law. But no one's ever heard that, and it's wide open to ridicule.

Rob Jenrick was doing a solid job navigating the morning media round until LBC asked whether a Cornish pasty would count. My heart sank a fathom. Is a pasty a substantial meal? Apparently yes, if served with salad and chips; but not without. Are pasties something Tory veterans of the coalition years want to be discussing again? No thank you. Fortunately for Jenrick, he was not involved in the 2012 Budget debacle over the so-called pasty tax, but I was and I still bear the scars. I love them, but I never want to talk about them again.

Someone put it about that I'm the source of an anonymous quote in the *Telegraph* saying there's an 80 per cent chance of a national circuit breaker within four weeks. Not true – I'm in favour of tougher local measures to avoid a national lockdown. I actually think I've made progress on this with Boris. At our early morning catch-up I showed him an outline of next week's circuit breaker in Northern Ireland. He said we should impose this in the worst areas in England, though without the school closures. I capitalised, telling him we must drive this through – no half measures – or the NHS will be overwhelmed. We have already lost a week.

What I don't need is a rear-guard action from the Treasury, who are briefing against any new measures.

'I need to go hard on "delayed action means more economic pain", I told Damon in frustration.

THURSDAY 15 OCTOBER

I announced that London and a few other places are going into Tier 2 from Saturday.

The original draft statement was quite bullish on vaccines, but No. 10 freaked, ordering me to delete anything that made it sound as if we think vaccines are the way out. This really annoyed me, *because they are the way out.* Since that's our strategy, it's ridiculous to be told I can't say it.

Even Jim thought the original version was too punchy (or 'bombastic', he put it. Ouch.) '"Mass vaccination centres" sounds too "Bill Gates microchips", he warned. He thinks phrases like 'at speed' make it sound like we're rushing it. He thought it was in danger of becoming 'fodder for the David Icke brigade'.

So I told No. 10 I'd take the vaccines stuff out on this occasion, 'but since that's our strategy it's hard not to repeat it'. Perhaps No. 10 should spend more time and effort getting the Chancellor to support the government position on suppressing the virus? I will not be blown off the vaccine drive by the sceptics – in No. 10 or anywhere else.

As for Tier 3, it's as clear as day we need to put Liverpool and Greater Manchester in. The data doesn't lie. The figures are shooting up. I spoke to Joe Anderson, the Mayor of the City of Liverpool (not to be confused with the Mayor for the Liverpool City Region – unbelievably, there are two overlapping mayors). Joe is being incredibly reasonable and working with us well.

But Burnham is cutting up rough and 'leaking like a sieve', as I put it to Helen Whately. He went in front of the cameras on the steps of Manchester Central Library, claimed the region was being treated as 'canaries in the coalmine', refused a local lockdown but called for a national one, and asked for more money than Liverpool despite the measures being the same. His degree of politicking is outrageous – and we'll see the damage it does if we can't get him over the line.

The view ahead looks horrible. France, which is only a week or two in front of us in the trajectory, has had over 30,000 infections in twenty-four hours. We're a shade under 20,000 and SAGE has said the R rate's now up to 1.3–1.5. Infections and hospital admissions are above the worst-case scenario and deaths are heading for that territory within two weeks.

FRIDAY 16 OCTOBER
Boris has been studying what they did during the plague and messaged this morning about how tiering worked in the old days.

'In 1606 the Privy Council decreed that theatres should be closed if deaths from plague exceeded thirty per week,' he told us.

'Not sure about these fixed thresholds,' I replied warily, given the debate we've been having about whether to formalise when an area goes into measures. I tried to imagine how it would feel to be very ill with Covid, knowing that if you didn't make it, part of your legacy would be to plunge an entire area into lockdown.

'Plague orders had a lot of similarities including isolation, contact tracing, quarantine for new arrivals, a ban on people meeting in groups. Penalties for breaking isolation a bit stiffer however,' the Prof replied helpfully.

Thankfully this was the end of the history lesson.

SATURDAY 17 OCTOBER

Woke up to another briefing against me from No. 10, this time in the *i*. Apparently 'Matt Hancock is the only person here who thinks there is actually going to be a vaccine … It's a running joke with other departments.' If so, I'm happy to own it. I'm certainly not going to let it deflect me from pushing vaccines at maximum speed. Thank God I banned the team from talking to No. 10 about the rollout. They just trash it.

The new rules putting London and other places up a tier came in at midnight, but the app only started updating users at 8 a.m. Apparently the Cabinet Office told the app people not to send alerts at midnight in case they woke everyone up. Sigh. I think most phone users have cottoned on to silent mode!

Joe Anderson gave me the awful news that his brother died of Covid last night. He's going to point to his loss to reinforce the message of just how dangerous the disease is. 'Stick to your guns on Manchester,' he urged. Welcome support from an unexpected quarter.

Had a bit of a counselling session from Nadine this evening. She told me to 'be bold' and wants me in full attack mode like I was when I took apart Great Barrington. 'You need to do it more often. You are too nice too often,' she told me. Yes, but it's important to pick the right fights. We need our MPs onside.

SUNDAY 18 OCTOBER

The *Telegraph* found out that I intervened to get Blair out of quarantine when he came back from the White House and is having a go. I make no apology: Blair may no longer be in government but he's a former Prime Minister and was quite clearly on diplomatic business. Even junior ministers are exempt from quarantine for such purposes.

The *Observer* also had a weird story about the department agreeing to give the police contact details for people who fail to self-isolate, which they've whipped into a privacy scandal. The whole thing was news to me. On enquiry, it turns out that officials unilaterally agreed the policy with the Home Office. Nobody thought to run it by ministers. So frustrating.

Cummings says he was told all the data given to the police would be anonymised (though I'm not sure how that would work) while the Prof says nobody told him or consulted him. I'm furious this went to Cummings but nobody bothered to ask me. It's another example of how he screws up lines of accountability: it's my head on the block for a decision I wasn't a part of. I reminded private office: big decisions like this *need to come to me*. He's an unelected adviser and this isn't how democracy works.

MONDAY 19 OCTOBER

Patrick Vallance seems almost as nervous as Downing Street about talking up vaccines. He's told the National Security Committee in Parliament that he doesn't think they will be in widespread use before next spring. I stand by my view that things will happen more quickly. And it's about delivery risk: if no one in the NHS thinks they'll be here any earlier, we won't be ready if we defy expectations and get there sooner. It's a happy irony to be worrying about the best-case scenario on something, having worried about worst-case scenarios all year.

For now, the virus is out-running us. We announced 18,804 new cases and eighty deaths today and we've got 592 people on ventilators. We've put more regions into Tier 3 and Wales has announced a two-week firebreak lockdown. How long can we hold off from a full national lockdown?

On the upside, we're making real progress on Moonshot. Trials of rapid tests are starting in hospitals then going into care homes. We've got 20 million kits on order.

Jim has been doing some thinking about vaccine distribution and worries that it may look as if we're prioritising people who vote Tory, which we certainly are not. He fears there could also be a BAME dimension to this, because many BAME communities are comparatively young. I think what he's saying is that if we're not careful, we may be accused of racism, however ridiculous that suggestion would be. To cover our backs, he suggests we ensure we secure strong justification for all our decisions from trusted third parties, and be ready for any kind of judicial review. Wise.

TUESDAY 20 OCTOBER

Talks with Burnham have broken down, and the PM announced Greater Manchester will go into Tier 3 from Thursday. Burnham walked away over a demand for £5 million more cash than Liverpool got. He only wanted it so he could crow that he squeezed more out of Boris – and I'm sure he preferred the local lockdown to be imposed so he didn't have to sign up to it. It's such awful, negative politicking. We should have imposed this last week when we acted on Liverpool, and not given him the space to play politics with people's lives.

Before the PM's announcement, Andy was outside the Bridgewater Hall doing one of his al fresco briefings when Sir Richard Leese, the council leader, showed him a text message tipping him off. Burnham went full drama queen for the cameras, feigning shock and horror. 'It's brutal, to be honest, isn't it?' he said. It's just such obvious game playing. I hope no one falls for it.

WEDNESDAY 21 OCTOBER

DCMS is lobbying for a relaxation of the rules on Remembrance Sunday so people at the Cenotaph, including the royals and the PM, can sing the national anthem. Of course we should say yes! It's a bit like keeping professional sport going – very small numbers but highly symbolic. It's the kind of thing Boris really cares about and sends out a positive message that some things are bigger even than this disease.

THURSDAY 22 OCTOBER

Jim is still very worried about the anti-vax nutters. He thinks we should try to introduce a public health sanction on publishing disinformation, perhaps tacking something on to the dreaded 1984 Act. He says companies like Twitter and Facebook are still blasé about their responsibilities because they don't think we really have the power to take any action against them. I've got another meeting with the social media companies coming up, during which he thinks I should say I'm prepared to use emergency regulation if necessary.

He also asked me how to deal with what he called an 'eccentric request' from No. 10 to switch the branding on entrances to Test and Trace sites from the NHS logo to the HM government one to look more authoritative. He asked whether to 'roll with it or tell them to take a jump?' Frankly I'm surprised. Why do they want to own something they currently consider a mess? Actually it's a good sign, suggesting they are confident it's heading in the right direction. Either way, I won't let them steal it. By way of compromise, I suggested we use both.

Late message from JVT, who says we've 'rescued the national anthem', i.e. won the argument that the risk posed by singing 'God Save the Queen' at a socially distanced outdoor remembrance service is acceptable.

'Great man,' I replied.

Boris damned Dido with faint praise at the press conference, saying only that Test and Trace helps 'a bit'. Not helpful.

FRIDAY 23 OCTOBER

Burnham has achieved what every true socialist craves: a fawning profile in *The Guardian* – 'king of the north', 'future PM', 'his eyelashes' etc. Recently he's been acting more like a pumped-up Peter Soulsby.

SATURDAY 24 OCTOBER

Mounting concerns over clinical trials of new treatments for conditions other than Covid. In theory, it's business as usual for trials of drugs for cancer, dementia etc. In practice, nobody is volunteering, I suppose partly because they're trying to stay away from hospitals and partly because the NHS is so focused on Covid. Jim thinks the whole clinical trial system is 'broke'.

He thinks there is too much reliance on goodwill: insufficient alignment of interests, too much clunky and duplicative bureaucracy and no data standardisation.

Added to that, he says, the Vaccine Taskforce is set to take up 'a HUGE amount of the critical and shockingly limited research nurse capacity' as they trial three to four vaccines over the next few months and measure the effects of any we roll out. He is extremely worried about the impact on life-saving research and suggests that we make 'opting in' to trials the default for patients unless they specifically opt out, taking the pressure off recruitment.

'We've been obliged to make many changes to suit Covid, many of them quite enlightened,' he pointed out, asking my view. He rightly says that there is a big bottleneck here with huge implications. He thinks it's justified to keep the research show on the road. I strongly agree, but it will take work and we will need the Prof onside.

Downing Street has started talking about Christmas. Yesterday they briefed the lobby that we 'could be able to get some aspects of our lives back to normal' by then. Vaughan Gething claims the firebreak lockdown in Wales is the best chance of making that happen. How to manage the festive season is a very sensitive question.

Damon alerted me to a bloke called Rocco Forte calling for my head in tomorrow's *Mail on Sunday*. 'Who is Rocco Forte?' I replied. I've genuinely never heard of him. Apparently, he owns some hotels and donated to the Brexit campaign. Oh.

SUNDAY 25 OCTOBER

Poor Dido is being blasted by the lockdown sceptics, who have decided she's to blame for everything they don't like about our response to the pandemic.

The backbench veteran Sir Bernard Jenkin has publicly called for her head, saying she 'should be given a well-earned rest'.

That was as diplomatic as he got in a full-frontal attack at the 'vacuum of leadership' at Test and Trace, which he thinks is 'destroying public confidence and compliance'. He thinks there's a 'spaghetti junction of command and control' at the top of the organisation and says Dido should be moved on to focus on 'lessons learned', i.e. put out to pasture. It's an irony that the central problem in testing throughout has been Cummings's long screwdriver.

To their credit, Downing Street launched a rear-guard action to try to take the heat off Dido by briefing that we're thinking of reducing the fourteen-day self-isolation period for people coming back from abroad to seven days.

Amid the chaos, they forgot to tell either me or Grant Shapps, who went nuts.

The Cabinet Office apologised, saying they'd been preoccupied by trying to stop the Sunday media totally unreasonably calling for Dido's head on a plate, with some success. Given the ferocity of the ad hominem attacks, I very much doubt that is much consolation to Dido. I told them that we need to back her all the way. 'The worst of all worlds is a wounded Test and Trace,' I added.

The Cabinet Office seemed genuinely taken aback by the hostile media coverage and asked if I'd been in contact with her. I reassured them that we have spoken and she is phlegmatic.

The seven-day average for cases is over 15,000 and curving steeply up. 'Ugly' was the Cabinet Office reaction. Patrick says none of it is looking good and a lot of hospitalisations and deaths are inevitable.

'We don't have much time to correct,' he added.

My daughter's birthday. It being a Sunday, I'm home to celebrate.

TUESDAY 27 OCTOBER

Could Labradors be our secret weapon against the pandemic? A bizarre and cheering morning finding out, watching disease-detecting dogs on the concourse at Paddington Station demonstrate what they can do on a crowd that included the Duchess of Cornwall. I smiled respectfully at all the right moments, but inside I was panicking. I couldn't stop worrying that the mutts might pick out Camilla, or indeed me, as having the dreaded disease. 'Please, please, don't do that,' I willed silently. Luckily the Labs didn't let the side down and correctly identified the man with the T-shirt that had an infected patient's scent on it. I was impressed.

These dogs can pick up the scent of Covid just like they pick up the scent of drugs. They're not 100 per cent accurate – but you can now use one of our new lateral flow tests to double check. I want them at airports and train stations to sniff out super-spreaders.

The department's briefing was: 'Evidence base too thin.' It's absurd. Just because they aren't conventional, officialdom can't see the point. I've pushed it and asked Jim to follow up. They'd certainly be cheaper than Moonshot.

WEDNESDAY 28 OCTOBER

The trajectory for hospitalisations is horrendous. I circulated a graph to the ministerial team showing we're on track to fill up all NHS beds by 17 December. Nadine responded with a four-letter word, followed by: 'We have to lock down.'

I spoke to the major health bodies: the royal colleges, the NHS Confederation, the BMA and the RCN. I took their view – all thought we need to do more – and encouraged them to push for action.

The direction of travel is clear. Macron's announced a lockdown for France until at least 1 December, and Merkel's ordered Germany to do similar. Ed Llewellyn in Paris thinks we should reach out to Macron and offer to treat some of their cases. Fantastic idea. I shared an office with Ed for five years in opposition, and he's a brilliant, creative diplomat. Because our problem is regional, we still have spare capacity in areas where cases are low. I messaged Boris suggesting it, but no reply.

We're continuing to think about Christmas. I talked to the devolved Health Ministers about coordinating. They all wanted to bat it up the chain to their First Ministers. Understandable – their bosses see diverging from England as a badge of honour, so figuring out a Christmas truce among devolved nations will take endless diplomacy to navigate the separatist politics.

THURSDAY 29 OCTOBER

We're putting so many new areas into Tier 3 that it'll soon be a national lockdown in all but name. SAGE warned that every family Christmas gathering will be a potential 'super-spreader event'. Everything is now geared towards saving the festive season. I am incredibly frustrated. Had we brought in tougher tiers three weeks ago, as the Prof and I were arguing for, we wouldn't be in this position. And for goodness sake, why aren't we pushing harder on ventilation as well as masks? We have known since a Spanish study proved it in the summer that Covid spreads more like smoke than droplets – yet the comms is still geared to masks, which are less important than ventilation.

FRIDAY 30 OCTOBER

A day of high drama and farce. Things started promisingly enough, with Simon Case and I talking battle plans ahead of a crunch meeting with Boris over the case for a national lockdown. Unfortunately, we were derailed by Cummings's continuing insistence that ministerial meetings are held by Zoom. I wasn't too fussed about this – we are used to it by now, and clearly it makes sense to reduce the risk of infection – till I spotted Rishi slipping into the PM's office. Meanwhile Simon was ninety miles away, struggling to hear any of it on 'terrible rural broadband'. Luckily he still had a strong enough signal to WhatsApp. 'Rishi is in the room, contrary to Cummings's stupid rules – so the PM will be under enormous pressure not to do enough once again,' I texted furiously.

To my surprise, the Cabinet Office reported that the Chancellor had already resigned himself to the national lockdown. Apparently his only question (and a fair one) is about non-essential retail – where obviously we have little evidence of transmission either way. He thinks it would be better to do something in secondary schools, where we know transmission takes place, instead of closing all shops, where we just don't know.

I can live with that, though I'm more worried about a rear-guard action from HMT to persuade Boris not to lock down. This has screwed us all over too often.

The Cabinet Office replied that when they spoke to the PM earlier today, he actually seemed less convinced than Rishi of the need for action and was really kicking back.

This was ominous and underlined the need for me to be in Downing Street, rather than making the case as a disembodied (and easily muted) head on a screen. They agreed that it is impossible to operate like this.

'It is humiliating and counterproductive,' I replied, asking them to override Cummings's rule. Surely any self-respecting official should see that the government functions more effectively with the right people in the room for the big decisions. It's even more bizarre than usual because Dom basically shares my view on this issue.

Against this extremely unsatisfactory backdrop, we agreed that all we could do at that particular meeting was confront Boris with horrible data then have a proper meeting on action later.

This afternoon I was called to a meeting of Covid-S, the strategy group chaired by the PM. This time it was in person in the Cabinet Room, and the only ministers invited were me, Rishi and Michael Gove. What followed was an hour and a half of intense discussion. My central argument was that we must learn from history, not repeat it. At the end: victory. Boris took considerable persuasion, but eventually he grudgingly accepted the stark, painful facts: that cases, hospitalisations and deaths are all rising exponentially and the NHS will run out of space unless we act. The upshot is four weeks of lockdown from next Thursday then back to souped-up tiers. Full announcement on Monday.

I had not even made it back to the department when I got a message from Steve Swinford at *The Times* asking me to call him as he was 'picking up some suggestions on your position re. national lockdown'. Then similar from Gordon Rayner at the *Telegraph*. How much have they heard? Who from? I batted it over to Damon.

Having won the lockdown argument, I was exhausted but elated and literally ran up the stairs to my office, stopping off at the seventh floor to see the Prof, who'd fought hard alongside me via Zoom.

'Well, thank God we got that,' I said.

'Secretary of State, you've saved many lives with what you've done today,' he replied.

After all the tension, this caught me up short.

'Well, I don't feel particularly good about it,' I replied falteringly.

'No, I imagine you feel like a general after winning a battle when there are bodies strewn all around you. But you've done a great thing,' he said – a reference to the famous Wellington quote after Waterloo: 'Nothing except a battle lost can be half so melancholy as a battle won.'

As I headed off to Suffolk, I finally relaxed. We took the children for a curry at Montaz in Newmarket, where the staff seemed excited to see us and were so kind and welcoming. It was horrible to think they were going to have to close again on Thursday and I couldn't tell them.

I really, really wanted to forget the pandemic, just for half an hour, and was doing my best to ignore my phone when Robert Peston's number flashed up. We were only halfway through the main course. I glanced at it surreptitiously, hoping the kids wouldn't see me – and almost choked on my chapati.

'I understand that this pm you, PM, Chancellor, CDL [Chancellor of the Duchy of Lancaster, Michael Gove] met. Am told 99 per cent likely there will be a full national lockdown from next Wed or Thurs,' Peston said.

So the cat is out of the bag – already! Furious, I forwarded the message to my SpAds and No. 10 comms. Who told Peston? How on earth had it leaked already? Only a handful of people knew!

By the time I got home, I had an enraged Boris on the phone saying his media people had told him hacks were pointing the finger at me.

'Whoever is telling you that is lying to you,' I replied furiously. He should know as a former journalist that no hack will give up their sources to anyone. Then he said he has to decide if what's been briefed will happen. 'I don't care what you do so long as we stick with the lockdown,' I said, 'You can't let outrageous behaviour like this cost any more lives.'

How had this happened? My money is firmly on Cummings via his acolytes. The agenda? To bounce the PM into announcing the lockdown sooner than later and stop him U-turning. If they got me sacked into the bargain, that would be a bonus.

By now I was being bombarded with calls from journos. I ignored them all. I texted the PM to say that obviously the accusations against me were untrue and 'I can prove if necessary'. This leaking is corrosive and completely counterproductive.'

Half an hour later he messaged asking me and Damon to bring our phones into Downing Street on Monday.

'With pleasure,' I replied coldly, following up with a long message telling him categorically that I don't leak and neither does Damon. Peston wouldn't have texted me asking for confirmation if I was the source. Plus: *cui bono* – it's not like I benefit from this information being out early. 'I'm taking a huge amount of flak to do the right thing and protecting you in the process,' I said.

'Understood, everyone overwrought,' he replied soothingly, but with Cummings dripping poison in his ear, I very much doubt that will be the end of it.

So after all our efforts, everything hangs in the balance. Either the PM has to rush into announcing and confirm the lockdown or there's such a backlash, especially from our truculent backbenchers, that he bottles it again. It would be a huge mistake if that happens.

Later Simon Case sent me tomorrow's *Mail* front-page headline: 'National lockdown next week'. He added a row of question marks and a dark warning that collective discussions will be much harder (i.e. less frequent) now.

'It's a fucking disgrace,' I replied. 'I hope you have a full inquiry.' It's offensive he's even suggesting I'm responsible for this sort of behaviour.

As lockdown approaches, I should be focused on getting the new measures right, testing, and the vaccine to get us all out of this nightmare. Instead I'm fighting for my political life. This is no way to run a country.

SATURDAY 31 OCTOBER

I hardly slept. The lockdown sceptics are going crazy. Nadine, who plays a key role in trying to manage Tory backbenchers, told me there was a mood of 'slowly building hysteria'.

Then confirmation this morning that the timetable for the announcement would be crunched, with Boris holding a press conference this afternoon. The start date is still Thursday.

We spent hours on the phone to ministers and MPs – a weekend's work crammed into a few hours – with Allan sending them graphs showing the facts for their area and what would happen if we did nothing. I briefed Labour, who are onside. Jonathan Ashworth deserves an honour for doing the right thing for the country. Consternation from friends about how it all came out. Jim described it as 'the fastest leak since Nick Clegg was on world-record form' – he was notorious when we were in coalition. Nadine was raging, telling me the culprit 'needs putting in front of a firing squad'.

'You're telling me,' I replied.

As if the day could get any worse, arch-lockdown sceptic Steve Baker went into No. 10 to see Boris and let rip. This could have ended very badly indeed. To his credit, Boris talked him round, to the point that Steve even posted a helpful message on Twitter, saying everyone should 'listen carefully to the Prime Minister'.

'We all need to think forward several weeks to the circumstances we could face,' he said.

The press conference was originally scheduled for 5 p.m., but amid all the chaos it was closer to seven by the time Boris, the Prof and Patrick got to the lecterns. First the scientists presented the data in all its starkness, underlined by the 326 deaths in the past twenty-four hours, the highest number since 29 May. The PM followed and gave it his all, warning of thousands of deaths a day if we don't do more.

'The over-running of the NHS would be a medical and a moral disaster ... Now is the time to take action, because there is no alternative,' he declared. No more contradictions and half measures today. He is such a communications bulldozer: when he's pointing in the right direction, he just ploughs through.

Lockdown will be a little lighter than last time because we've got better evidence about what works. Outdoor exercise will be encouraged and schools will stay open, but otherwise it is full-on.

'Well,' I replied to a message from Jeremy Hunt after Boris had fin-ished. 'You wanted a sense of where things are up to!'

'Sense you have won a big victory,' he replied.

After the flak I've taken over the past twenty-four hours, I don't feel triumphant, but hopefully we've avoided a complete collapse in the NHS and those Lombardy scenes in our hospitals.

NOVEMBER 2020

SUNDAY 1 NOVEMBER

'The optimist returns!' Boris cried, surveying a graph showing a tiny dip in the R number in the past twenty-four hours. Last night's storm had subsided and there was no mention of leak inquiries, but he was still far from reconciled to the lockdown he had so grudgingly authorised. His lingering doubts were fuelled by a long phone call with Professor Carl Heneghan, who did his best to persuade the PM that the death modelling is wrong. As he was listening to Heneghan, periodically grunting his agreement, he was simultaneously WhatsApping me and the Prof, sharing links to the supposedly flawed data.

Poring over the latest figures, he continued to fret that we will be accused of 'blinking too soon'. Simon Case and I, who were fielding his messages, kept our cool and waited for him to move on. Later Simon called me and said he'd better have a briefing on the vaccine rollout plans. I said by the end of the week I'd be ready to present them to him and then to the PM. They're pretty well baked now – but I've still got to protect them and make sure there's no interference or meddling from Downing Street. It's no way to work, but I don't want Cummings to mess it up.

I spent most of the day dealing with questions about the rules. Nadine had done an amazing job with backbenchers and says the majority of our lot are now onside. Less encouraging was the discovery that Cummings is deliberately ignoring my calls and messages. It is extraordinary. We're in the middle of a national crisis in which hundreds of people are dying every day and, whether he likes it or not, I'm in charge of the health service. Yet he now won't talk to me. It's pathetic, petty and downright irresponsible.

MONDAY 2 NOVEMBER
Boris is fascinated by a grand experiment taking place in Slovakia, where the government is said to be making the entire population take a Covid test on the same day. It's a massive operation involving 8,000 soldiers, 15,000 medics and 5,000 testing stations. Slovakia has a tiny population (just 5.4 million), so it would be hard to scale, but it will be interesting to see how it plays out.

TUESDAY 3 NOVEMBER
Finally some movement on social care reform. Given that it was a manifesto pledge, Boris is trying to get it moving, knowing how important it is to so many people. Senior advisers from Nos 10 and 11 met today to try to thrash out a way forward. Munira Mirza and Cummings represented the PM, Liam Booth-Smith represented the Chancellor, and Emma Dean represented me.

Emma says Boris is 'holding firm at the moment' that it has to happen.

'Yes, it does,' I replied immediately. I told her we absolutely must keep pushing for the implementation of Andrew Dilnot's recommendations, which are now almost ten years old and needed more than ever.

Meanwhile I think someone's trying to smear me. First I'm falsely accused of being in a Commons bar after 10 p.m., then I'm falsely accused of leaking, and now *The Sun* wants to know if I went to have a haircut with Michael Gove at the weekend. Nothing to declare there: Michael and I have shared many good times together over the years, but our relationship does not quite extend to joint trips to the barber. However, the drip-drip is concerning and is getting so tiresome. Later one of my allies received a message from a Sunday newspaper journalist saying, 'We need to talk about who is framing Matt at some stage...' I think I can take an educated guess.

There's a leak about the vaccine rollout starting in early December. Obviously this is my hope – and I'm setting the system up to be ready – but it's hugely risky and may not even happen before Christmas, so I messaged Raab asking if he could play it down on tomorrow's morning media round. 'We have always said the best-case scenario is a vaccine in December and so are preparing in case, but it is emphatically not our central expectation and no vaccine is certain,' I told him.

I think he'll be helpful.

What No. 10 really wants to announce is a new 'test and release' scheme to reduce the length of time people have to self-isolate. They're getting irritated with Dido for taking so long to make it happen. She says it will be another two weeks – there are changes to the app needed and other technical fixes – prompting a sulk from Cummings, who says that in that case, we might as well not bother. In normal times, driving through a major change in two weeks would be regarded as warp-speed.

I'm seeing Simon at the end of this week to talk about plans for the vaccine rollout – a very important meeting.

The presidential election is under way. I can't stay up all night to watch results coming in but am desperately hoping for a Biden win. Trump has been so awful in this pandemic. It would be such a relief to have some rationality in the White House and to restore some Western leadership and resolve.

WEDNESDAY 4 NOVEMBER

The job today was to win the Commons debate ahead of the vote on Covid measures. I knew I'd be time-constrained summing up, and after responding to all the MPs who'd spoken, I would only have about 200 words to win over anyone still sitting on the fence. I told my team they had to be the best 200 words ever written, reminding them that the Gettysburg Address was only 272. They did a decent job, though I doubt my speech will go down in history. Unhelpfully, the PM sauntered out of the Chamber just as Theresa May got to her feet to speak, which looked disrespectful and won't have done us any favours. All the same, we won the vote convincingly: 516–38 – although with an ominous thirty-four Conservative MPs against.

Feeling pleased enough with how things had gone, I headed back to the office. I had barely sat down when the Prof rang, quietly informing me that there's a new drama. After reflecting on the Commons debate and the scale of the majority for the measures, he mentioned that there is a problem with mink in Denmark. There's new evidence of the disease incubating in these farmed animals and, crucially, a new variant going back from mink to humans. Worse still, it may be resistant to any vaccine.

I asked him whether we should immediately shut the travel corridor between the UK and Denmark. Ever mindful not to step out of line, he said that this would be a call for ministers, but his clinical view was that acting immediately on a precautionary basis 'wouldn't be disproportionate'.

I called Grant Shapps, who agreed. 'If it puts the vaccine project at risk, let's get on with it,' he said. So, with his support, I called Michael to set up a formal meeting in the morning and asked for a briefing on my desk for 8 a.m.

THURSDAY 5 NOVEMBER
'How many mink are there in the UK?' Emma Dean asked anxiously.

Thankfully, none in captivity: fur farms have been banned since 2000. There are quite a lot in the wild, but they steer clear of humans. In Denmark there have already been twelve cases of the virus jumping from the animals to humans, and they are culling all 17 million of their farmed mink. Denmark is going into lockdown: this type of zoonotic disease is not to be messed with. The chief vet here is following up to see what it might mean for wider species mutations and risk. The result:

we're going to close the travel corridor with Denmark and effectively shut it off to all travel – including for lorry drivers. I've been warned that it could lead to a short-term shortage of some meat but decided to press ahead anyway. I'd prefer to skip a rasher of bacon than run the risk of, effectively, a whole new disease arriving from Denmark.

The decision made, it was up to Grant to announce, so I spent much of the morning dealing with an urgent parliamentary question about how Covid regulations affect the law surrounding assisted dying abroad. The issue is whether voluntary euthanasia could be classed as a 'medical procedure', for which people can travel freely. What a heart-wrenching debate and what irony: to protect the living, we've brought in measures that could prolong the suffering of the dying.

FRIDAY 6 NOVEMBER

Ahead of the announcement, I asked Simon Case whether the PM had been fully briefed on the Danish mink scenario. 'Yes! Bizarre and worrying,' he replied. I told him we are not taking any chances. The new strain has four different spike proteins and does not appear to respond to neutralising antibodies.

Jim represented the department at a G7 meeting, sending me periodic updates (Canada 'clearly struggling with testing'; US 'short of gloves and gowns'; Germany grappling with older demographic; France reducing quarantine from fourteen days to a week 'to make it more acceptable' and also has a national curfew but is 'not sure if it's working').

I suggested we reach out to the Americans and offer to help with their PPE crisis: we've now got more than we know what to do with. 'From memory, £30 billion on order, and something like £20 billion delivered already. Rishi would be happy if we could sell a few,' Jim replied.

As his turn approached to speak at the meeting, Jim reported that everyone was 'very glum'. I agreed that he should try to strike a more positive note and could at least be upbeat about the vaccine and mass testing.

I'm taking the G7 chair next year and want to put the rocket boosters under it. I've sat through enough boring G7 and G20 meetings and don't want to preside over any more. The whole set-up only really works when there's a substantial issue to discuss. I've asked Jim to think about how we can liven things up.

Simon Case called to discuss whole-population testing. Downing Street wants to appoint a general to oversee it and report daily to COBRA. That's fine if we can work out how responsibility for mass testing would fit with responsibility for the existing testing system. We've told the Cabinet Office that whatever they do, they must not dither or do anything that undermines Dido.

Later this afternoon Simon and I had our long-planned meeting to discuss the vaccine rollout. I was unusually nervous, because we don't have time to muck about. I want to protect the project against massive central interference and I want the centre to have confidence our plans are ready. I needed to convince Simon that everything is in place and Downing Street can just press go. Due to Covid rules, I could only take one official, but I had four others lined up to contribute by Zoom, each tasked with explaining different aspects of the rollout. One was due to talk about vaccine supplies; another, delivery to the NHS; a third would explain our plans for deployment through hospitals, GPs and pharmacies; and a fourth would set out how we plan to reach individuals and groups who can't go to vaccination centres. Ahead of the meeting, we spent an hour putting the finishing touches to our presentation and trying to anticipate tricky questions. We were all on edge: it was the culmination of months of groundwork.

As I walked into the grand oak-panelled Cabinet Secretary's office, feeling as prepared as I could be, I noticed that the big screen was not switched on, and there was an IT man fiddling around with cables under the boardroom table. I was surprised: we've all been using Zoom for months now and everything usually works fairly seamlessly. I was just beginning to wonder whether the meeting would have to be postponed when – bingo! The screen burst into life. There was my team, pens and paper at the ready. There was still no audio, but diaries were tight and the clock was ticking, so I launched into a high-level introduction while the IT guy continued to work his magic.

Glancing up at Simon, I could tell that my opening words were going down well, so I galloped through my part of the presentation before handing over to officials. 'And now, over to Maddy, to talk us through the first section!' I concluded cheerfully.

Simon and I looked up at the screen and could see Maddy's mouth moving, but there was still no sound. I scoured the room for the IT guy, but he had vanished. What to do?

Rescheduling the meeting was not an option: coordinating diaries would take ages. There was nothing for it but to deliver the rest of the presentation myself. Gulping hard, I threw myself into it, desperately trying to remember all the points my team were due to make.

Simon seemed impressed. He and James Bowler, his replacement on Covid at No. 10, asked some decent questions, all of which we'd prepared for.

'Well, you certainly seem to be on top of it all,' he said encouragingly. 'You better present it to the PM.' And that was that. A win – despite having to fly solo. I practically waltzed down Whitehall. We are ready to roll.

SATURDAY 7 NOVEMBER

Biden has done it! I heard the news as I turned the radio on in the kitchen, before the rest of the family had got up. I lay on the sofa and, somewhat to my own surprise, I burst into tears of relief. Finally an end to the Trump madness. He has been such a disaster for the western values I hold so dear. After a couple of minutes, I pulled myself together and put the kettle on: a very British celebration.

Boris thinks Dilyn had coronavirus. The mink crisis had clearly got him thinking about pets, and he is now convinced his dog had the disease around the same time as he did.

'Would there be any point in getting him tested for antibodies?' he enquired.

There was a long and awkward pause while Patrick and the Prof tried to work out whether he was joking or whether we needed to summon the chief vet to provide a considered response. I grappled with the mental image of some hapless Downing Street aide manhandling Boris and Carrie's wayward mutt while someone in a white coat extracted a blood sample. For a while, we just left the message hanging there. Eventually the Prof broke the silence.

'I don't know if the human antibody test would be suitable,' he replied diplomatically. 'And there's not much evidence of dogs coming to much harm. In my view, neither you nor the dog pose one another any risk (from a Covid point of view).'

'You've clearly never meet Dilyn, Chris. That dog poses a clear and present danger...!' said Simon, with three emojis: dog, virus, red card.

'I think our dog got it as well in April,' Patrick chimed in. He said the chief vet thinks dogs are 'very very low risk'.

'Cats can get it. And don't get a ferret,' he added helpfully.

I stared at the ferret thing, thinking, 'Have I somehow managed to miss a whole new risk category? Christ. Britain has millions of ferrets!"

'Seriously, are we going to have to do something about ferrets?' I asked anxiously.

'Reverse?' suggested Simon.

'Terminate?' I replied grimly.

Patrick still seemed unsure of how much of this was in jest.

'Ferrets can catch it, that's all,' he said, adding that intensively reared mink are the big problem. Reassuring.

SUNDAY 8 NOVEMBER

Remembrance Sunday. The Queen travelled back to London for the first time since March to lay a bouquet of white and lilac orchids at the grave of the Unknown Soldier at Westminster Abbey in a poignant private ceremony.

The *Sunday Times* has done a hatchet job on Kate Bingham,

---

* It's 500,000 – I checked. Quite a few are pets. There's no accounting for taste...

revealing that she spent £670k of taxpayers' money on PR consultants. They've discovered that she hired eight full-time spin doctors from an outfit called Admiral Associates. I'd been pretty cross at some of the briefing, but I had no idea it was at public expense.

'Who the hell signed this off?' I asked the team. Blank faces all round.

Turns out the contract went through the Department for Business, Energy and Industrial Strategy, not us, which meant we had no opportunity to block it. I've genuinely no idea what she was thinking: we have plenty of brilliant comms people who would have been more than capable of handling it for her.

Over in the States, after a lot of nonsense about 'electoral fraud', Biden has officially been declared the winner. Trump is not taking it well and won't concede. How embarrassing – and appalling – to be such a sore loser.

Global coronavirus infections have passed 50 million cases.

MONDAY 9 NOVEMBER

Kate's now the target of a massive media pile-on. I don't like the fact that she hired PR people, but she doesn't deserve the ferocity of attacks she's getting.

'Who's dumping on her?' I asked Damon.

'Lots of people,' he replied darkly.

One lobby hack called him last night to say they're reporting that both No. 10 and the department have lost patience with her. Journalists want to know whether I still have confidence in her. Well, yes I do. It's about perspective. Some of her interventions haven't been helpful, like trying to block my insistence that we buy enough vaccine for the whole population, but she has done a fantastic job with the vaccine contracts, and we've got to protect her. And there's more: how will we ever get amazing people to give massive public service in the country's hour of need if they're treated like this? I told the team to give it both barrels.

Much more importantly, Pfizer has announced its vaccine is 90 per cent effective. So far, we have 40 million doses on order.

Boris and I are on the same page in managing expectations, because we don't yet have the safety data, and he warned at the press conference that it's 'very, very early days'. Perfect. The Prof agreed that we need to handle it carefully but says that if this one works, others probably will. He thinks spring 2021 looks much brighter.

'Medical science is great,' he said to me afterwards.

JVT response was that he's 'a bit excited', which is his way of saying that he's very excited indeed.

My own enthusiasm was tempered by a warning shot from George Osborne about how we manage the rollout. 'Make sure you've got a clearly understandable plan – because nobody is going to accept being at the back of the queue,' he said.

'100 per cent,' I replied.

I sent him a link to the JCVI's advice on priority groups, which are primarily based on age.

'That's all fine – except I'm last in line (along with half the population), and if people in their forties are getting the vaccine in Germany or France or whatever and I'm told to wait for many months, that won't be good,' George pointed out.

Yes and no: the debate in Germany right now is why Britain has so many more vaccines on order than they do, given that they invented it. George wanted to know what had happened to our 'plucky Oxford vaccine'.

'Soon…' I replied.

I've now got another Perm Sec specifically for testing. We need to manage the optics of this appointment carefully. I told Damon to ensure the press don't interpret it as Dido being undermined – when in reality it's more backup for her.

TUESDAY 10 NOVEMBER

After months of working it up in secret, today I presented the vaccine rollout plan to the PM. I've rarely seen him as enthusiastic. Finally I think he realises this really is going to happen.

'Can we go faster?' he boomed, banging the table.

'Prime Minister, I am always asking my team the same question. We are going as fast as humanly possible,' I replied.

As expected, the price of success is that No. 10 has gone from not believing the vaccine will happen to getting completely carried away. Yesterday they started putting it out that '10 million people' could get the jab before Christmas. The figure is from an out-of-date contract – and is disastrous for the very careful expectation management we've been doing. It was never the plan, is never going to happen, and Damon spent half the day trying to kill it.

Potential trouble ahead with a faction of Tory MPs who still think everything we're doing on the pandemic is an overreaction. They've set up a 'Covid Recovery Group' to campaign for 'living with the virus'. I fear we are going to be hearing a lot from them.

Interesting moves afoot in No. 10 tonight. *The Times* and *Mail* both report that Boris wants to appoint Lee Cain as his chief of staff. Apparently it's causing major ructions…

WEDNESDAY 11 NOVEMBER

All hell has broken loose over the proposed Lee Cain appointment, and he has walked out. Apparently there was a big showdown, with members of the PM's inner circle taking different sides. It's a dramatic setback for Cummings, and there's lots of speculation today that he might also go. I tried to steer well clear but had a very weird encounter with him in Parliament by Speaker's House this afternoon. At first I didn't even recognise him. I was walking through the courtyard after PMQs and saw a guy dressed like Noel Gallagher, shambling along in a ridiculous hat and raincoat. I assumed it was some civil servant.

'Matt!' he said. I looked up and it was Cummings.

'How are you, Matt? Great to see you!' he said with uncharacteristic levels of enthusiasm.

'Very well thanks,' I replied warily, thinking, 'Why are you in Parliament? You hate Parliament! And why are you being nice to me?'

Wanting to say something polite, I thanked him for giving me an extra SpAd – something I've been pushing for since the beginning of the pandemic. He looked completely blank. I walked away feeling un-settled. He's ignored my calls and texts for weeks, done his best over a long period of time to get me fired and suddenly he's hanging around in Parliament, dressed like a roadman, being friendly? Very odd.

The daily press conference focused on the vaccine rollout. JVT re-vealed that he has told his 78-year-old mum to get ready to be called forward, along with everyone else in priority groups. The headline in tomorrow's *Metro* is a classic: 'Van-Tam: Jab for Mam'.

JVT said he hadn't planned to talk about his mum in this way; it's just what he usually does when he talks to patients. 'None of it was staged. When I advise patients I often say this is what I would do for my mother/child/sibling etc. As a doctor I feel it's the best advice you can ever give to any patient,' he explained.

Gove was tickled by the *Metro* headline and sent me an 'I ♥ JVT' message.

Irritatingly, Sir John Bell has been openly questioning how well the NHS will manage the vaccine rollout. Jim had a quiet word, explaining that we all have our concerns – of course we do! – but this not a sub-ject that benefits from being discussed in public. I texted him a similar message. He was suitably apologetic.

THURSDAY 12 NOVEMBER

An infuriating leak to the *Telegraph* about Moonshot, based on some departmental documents they obtained.

I am so sick of this. The story is mainly about mass testing, but there's a line in there about Boris's 'freedom pass' idea, which will be very controversial. I messaged Simon Case saying we cannot carry on like this. I know No. 10 has a lot on, but we need to find out where this stuff is coming from. I told Simon I'd formally request yet another leak inquiry, if necessary.

Late this afternoon I headed down to Dover for a *Question Time* special. The usual format had been adapted for a smaller audience and involved quick-fire questions to panellists.

Fiona Bruce asked if people wanted to see me being used as a guinea pig for the vaccine. Cue a sea of raised hands.

'So, you want to wait to see, basically, if Matt doesn't drop to the floor frothing at the mouth?' Fiona joked.

Fine! I have every confidence. We haven't cut a single corner, and I'm more than happy to oblige.

Rumours growing that Cummings will be out by Christmas. Wow. That would explain why he was being so weird when I bumped into him yesterday.

FRIDAY 13 NOVEMBER

Cummings has gone! Not just out by Christmas but gone now. I am elated and, more than anything, relieved for the sake of the vaccine and the country.

'Now we can actually build a government that works effectively,' I told Simon Case excitedly.

We talked about restoring proper processes and ensuring everything that should come to me does come to me, instead of being diverted to one of the many random groups Cummings set up to interfere/cut me out of the loop/attempt to control everything. My team – officials and advisers – are thrilled. He's been such a frightening, damaging, negative force for so long. There's some nonsense doing the rounds about him continuing to work on Moonshot. That certainly won't be happening. All he's done on Moonshot is thwart progress with his endless meddling, leaking and briefing. Why would we let him anywhere near it again? I am beyond relieved.

Just as George predicted, now the vaccine is within touching distance the special pleading from vested interests has begun. Cabinet colleagues are all arguing that their groups deserve priority: Eustice wants jabs for seasonal farm workers, DfE wants jabs for teachers, the MoD wants jabs for soldiers, the Home Office is arguing for jabs for police etc. The teaching unions are by far the worst, acting like they're somehow equivalent to NHS frontline workers.

Michael Gove, Rishi and I – the only ones with a full overview – all agree that the only way to approach this is by clinical need. There is no case for letting those who shout the loudest jump the queue.

SUNDAY 15 NOVEMBER

Boris has been pinged by the app. I sent him a sympathetic message and tried to make him feel better by saying that this shows the system works.

Meanwhile the *Sunday Times* thinks we've been dishing out multi-million-pound contracts to 'cronies'. Really? I'm absolutely fuming. I had nothing to do with testing contract negotiations. I've not been involved in either the pricing or the decision making behind who's been awarded government contracts. Any journalist worth their salt would know that all contracts have to be decided and signed off by the civil service – who are independent of me. Throughout the pandemic, the only contract I've been involved in is the Oxford AstraZeneca one – to ensure exclusive access. With all my years of experience as a politician and Cabinet minister, would I seriously just bung millions of pounds' worth of deals to my mates, just kind of hoping nobody would notice? I find this so galling: people have been working every hour to save lives, moving at lightning speed relative to normal times, only to be repeatedly accused of doing something dodgy.

I am torn over how to respond. Should I hit it hard and risk making it a bigger story, or keep my head down, since it's complete rubbish, and wait for it to go away?

Dido has been dragged in too, because of her tangential links to Randox. I sent her a supportive text. She is philosophical. 'Don't worry on my account. I recognise that all the noise this week is about bigger stuff than me,' she said.

I'm on *GMB* tomorrow, the first Cabinet minister to go on for months. No blanket broadcast bans in the post-Cummings era!

MONDAY 16 NOVEMBER

I survived the Piers Morgan mincer, emerging a little bashed about but much cheered by fantastic news about the Moderna jab, which has

94.5 per cent efficacy. Kate's been on it and we can get 5 million doses. Our original order was relatively modest, because the formula is so similar to AZ's, but these results are so impressive we'll secure some more now.

We've sorted out most if not all of the issues with the Covid app, which has hit 20 million downloads. Not bad!

TUESDAY 17 NOVEMBER

Hugo Rifkind has written a glowing review of testing in *The Times*, describing his own experience with the system as 'phenomenal'. I shared it with Dido to cheer her up.

'Lovely to see. I can't imagine who has done all that work… the Test and Trace elves?' she replied.

'You!' I said.

I am pushing hard to reduce isolation periods for people who test negative using lateral flow kits. Annoyingly, this needs cooperation from the MHRA, who are currently refusing to sign it off. Basically, they don't like the idea of DIY testing. It's so frustrating: their job is to define whether a test is effective, not dictate the circumstances in which it can be used.

In another frustration, HMT appears to be trying to play us off against Rob Jenrick's department over funding for social care. With the spending review looming, Helen Whately spoke to Rob about what we need, and he said the Treasury had told him to leave negotiations over the social care budget to me. She was taken aback, because it's the exact opposite of what the Treasury told us, which was basically to leave it to Rob! Very cheeky. I told Helen it sounds like the Treasury trying to divide and conquer. Social care funding is too important for such games.

WEDNESDAY 18 NOVEMBER

Something strange is going on in Essex and Kent. Everywhere else, cases are coming down – but there, still soaring. Nobody can figure out why. Local councillors think it's because people are breaking the rules, but Priti, whose constituency is in Essex, thinks something more sinister is afoot. She was sufficiently worried to call me after our Local Action Committee Gold meeting today, where we decided on which areas go in which tiers, to reiterate her concerns. She knows her patch extremely well and is very intuitive, so I was already taking it seriously. I've asked PHE for a full analysis of cases in those areas.

I sent Boris a chart showing the vaccine portfolios around the world by country, with the UK at the top of the league table. He loves that kind of thing, so I knew he'd be reassured. The only other places to have secured orders for at least five doses per capita are the United States and Canada.

Annoyingly, it won't be me who gets to sign the historic documents when the various vaccines are finally approved for use: for propriety and ethics reasons, it has to be a minister who hasn't been involved in procurement. I've delegated it to Jim.

'I am so spectacularly jealous of you being the minister who actually approves the vaccine, inshallah,' I told him.

Dido's the latest to be pinged by the app. I may start regretting we made it so efficient. So much so, some are now calling it the 'pingdemic'. Thank God the vaccine is almost here.

FRIDAY 20 NOVEMBER
I met my Slovakian opposite number to talk about their government's super-ambitious 'let's make the entire population take a Covid test all on the same day' initiative. He was astonished and very flattered that we might copy the idea. I have my reservations – not least that our population is more than ten times the size of theirs – but Boris is super keen. If we're going to attempt it, we'll need total buy-in from the MoD, but Ben Wallace, who has been consistently supportive throughout this nightmare, is starting to get annoyed by all the appeals for assistance from the armed forces, which have in fairness become a bit too casual.

He's continually fielding requests for squaddies to help with testing and other Covid-related stuff, and feels some in government may be taking advantage. He sent me a very stern message today saying he would NOT (his caps) authorise any more such requests until we can prove their added value.

My twenty-sixth press conference tonight. Key message: the vaccine is coming!

SATURDAY 21 NOVEMBER

The Slovakian scheme is on the skids. The PM has been talking to the Slovakian PM and is incredibly eager to give it a go. Safe to say Cabinet does not share his enthusiasm. Today's the day I had to get ministerial approval on the plan. It did not go well. Bluntly, they think it's crazy.

I set out the practicalities. Doing my best to ignore the increasingly incredulous expressions on the faces of the Zoom attendees, I walked everyone through what would be required: nothing less than the entire military and every part of the NHS that could be harnessed to the cause. The price tag? A cool £1 billion.

Knowing this one came straight from the top, I gave it both barrels. Boris has wanted to try this, and if it can shorten lockdown then it's financially worth it. But by the time I wrapped up I knew it was doomed.

George Eustice dismissed it as ridiculous. He argued that we should not go along with the initiative just because Boris wants to do it and has been making friends with the Slovakian PM. The Treasury said they wouldn't pay for it. Ben Wallace said the military was already deployed on other missions. There was clearly no point in arguing, so Michael Gove brought the meeting swiftly to a close, telling everyone that we'd review the policy and revert.

Somewhat reeling from onslaught, I picked up my phone to Emma.

'Well, that was a drive-by shooting if ever I've seen one. Shows the limit of the PM's powers, even in a pandemic. Cabinet government lives!' I said cheerfully.

Much too late, I realised I had forgotten to press 'Leave Meeting' on the Zoom. Around twenty ministers and officials were still on screen, listening to every word.

Recovering my composure, I messaged Simon Case.

'Unfortunately, the boss's mass testing proposal has just run into a brick wall,' I reported.

He asked whether they raised legitimate concerns or were just playing politics.

'Largely legitimate,' I replied. He said he'd break the news to Boris.

After giving Simon time to speak to him, I called the PM, who seems to be taking it on the chin. Looks like Slovakia-style universal testing won't be our way out.

AstraZeneca is on the brink of announcing its efficacy results. Sounds like they will update the Stock Exchange on Monday. For now, we can't breathe a word.

SUNDAY 22 NOVEMBER

I'm under fire from *The Observer* over Gina's appointment to the DHSC board. They've described her as my 'closest friend from university' (true – one of) but are also making a song and dance of the fact that she's a 'director of a lobbying firm'. It's completely misleading. The truth is that she hasn't been actively engaged with the company in question for years and every aspect of her appointment to the department went through all the proper channels. Everything that should have been declared was declared, and she was appointed after she proved herself during her stint as a volunteer just trying to do her bit for the country. Fortunately, there's enough other news around that the story hasn't run hard, but I couldn't help feeling that the department should have issued a more robust rebuttal.

Labour's suggested we should appoint a Vaccine Roll-Out Minister. I agree. As it happens, the PM had had exactly the same thought. If we choose the right person, it could work very well.

Pascal Soriot at AstraZeneca messaged offering a briefing ahead of the company's planned announcement tomorrow. Pfizer's also one step closer to delivery, having sent its clinical trial data to the MHRA. We only have days to get everything in place.

MONDAY 23 NOVEMBER

The results are officially in for the Oxford/AZ jab and it's 70 per cent effective, potentially rising to 90 per cent with the right adjustment to dosage. It is far cheaper and easier to store than the Pfizer and Moderna version. All very good – though Jim has received a tip-off that it may not get FDA approval in America. Quite why is unclear – vaccine nationalism?

Along with the devolved administrations, we're still working on how to manage Christmas. For once Sturgeon is resisting the temptation to tartanise the rules. At a COBRA, all four nations agreed: three households will be able to meet up indoors and outdoors for five days from 23 to 27 December, forming a kind of 'Christmas bubble'.

This evening Boris called about the Minister for Vaccine Roll-Out idea. I think he thought I'd be opposed to it, but I was enthusiastic. He suggested a junior Lords minister to do the job, but I said that wouldn't work – we needed a heavy hitter – and suggested instead that he gives the job to Nadhim Zahawi. Boris loved it. It helps me too: Nadhim and I wrote a book together years ago. Not only are we still close and talk all the time, but he's an incredibly effective minister and has been involved in vaccine procurement on the BEIS side since the start. Boris is going to call him, but it sounds more or less done and dusted. It's the best job offer in the world – the heavy lifting's been done and he just needs to get out there and be the face of it. He's hardly going to say no!

TUESDAY 24 NOVEMBER

I'm getting some credit for ordering the full 100 million doses of the AZ vaccine, overruling the 30 million recommendation from the Vaccine Taskforce. Grant Shapps generously gave me a shout-out for it this morning. This clearly annoyed BEIS, because they started putting it about that it wasn't true, briefing that they did in fact recommend ordering 100 million so I shouldn't get any extra plaudits. We asked them to check their records, and once they'd done so they retracted. Later Damon sent me a message saying Alok had 'calmed down'.

'Once he found out that it was true!' I replied.

WEDNESDAY 25 NOVEMBER

A stressful day working out how the country will be divided into tiers when lockdown ends. A load of MPs who think their rural constituencies are being unfairly lumped in with more populous Covid hotspots are very unhappy indeed. Nadine, who's been trying to assess the scale of the revolt, reports that the parliamentary party is 'in meltdown' and told me to 'prepare for hostile fire'. Local public health officials are winding things up, moaning that they haven't been consulted etc. The announcement's tomorrow, with a vote next week, so we need to pare some of the rebels off. My feeling is that it will be bumpy but fine in the end.

Rishi delivered his spending review, warning that the economic emergency caused by Covid has only just begun. The Office for Budget Responsibility thinks unemployment will hit 7.5 per cent and the economy will shrink by 11.3 per cent, the biggest decline in 300 years. Debt is forecast to be at its highest outside wartime. Economically, it is equivalent to a war. However, early fears that we'd be unable to service our debts have proven unfounded, with the Bank of England covering it. It was established in 1694 to fund a war. Now it's funded the Covid response. But the hangover is going to be painful.

THURSDAY 26 NOVEMBER

Boris came to the Commons to back me up as I announced the new tier allocation. From the Dispatch Box, I couldn't see all the furious faces behind me, but there were quite enough stony expressions on the opposition benches to leave me in no doubt about the scale of sacrifice people will have to make. Most of the country, including London and Liverpool, will be Tier 2, while large parts of the Midlands, north-east and north-west, including Greater Manchester and Birmingham, will be in Tier 3. Only the Isle of Wight, Cornwall and the Isles of Scilly will be in Tier 1. In all, more than a third of the population will still be under tough restrictions.

After the bloodletting in Downing Street, Boris is trying to restore order and has appointed Dan Rosenfield his new chief of staff. He's a great choice. Dan and I got to know each other when he was George

Osborne's private secretary and we nearly ended up having to spend Christmas together after getting stuck in a snowstorm. When George was Chancellor and I was newly elected, we went on a pre-Christmas work trip to New York just as a snowstorm hit the city. We were due to fly home on the red eye landing in London on Christmas Eve, but BA started cancelling flights. Pulling every string he could find, Dan somehow managed to get us onto an embassy minibus which ploughed through the blizzard to JFK. We got the last seats on the last flight out – everything else was cancelled till after Christmas. He's a man who can get stuff done.

FRIDAY 27 NOVEMBER

Even Dido's husband, John Penrose MP, is kicking off about the way the tiers have been allocated. He and Liam Fox have issued a joint statement saying they 'cannot agree' with the methodology. They claim their north Somerset constituencies are being 'punished' because of higher infection rates in Bristol.

But if we have to carve out every pocket of England with a lower infection rate than nearby towns and cities, the map of England will look like a dry riverbed – and certain MPs would still be moaning. Another backbench complainer was Conor Burns, who sent me a sheepish message apologising after some of his comments were quoted on the *Today* programme.

'They were aimed to protect my position in Bournemouth, where the hotel and hospitality sector are furious and I'm being accused of being a government lackey,' he explained.

So much special pleading…

The R number is inching below 1 for the first time since August. The lockdown is clearly working. And we've told hospitals to be ready for a best-case scenario of rollout of the vaccine in ten days. Here's hoping!

SATURDAY 28 NOVEMBER

Boris has put a sunset clause on the new tier system to try to head off the rebellion. The new regulations will now expire on 3 February.

I'm not thrilled, because it just means another tricky vote later. We're going to win – because Labour are onside – so why force ourselves through the painful process again in February?

SUNDAY 29 NOVEMBER
Infection rates remain worryingly high in Kent, yet people there are up in arms about being in Tier 3. I spent seventy-five minutes on a call with Tory MPs with Kent and Essex constituencies and came away slightly shellshocked. They're all furious. The real question is why the virus is spreading so fast there. We are trying to get answers.

I asked Helen Whately why she thinks people are so angry.

'Tough. My theories... people are poor (the wealth of west Kent disguises it); lots of key workers who cannot work from home; also can't afford to isolate; combined with low compliance...' she replied. She says some people in Kent don't think the virus is a problem, don't like facemasks etc.

No. 10 is getting increasingly twitchy about the looming rebellion. Boris has been hinting that the rules could be eased in December (no chance) and that MPs will have another opportunity to vote in January. He wrote a piece for the *Mail on Sunday* today, suggesting we'll be back to 'something like life as normal' by Easter. Classic Boris optimism – this time backed by medical science.

He's still pushing the 'freedom pass' idea. Emma Dean has been wading through a proposal to give people 'twenty-four hours of freedom' with a negative lateral flow test. She asked my view, which is that we need to look at it in the round.

'I'm not mad against, but it has to fit in with the strategy,' I replied.

I hit back hard at the idea of saying anything about this ahead of tomorrow's vote though. That would be madness! Our MPs are already in open revolt without throwing this grenade at them.

MONDAY 30 NOVEMBER
Another day spent largely working through the vaccine rollout plans. One worry is staff. There are huge regional variations in the numbers

of people available to get vaccines into arms. Officials say the north-east has only 11 per cent of the people we need, while London has 350 per cent of what's required.

'Christ,' I replied. We are going to need an army of volunteers.

Despite my reservations, the vaccine passport concept is gaining ground. Some MPs are already very exercised, stoked by libertarians across the political divide.

My SpAds asked if we can 'kill off the idea' or whether we have to leave it open as an option down the line.

'Play down. Nowhere near there yet,' I replied. They suggested saying, 'This is not something we are currently looking at,' but some-one somewhere is probably looking at it (certainly the Cabinet Office), so we'll have to fudge.

DECEMBER 2020

TUESDAY 1 DECEMBER

We finally have the vaccine! After my early morning meeting, Jim came into my room to tell me personally he'd just formally signed the Pfizer vaccine off. I was on my way out of the door to see the PM in Downing Street at 9.30 a.m. – perfect timing. I hugged Jim, drove to No. 10 and walked into the Cabinet Room, where the PM was standing behind his chair with Rishi, Simon and a few others dotted around.

'We have a vaccine! It's been formally approved!' I announced.

Boris danced a little jig, his jubilant moves giving every impression that he hadn't had much dance practice of late. We were all elated. We know this is the only way out. So many people feared it would never happen. But here it is, the first in the world, in under a year.

'When can we tell people?' asked Boris. I explained it's highly market sensitive, so not a word until 7 a.m. tomorrow.

From Downing Street I headed into the Commons, where I was brought back down to earth with a thud by the debate over tiering arrangements. The lockdown sceptics were in full cry, whipped up by Mark Harper, who was revelling in his late-life conversion from loyalist backroom fixer to fearless Covid freedom fighter. The PM was barracked from all sides as he opened the debate, while I sat there just wishing I could tell them all about the vaccine. Although we won the vote by a massive margin of 291–78, a rump of Tories (fifty-five backbenchers in all) voted against the measures, including the influential and respected chairman of the backbench 1922 Committee, Sir Graham Brady. I told Boris that he should take this seriously: when government relies on opposition votes, it hands the power to opposition leaders.

Now the vaccine is here, there's a new urgency to the debate over the merits of vaccine certification. On the morning media round, Gove said there were 'no plans' to introduce 'vaccine passports', but I know he is still very keen on the idea. Other than for international travel, where it's out of our hands, I'm against. I don't like the 'papers please' intrusion, and I just can't see it working. Far better just to drive up vaccination and keep the virus under control, then open up as soon as we safely can. Boris is torn between his instinctive opposition to state meddling and his impatience for the return of some semblance of normality.

Mid-afternoon I received a furious message from *Daily Mail* editor Geordie Greig that featured some very Anglo-Saxon language about the BBC. In the early days of the pandemic, the *Mail* ran a magnificent campaign to raise money for PPE. Readers were incredibly generous and gave millions. Now the BBC has run a snippy story suggesting that some face masks may have been made by Uighurs in Chinese detention camps. The *Mail* bought them from a third party checked and authorised by the NHS. If there's an issue, it applies to max 100,000 masks out of 40 million pieces of kit. Geordie asked if I would issue a supportive statement, to which the answer was 100 per cent YES.

Plans for tomorrow's announcement were almost derailed by BioNTech, who told a select group of hacks in Berlin that the MHRA have approved the jab. They issued a press release describing the news as 'embargoed until confirmed'. Extremely naive to imagine this incredibly market-sensitive hot info wouldn't leak. Cue a frantic operation our end to get them to retract it pronto. Here's hoping German journos are not as hungry as our own.

In a strange procedural quirk, later I had to seek official prime ministerial approval for the vaccine rollout. This involved a joyful meeting with Boris at 8 p.m. in the Cabinet Room. JVT came along and gave him a very short formal briefing, explaining that the vaccine is 95 per cent effective and has proven safe in trials of 20,000 people. At the end, Boris adopted his most serious voice and said, 'Yes.' I have absolutely no idea why this funny little ceremony was needed, but I think we all enjoyed it.

On the way out of Downing Street I bumped into Rishi, who gave me a man-hug and thanked me for pulling off the vaccine. I think he was more relieved than anything else: all the emotion in that building that we are finally on our way out of this thing.

Tomorrow is going to be massive.

'Let's not fuck it up' was Damon's parting shot.

WEDNESDAY 2 DECEMBER

I woke early because I was so excited. All the work we'd done – the effort to accelerate approval, the risks taken buying early and at scale, the agonising over who should be prioritised and the decision to publish the queue – was about to pay off. I'd challenged the team to deliver a vaccine by Christmas, and they'd come up trumps with almost a month to spare. I'm so incredibly grateful to everyone for all their hard work. Now it's about rollout.

I'd set my alarm at 5 a.m., leaving the house as quietly as possible for the BBC's New Broadcasting House. The announcement to the markets was due at 7 a.m. sharp. From the privacy of a green room in the bowels of the BBC building, my first call was to my counterparts in the devolved administrations. Ridiculously, we'd had to keep them in the dark about the impending announcement because we were worried about leaks. I did want Robin, Vaughan and Jeane to know before the rest of the world, though, so had asked them the night before for a call at 6.30 a.m.

They'd clearly worked out what it was about, but if they'd been briefed by anyone on a confidential basis they were all discreet enough not to say so. Over the past year we've built up a strong relationship as a quartet. We've all been through the same wringer, and all of us bar Robin (the only Ulster Unionist Party member of the Northern Ireland executive) have to deal with flak from our own political side. I now look forward to these calls as a kind of joint therapy. I told them that the vaccine had been formally approved and now the hard part starts: rollout. I said I wanted to start as soon as possible but only if all four nations could press go on the same day. We settled on Tuesday 8 December, giving us six days to get the first lorryloads of vaccine into the country and safely to their distribution points. It's a day later than I'd planned, but as Vaughan wisely pointed out, trying to manage a major operation over a weekend is asking for trouble.

After the call, I checked in with JVT to be absolutely sure of the details and the correct terminology, then at 7 a.m. on the dot the official announcement went out to the markets. Moments later I was on air telling the world. What an enormous privilege it was to deliver this wonderful news.

How fast can we do this? How long will it take to vaccinate the most vulnerable groups? This is what everyone wants to know, but for now we don't have those answers. Manufacturing vaccines is a biological process in which all sorts can go wrong. I haven't even shared the draft schedule with No. 10 – it's too contingent, and it would probably just leak. I'm determined not to let expectations run out of hand in all the excitement, but it's hard not to get carried away when you can see some light at the end of the tunnel.

By the time I finished with the broadcasters and headed into Downing Street for the PM's daily meeting, I was exhausted but happy.

We discussed Day 1 plans. Boris said he wanted to do the press conference and he wanted Simon Stevens by his side, so people understand that the NHS is handling the rollout. In truth he also wanted Simon in front of the cameras so that this is on his shoulders too. Meanwhile the Prof very gracefully delegated his slot to JVT, who has done most of the heavy lifting on this one.

Unfortunately, Boris's good humour did not last long. By mid-afternoon, I was just finishing answering questions in the Commons when I got a series of texts on the front bench from an increasingly desperate-sounding Emma Dean, saying he was 'going mad' on a Zoom about the rollout with No. 10, the Cabinet Office and Nadhim.

I was meant to be in the meeting, but there were far more questions than the usual hour's-worth and the Speaker was understandably allowing everyone to ask. It should have been a joy – all the questions were congratulatory in tone – but I was getting increasingly frantic texts from Emma that I saw each time I sat down between questions.

'Really need you on this call,' she appealed.

'On my way,' I finally replied, as I answered the last question and rushed out to my waiting car to take me the 300 yards to Downing Street. 'What's going wrong?'

She said Boris was being wound up by his team. He wasn't happy that we're launching on Tuesday, not Monday; wasn't happy with the timeframe for vaccinating care home residents; wasn't happy about the way we're working with the devolved administrations; and had a bee in his bonnet about the use of wholesalers to get the vaccine to GPs.

Poor Nadhim was valiantly 'trying to hold it together', as Emma put it – but he's only been in the job a couple of weeks and understandably isn't across all the detail yet.

'Oh FFS,' I replied, urging Louise, my incredible driver, to get me there before it all disintegrated. I finally made it to the Cabinet Room and could reassure the Prime Minister we would go as fast as possible. We would take away all of his challenges and see how much faster we could go. But I'd already pushed the team to go as fast as possible, and they were highly motivated to anyway. His intentions are good but, I wish he'd take a moment to congratulate the team and keep their morale up, not lose it like this. It's going to be a long old slog.

Then more trouble when the European Medicines Agency suddenly went all sniffy about the speed with which we authorised the vaccine. In an unbelievably irresponsible intervention, they suggested we'd prioritised speed over public confidence. I can't think of a more reckless thing to say. Not only was it completely untrue – we have painstakingly followed all the usual safety steps, the only difference being that the scientists have run various trials in parallel rather than one after another – it also risked doing exactly what they were accusing us of: undermining public confidence. Luckily nobody sensible was listening, not least because we'd organised a press conference fronted by June Raine, chief executive of the MHRA, Wei Shen Lim from the JCVI and Munir Pirmohamed from the Commission on Human Medicines, who explained how they'd managed to authorise it so quickly without cutting any corners. June was simply magnificent – she has a rare ability to combine detail with clarity, explaining how we can be sure the vaccine is safe.

Finally, a lovely message from Nadhim.

'What a day! You are a hero,' he exclaimed, with a bunch of bicep curl emojis in different skin colours.

'Big team effort,' I replied, because that is what it is.

THURSDAY 3 DECEMBER

A cloak-and-dagger operation to get the first vaccine consignments into the UK. It's hard to put a figure on the value of a lorryload of life-saving treatment needed by the whole world, so we weren't taking any chances. Imagine if rogue actors or hostile states got wind of the delivery and tried to hijack the vehicle or seize the goods? There were five possible routes in: by sea to Dover; a longer sea route; through the Channel Tunnel; on commercial air freight; or, as a last resort, by military jet. Only a handful of people were privy to which route we chose, and all were sworn to secrecy.

Throughout the day I was sent updates on the physical progress of the first consignment: 800,000 doses of the vaccine. I asked for a picture and was shown two small crates containing the −60 degree freezers, mounted in an unmarked lorry. For something so important, it looked completely unremarkable.

At lunchtime, a drama: in hushed tones, officials told me that the team was switching route 'as a precaution' following a credible security threat. It was amazing work by our intelligence agencies and the private-sector company who first spotted it, and just goes to show that we were not being paranoid.

The team reassured me that the change of plan would only delay delivery by a few hours. Then, mid-afternoon, came confirmation that all 800,000 doses were safely in the UK. Relief! The Northern Irish delivery was on the ferry to Belfast; the English/Scottish delivery was being escorted to its secret warehouse, where it will settle after the journey; and the Welsh delivery had already arrived at theirs. All four consignments were awaiting clearance by the regulator. Inspectors had to check the vaccine hadn't come to any harm in transit. Finally the all-clear: our vaccines were ready for deployment! Over the next few weeks we'll repeat the whole exercise for the delivery of millions more doses.

As news spreads, we're beginning to get sheepish requests from VIPs around the world. A Middle Eastern diplomat reached out to Nadhim asking if we would be willing to send 400 shots for the royal household. Nadhim sounded embarrassed and asked my advice. He assumed we'd have to find a polite way of saying no. In fact, I'm up for these small diplomatic efforts – so long as the Foreign Office agrees of course. Done appropriately, it pays dividends for international relations. Nadhim sounded relieved, saying that the King himself is asking.

Earlier, Gavin Williamson got somewhat carried away on LBC Radio, claiming that we got the vaccine first because 'we've got the best medical regulators'. Ever-patriotic, he described them as much better than the French, Belgian and American regulators. Warming to his theme, he trumpeted that it all comes down to Britain being 'a much better country than every single one of them'. The minute I heard it, I knew it would cause trouble. Sure enough, as soon as the Americans woke up, the US media wanted to know what Anthony Fauci had to say about it. Under pressure, he suggested our approval system is in fact inferior to theirs. I listened with my head in my hands, because what we absolutely do not need at this stage is people worrying that the vaccine isn't safe, and why, oh why, did Gavin go there?

Thankfully, many angsty phone calls later, Fauci retracted his statement and apologised.

Former US Presidents Obama, Clinton and Bush have all said they'll have the vaccine – on live TV if necessary – to boost public confidence. JVT and I discussed whether we should do anything similar or whether it would be better to wait our turn, to underline the value of the clinical prioritisation. We decided to see how it goes. Plenty of high-profile public figures, including Sir David Attenborough and the Queen, are in the first tranche anyway due to their age and are much more persuasive than we are.

FRIDAY 4 DECEMBER

The first big setback: Pfizer's got an issue with its production line. The vaccine isn't brewing as fast as they'd like, and the European Medicines Agency won't sign off a second production line in Belgium. It means we are unlikely to get the 10 million doses we're due to receive before the end of the year, and production estimates for early 2021 are being scaled back. I'm nervous, but we did expect glitches, which is why we're being coy about numbers. Thank goodness we didn't let the plans go public.

Thanks to the November lockdown, the R is under 1, but we're back in the tier system, which is messier than I'd hoped. With Christmas coming and the excitement around the jab, I'm worried about complacency.

SATURDAY 5 DECEMBER

Now the vaccine is here, we're understandably under growing pressure to tell people when life will get back to normal. Clearly the speed of the rollout will determine that date. It's impossible to know, but if we can get all vulnerable people vaccinated by February, we could start to loosen restrictions by the end of March. I say this to try to give a sense of hope but also realism: the vaccine won't sort this out by Christmas.

Yesterday Bahrain became the second country in the world to approve the Pfizer jab. Meanwhile Russia has announced it has delivered its Sputnik V vaccine to seventy clinics. The name makes it sound alarmingly like rocket fuel.

'Does it work?' I asked JVT.

'We have absolutely no idea' was his considered reply.

SUNDAY 6 DECEMBER

Blown off-course by a storm. Bad weather over in Northern Ireland has delayed distribution, throwing our whole timetable into doubt. We have to be so careful that the vaccine isn't bumped around on ships and lorries: if it is destabilised, it literally becomes ineffective. Whatever happens, I'm determined the rollout must start on the same day in all four nations so everyone can see it's a fair, united effort. If that means it takes an extra day, so be it.

Tonight, in my huge weekend box, I found a submission from Jenny Harries saying the JCVI wants to add 900,000 more people to the clinically vulnerable list. The difficulty is that this would also add them to the vaccination priority list. A very tricky situation: we can't mess around with the queue at this stage. I'll talk to her about it next week. There must be a solution.

Helen Whately says care home staff are 'desperately tired and feel forgotten again'. I was upset by her message: I am only too aware how hard these teams work and how difficult the job is at the best of times. Given they will get the vaccine in the first tranche, I hope that will give at least some indication that they are highly valued.

MONDAY 7 DECEMBER

One day to go. Simon Stevens says tomorrow will be a 'decisive turning point' in the battle against Covid-19. He's right. He has also said that the 'majority' of vulnerable people will receive the vaccine in January and February 2021, which I think is realistic.

NHS comms expert Simon Enright, who's handling the media on this, ran me through the plans. The first patient will be a ninety-year-old lady in Coventry. The second patient is from Stratford-upon-Avon and is called William Shakespeare. Nice!

This afternoon I went to King's College Hospital to check everything is in place for day one. I was escorted to a non-descript room in which there was a freezer no bigger than the kind a large family might have in their garage. On the front, in electronic red letters, it read: –60. Inside were 10,000 tiny vials. I was suddenly hit by an overwhelming urge to pick one up in admiration, which would have been a complete no-no. They were cryogenically frozen and needed to stay that way. Besides, having had frostbite once – during a trek to the North Pole – I didn't fancy putting my fingers through that torture again.

TUESDAY 8 DECEMBER

A huge day. The thrill of the first jabs going into arms – then a terrifying late-night development that could bring the entire vaccination programme screeching to a halt.

Everything had been going entirely to plan. Shortly after 6 a.m., while I was still getting dressed, I received confirmation that the first person had been inoculated, and I hurried off for the morning media round.

Gina and Damon accompanied me to the broadcast studios and both told me off after I failed to use the phrase 'first in the world' during my first interview on Sky. 'You need to relax' was Gina's advice, by which she meant: 'Stop being so buttoned up.' What she did not mean was that I should lose it altogether, which unfortunately is exactly what happened later. I was on my own in a dark windowless booth, answering questions from *GMB*, when they played the video of Margaret Keenan getting her jab. I hadn't seen it before and was suddenly overwhelmed by the magnitude of it all. I completely lost it, blubbing away, battling to regain my composure as tears streamed down my face.

'For Christ's sake, pull yourself together,' I told myself desperately. There were five-four-three-two-one seconds to go and then the camera was back on me, my microphone was live and my watery red eyes were there for all to see.

I'd just had time to scrub the streaks off my face, but when I tried to answer the next question, my voice came out in a weird sort of croak. Feeling completely unprofessional and exposed, I staggered through the rest of the interview and bolted out of the booth. Gina said at least I'd shown how I felt. 'So long as they don't think it was faked,' said Damon. 'Far from it,' I said. 'You should have seen me while they were playing the tape – I'd completely lost it.' Fortunately, the nation had not witnessed any heaving sobs, but I had lost my dignity. On the way to the car, I thought about what Damon had said and worried there might be criticism from certain quarters – those who'd say I'd done it for the cameras. Of course I didn't. But maybe I shouldn't have been so embarrassed. All too often, politicians feel they can't show any emotion. That's all wrong. I'm not saying cry at the drop of a hat, but when something affects us deeply, we should be able to show our true feelings – not hide them out of fear.

Next up was a bizarre, long-planned video call with my Chinese counterpart, known to the Foreign Office as 'Minister Ma'. I updated him on the rollout announcement, but that was as substantive as our discussion got in what was a laughably Potemkin meeting.

He was sitting in a grand hall surrounded by dozens of officials, and all his responses were impeccably formal, telling me absolutely nothing new. For half an hour, we skirted around each other like two goldfish in a tank, before thankfully we were both called away.

Since summer, Cabinet has been held in the vast Locarno Suite in the Foreign Office, the closest place to No. 10 with a room that can accommodate all twenty-two of us, as well as the Prof and Patrick, with the requisite two-metre distance between participants. As I strode through the ornate marbled hall from my weird China call, I received good news: research published in *The Lancet* has concluded that the Oxford/AstraZeneca vaccine is safe and effective, giving good protection. The majority of those involved in the research were under-55s, but there is evidence it will protect older people too. The *Lancet* publication also presaged the Pfizer approval, so this is looking pretty good for Oxford. It meant I could brief colleagues that the rollout has begun and the Oxford jab should be coming very soon.

One of the lovely things about today was all the messages of support – from as wide a range of people as Laurence Fox to Andy Burnham. Meanwhile the virus continues its relentless march. We now have a triple challenge: stopping the spread, rolling out the vaccine and expanding testing. Boris is worried about keeping the four nations aligned in the run-up to Christmas and has tasked Michael Gove with dealing with Sturgeon. Sooner him than me. I've decided the rules around Christmas are too tricky to handle, so I'm leaving it to Michael to negotiate.

Utterly exhausted, I headed home for dinner, telling myself that I should relax. I even allowed myself a glass of wine. I was on my way to bed when my phone rang.

I glanced at the time: 11.43 p.m. Nobody rings at that hour unless it's bad news, least of all the Prof, whose number was flashing ominously on the screen.

In that calm, professorial voice of his, he explained that three people had had a serious adverse reaction to the vaccine. One had nearly died. All three patients are receiving the best care, and two are definitely going to be OK. As for the other: who knows.

What did this mean? What is the risk? Are we going to be able to carry on?

Without precise figures, and still on the phone, the Prof and I tried to calculate the statistical risk. We vaccinated 4,000 people today. If three out 4,000 had a massive reaction, then that's 38,000 out of the whole population. And 38,000 is an awful lot of people.

'Jesus Christ,' I thought, feeling physically sick. We may well have to halt the entire vaccination rollout. That would be a disaster.

'Perhaps all three have a history of anaphylaxis?' I asked hopefully.

'If so, then we may be OK,' the Prof confirmed. 'If that is the case, then all we need to do is change the advice for such patients and carry on.'

'When will we know?' I asked desperately.

'I've given them until 6 a.m. to get back to me on that, then we have to decide if we stop vaccinations tomorrow,' the Prof replied.

'OK. Call me any time,' I said grimly.

Still feeling nauseous, I slumped into bed, with my phone switched on next to me, knowing I would not get a wink of sleep.

WEDNESDAY 9 DECEMBER

At 5.30 a.m. my phone went: Natasha.

'All three had a clinical history of anaphylaxis,' she said immediately. 'CMO recommends that we change the protocols this morning to say anyone with a history shouldn't take this vaccine, introduce a fifteen-minute wait after vaccination to monitor people, restrict the rollout to hospitals for the next couple of days and get on with it,' she said. 'Are you happy to proceed?'

I can't remember ever being so relieved in my life. 'Go ahead,' I instructed, thumping the air. I told the team that we needed to be completely open about what had happened. No secrets or cover-ups. That is the golden rule of confidence building. Nothing else today was on the scale of that easy decision, taken at 5.30 a.m.

Two reports did make interesting reading. The first, a series of papers written for SAGE, attributed the resurgence of Covid cases to people going abroad during the summer. It reinforced what I've always suspected: we should be tough on travel, even to places where cases are low. The second, more tentative, suggested Covid-19 was circulating in Italy in November 2019, far earlier than previously admitted. I've no idea if it's true, but it's certainly food for thought.

THURSDAY 10 DECEMBER

Hospitals in Kent are really beginning to struggle. The ingrained culture of secrecy in the NHS is making things worse. Gareth Johnson, our Dartford MP, messaged me last night claiming that hospitals had been told they should not reveal the pressure they're under, a policy which only plays into the hands of the many people who think we're inventing this crisis. Hospital CEOs say the directive has come from NHS England. Gareth asked what the rationale is for the omertà and whether the policy can be changed. He says that 120 out of 400 beds are filled with Covid patients.

'We need the NHS in Kent telling it as it is!' I replied. How is it remotely helpful to pretend things aren't difficult?

Thankfully by the end of the day there were no more serious adverse reactions to the jab, so we've decided to expand the rollout to GP services next week, all being well. From there, we'll move on to pharmacies, sports centres, conference halls etc. We're now well into the tens of thousands, and people love it. Social media is full of enthusiastic tweets about people getting their jabs.

JVT and I discussed our own plans. Given how well it's going, we've decided to wait in line. There's no need for us to take it to show confidence, and we'd be criticised for queue jumping.

After weeks of arm twisting, we've finally persuaded the Treasury to agree to £500-a-head payments for people who are told to self-isolate. The idea is to make it easier to do the right thing. Getting it past the Treasury bureaucracy has been an absolute nightmare, but I think it will make a huge difference to compliance.

This evening I went for a quiet dinner with Nimco. The only place we could find open was in the garden of the Four Seasons Hotel in Park Lane. Not my natural haunt, but we've shut down most of the others.

Even in death, mink are causing a nightmare. The Danes think the decomposing carcasses of culled animals may have contaminated the groundwater. Yuck.

FRIDAY 11 DECEMBER

Fridays are typically quieter in Westminster, so I took the opportunity to film a series of Christmas and New Year messages for the department with Lauren from the parliamentary team. Midway through this cheerful exercise, I was interrupted by a phone call from JVT.

'I think I know what the problem is in Kent,' he said bluntly. 'I need to come and see you about it. Genomic testing has found a new variant. It must be spreading much faster. It's obviously now across Kent, Essex and London.'

For the second time in three days, my stomach lurched. At least this explained why the Kent numbers had been so stubbornly high.

'This is a disaster,' I replied. I fired questions at him: How much do we know? When did it first appear? Will the vaccine still work? If the November lockdown couldn't keep it down, what will?

'I don't know,' JVT replied honestly. He asked me to give him the evening to find out more. Taking a deep breath, I asked Natasha to fix a Zoom for early tomorrow afternoon and tried to return to my task. It was impossible. Trying to create upbeat, grateful Christmas messages when I now knew there was no chance of a normal Christmas felt almost insulting. I attempted to keep recording, but my heart wasn't in it. Later the team told me the footage was unusable – apparently the news was written all over my face. I couldn't hide my disappointment.

The new variant reinforced my determination to derail a Department for Food, Environment and Rural Affairs proposal that would allow seasonal workers from eastern Europe to continue coming here to work on farms. It is complete madness, especially given the mink scenario. Seriously, why don't they just hire local people and pay them more? The clinical advice is that letting in so many foreign labourers could set our vaccine programme back six months. DEFRA duly fell into line.

On my recommendation, Jim Bethell has been talking to George Osborne about how to make a success of the G7 summit when we host it next year. George's advice is to keep the agenda tight and pay proper attention to the atmospherics: choose a good venue like a country house hotel; make sure bits of the summit are held somewhere with a cool vibe; and don't forget to give them all a gift. The Germans once gave me a whole dark-chocolate Brandenburg Gate; the French, something from Hermès. Last time we hosted, we gave the leaders Burberry scarves.

'Perfect,' I replied. 'Let's make the focus "protect the west from the next pandemic".'

Later Jamie alerted me to an article in the *i* newspaper by Stephen Bush saying my approach to the pandemic has been vindicated while the Chancellor 'called the whole thing dead wrong'. Nice for me, but a bit harsh on Rishi. Jamie may have left, but he's still looking out for me and asked how my relationship with Rishi is doing, to which I replied – truthfully – that it's in a great place.

'Make sure you're being as nice and supportive as you can to him, even if HMT are being twats,' he replied. Good advice. While Rishi and I haven't always agreed, he has done a terrific job protecting the economy.

Finally, a text from Damon, informing me that someone spotted me at the Four Seasons Hotel and has told the media that I was quaffing champagne.

'Am I OK to say you didn't buy champagne? The idiot is saying it cost £3.5k,' Damon asked.

Er, yes. I would never spend £3.5k, or even a fraction of £3.5k, on champagne, and I am certainly not feeling remotely celebratory.

SATURDAY 12 DECEMBER

The whole Christmas plan is disintegrating.

I woke up to hear Professor Linda Bauld, an expert in public health at the University of Edinburgh, labelling the proposed relaxation a 'mistake' because people will travel from high- to low-prevalence areas to see relatives. Later Vaughan Gething chimed in to suggest that if cases remain high, we may have to change tack – blowing apart the UK-wide consensus. And this is before we go public about the new variant.

At 2.30 p.m. I logged onto the Zoom with JVT. It turns out that PHE has been tracking the new variant for some time – as they do with many others – but were not seriously worried until they put two and two together with the cases rocketing in Kent. It now accounts for almost all new infections in the area. There's a possibility it started in France, but that's now irrelevant. The Prof thinks it's unlikely to be any more deadly but it may well be more transmissible.

With a sinking feeling, I told the others that we must publish the details and inform the WHO. I know there will be huge consequences: just look what the mink variant did to Denmark, and what has happened to South Africa, where a new variant was detected in October. Macron now has every excuse to close the border at Calais, and the rest of the EU will swiftly follow. If the new variant evades the vaccine, we are all well and truly stuffed.

These formalities agreed, I called Boris, who was surprisingly sanguine. He seemed somehow resigned to the misery we will have to inflict on everyone.

'It's going to make Christmas very difficult,' I said.

'Christmas was already going to be very difficult,' he replied philosophically.

Later a GP friend got in touch to tell me that younger care home workers are reluctant to have the vaccine. Understandably, operators are worried about their legal position. What if an unvaccinated carer brings Covid into a home and infects a resident? Could the company be held liable? I messaged Nadhim, saying we needed to discuss. 'Clearly we can't mandate,' he replied, meaning: we can't force care workers to have the jab.

I'm not so sure. If you want to work with the most vulnerable people in our society, surely you have a duty to be vaccinated? This is why the hepatitis B vaccination is already mandatory for doctors. People will have strong views on both sides, but I know where I stand.

Separately, I asked Nadhim if he thinks we made the right call when we said we won't pile vaccines into Covid hotspots. It's been bothering me.

'Yes, because of the fairness argument,' he replied, adding that if we'd approached this geographically, great swathes of the country would be left without any vaccine at all.

SUNDAY 13 DECEMBER

All hell is breaking loose over Christmas. Damon says Tory MPs are 'already furious' at the prospect that everything will be cancelled. Pretty much everyone else is saying it would be insane to press on as planned. According to Helen Whately, the situation in Kent hospitals is dire and it's not at all clear how they will cope over the next few weeks, even without the Christmas easements.

'I don't see how we can have them,' is her gloomy verdict.

Ever eager to throw in his tuppenny worth, Chris Hopson of NHS Providers publicly appealed to us to 'think really carefully' about the festive season, which is his way of signalling that he'll be on the radio every single day complaining about how awful everything is unless we change course.

I asked the Prof whether he thinks there is any way we can stick to the original plan. Basically, no.

'The problem is that we'd be taking a risk from an already very high base,' he said.

If we have to U-turn, hopefully the Kent variant will reduce the backlash. His worry is that if there is any suggestion the vaccine doesn't work for the new strain, the right-wing press will start arguing that we should just let the virus rip.

'That's why we reassure on the vaccine,' I replied. There's no evidence the vaccine doesn't work.

Susan Hopkins at PHE is tearing her hair out that they didn't pick up the clusters earlier, given they have known about the new variant since 20 September, though to be fair to them, they could not have known back then how significant it would become.

The good news is that the vaccine rollout is going from strength to strength. I think we might be able to jab as many as 2 million people by Christmas. When I publicly suggested as much, Simon Stevens kicked off. In a patronising message to Damon, he sniffed that there is 'no version of reality' whereby 'several million people will receive the vaccine before Christmas', saying that whoever put this about (i.e. me) 'might want to urgently undertake some course correction before that inevitably becomes clear'. According to Damon, NHS England now want to 'distance themselves a bit' from the 'millions line'. Very bad idea.

'We must NOT look like there's any separation,' I said firmly. I can just see the 'government split' headlines. I may have not stuck to my own adage about under-promising and over-delivering – Simon's got a point – but it's for me to clear this up, not for NHS England to brief against.

I'm doing the morning media round tomorrow and asked Nadhim his advice. 'Do you need to say a number?' he asked, adding that we've done 100,000 so far.

'I don't need to, but I've got so much shit to shovel it would be nice to have some cheer too,' I replied.

His response was three heart emojis and a bunch of praise.

'This job would have burned out the best of us,' he said, kindly.

MONDAY 14 DECEMBER

Amazingly, this morning I managed to row back from my 2 million comment without any fuss. Another minor screw-up sorted. At least it was only on the comms.

Then later I announced the new variant in a statement to Parliament. The reaction wasn't as sensible as I'd hoped: even normally reasonable MPs like Greg Clark and Damian Green are going tonto. Everyone can see Christmas falling apart, and judgement is going out of the window. In a sign of Downing Street nerves, Michael Gove summoned me to the Cabinet Office to ask whether we can go any faster with the jab. Er, no. We're already going all out. I've already answered these 'daft laddie' questions. The pressure to accelerate is immense. The next few days are going to be very rough.

TUESDAY 15 DECEMBER

Boris is digging in over Christmas, saying the rules will still be relaxed.

He's urging people to keep their celebrations 'short' and 'small'. It's not going down well. The healthcare sector is going ballistic, with multiple stakeholders piling in to say it's 'rash', will cost many lives etc. The attacks feel coordinated – I don't know by whom.

Last night's meeting with Gove turns out to have been a rehearsal for an hour-long grilling by the PM. It boiled down to a dozen different ways of asking us to speed up. Once again: we're going as quickly as we can. The only question is how best to motivate and how to set expectations.

'Whatever we do, we must not over-promise. Please, *please*, let's not do that,' I appealed, somewhat humbled by my own mistake on this front this week. Far better to keep expectations low, then knock it out of the park. Boris grunted, leaving me none the wiser about whether he was taking any notice. Not over-promising would, after all, require him to change the habit of a lifetime.

At lunchtime, I was furious to discover that someone in No. 10 had killed off a statement I was due to make in the Commons about mental health, setting out some very long-awaited reforms to care for the most vulnerable patients. I got straight on to Dan Rosenfield, pointing out how important it is (the law hasn't been changed for forty years!). I've gone to great lengths to make sure this work continued throughout the pandemic, so the thought of it being pulled at the last minute is galling.

'Grateful for your help reinstating,' I messaged.

He blamed Brexit legislation for taking up parliamentary time and offered to find another way to push it, e.g. at PMQs.

'That would be a total travesty,' I replied grumpily. He batted me off to the Chief Whip, who promised it first thing in the new year.

WEDNESDAY 16 DECEMBER

The consensus with the devolveds over how to handle Christmas is falling apart. Wales and Scotland are both tightening up their rules, although characteristically, in different ways to each other. The boss is trying to hold the line, saying we won't criminalise people who made plans based on the five-day relaxation announced in November, but emphasising that three households over five days is the maximum, not the target. We issued a lot of other guidance in the hope that people will minimise social contact, but I am not optimistic.

Later we worked our way through the country, assigning tiers. It was the sort of meeting that simply couldn't have been done a few years ago: eighty-five people on a Zoom with another dozen socially distanced in my office, experts from each part of the country, ministers from other departments and observers all looking at a very high-quality set of graphs and slides of what is now very rich data. Many places moved into stricter tiers, but there was one bright spark: Herefordshire, where there are hardly any cases, will be moved into Tier 1. For some places, though, three tiers are not enough. We need a tougher Tier 4 – but I can't get it agreed.

To Jens's relief, Germany will start rolling out the Pfizer BioNTech vaccine on 27 December. He's been increasingly stressed and miserable: it's a German vaccine, for Christ's sake, yet they're not getting it first. I can only imagine the grief we'd get if the tables were turned and a British vaccine were given to the Germans first. It makes me even more grateful we insisted on the exclusivity clause for the Oxford AstraZeneca vaccine.

THURSDAY 17 DECEMBER

I'm wrestling with how to keep schools open if Cabinet colleagues won't support mass testing. Yesterday I took a really aggressive call from Gavin Williamson in which he made it quite clear he could not support the policy, on practical grounds. When he had finally blown himself out, I messaged No. 10 warning them that I can't make this work against his very clear opposition. I hadn't entirely recovered from this frustrating exchange when I got a bollocking from Ben Wallace, who clearly feels his troops are being overused and now says he won't sign off any request from the Education Department for military help – not that it sounds as if Gavin wants any.

'I will send in planners, but we are not repeating the failed Liverpool experiment,' he said sternly.

He was referring to a pilot scheme on Merseyside involving mass testing and testing close contacts of positive cases every day for a week. Overall, the analysis I've seen is that it was actually quite successful, reducing transmission by a fifth.

When I pointed this out, he hit back that it had involved a huge number of soldiers running around testing people who weren't in the worst hotspots, after which there was shoddy follow-up by Test and Trace.

'Next time you all want to use troops I am going to require much clearer defined outcomes,' he said, leaving me feeling like a soldier who hadn't bothered polishing his boots.

All this would be easier if Dido wasn't under so much pressure at Test and Trace. Yesterday she messaged saying she is really worried we are pushing things too far and that what is being discussed 'is un-doable'. She fears any expansion to the testing programme at the moment risks undermining what we are already doing.

Adding to the list of unhappy colleagues, Nadine is in high dudgeon about being inadvertently left off a conference call about Christmas plans with various Tory MPs. She's told Allan that she is 'hugely insulted', which is obviously not how I want her to feel.

All of this was a grim start to a day dominated by the announcement of the new tiers, which effectively cancel Christmas. Worse for me, they also scupper Martha's birthday dinner tonight, which was set to be our first night out in months. I feel terrible about it, but I don't have any choice.

The only bright spot was announcing moving Herefordshire down to Tier 1, to the delight of everyone in Jesse Norman's constituency. Later he sent me a hilarious gif of football-style celebrations. I've come to hate the tiers: they do reduce the pressure in places where case numbers are low, but the boundaries are impossible to draw sensibly, and the whole thing doesn't keep us together as a country. I hadn't appreciated how important that is.

The Kent variant is still a huge worry, but while we're jabbing like fury pretty much everywhere else, ironically, we seem to be failing there. Tracey Crouch, the MP for Chatham & Aylesford, forwarded me an angry email she'd received from the oncology department at Maidstone and Tunbridge Wells NHS Trust complaining that vaccine supplies there are 'a distant dream'. The hospital is inundated with Covid patients and is on Black Alert Level 4, meaning they've been forced to cancel all planned operations, yet apparently none of the medical staff have been offered jabs. Worse, they're not being given any information about likely timeframes. Apparently there's another hospital in the area where even admin staff have been offered vaccines. Whoever wrote to Tracey labelled the situation 'preposterous', and they're right. I messaged Nadhim, saying we need to pile vaccines into Kent. He replied that his team will do all that's humanly possible. 'Keep the faith,' he said – which I am.

Betty Boothroyd called the office via a public line, asking if there's any way she can get her jab soon. She's ninety-one and very vulnerable. I called her back myself as I was in the car home on Park Lane. I'd never met her, but she's something of a hero of mine. As Speaker, she was a real trailblazer for women in politics. I said yes, we can get you your jab – given her age, she's entitled to it – but the deal is you have to have it on camera. She readily agreed. It reminded me just how worried and vulnerable nonagenarians are – even the most forthright of characters. I gave her number to Nadhim, who is going to fix it.

Later JVT called. He and the Prof have been thinking. They have worked out that since the first dose of the vaccine gives about four times as much protection as the second dose, the best way to save lives might in fact be to give the first dose to as many people as possible as fast as possible and then delay the second. They don't think this will harm the end protection – in fact it might even make it stronger – but in the face of this huge second wave, and obviously limited supply, giving a first dose to a new person would be much more life-saving than giving a second dose to someone who's already had their first.

This approach hasn't been clinically trialled, and is not what the formal authorisation says, but JVT and the Prof think it can only do good.

'What do you think?' he asked. 'Can we make this fly?'

I thought about Betty Boothroyd, who'd have her second jab delayed. She wouldn't like that, but it would allow someone else her age to get a first jab sooner. The logic is impeccable.

'If it's based on your scientific advice and it will save lives, we can sell it,' I said. 'Given the massive sacrifices people have made already, people will buy this.' Actually, I'm excited – this way, we can protect more people.

Abroad, Emmanuel Macron has tested positive shortly after a meeting with other European leaders, meaning they all have to self-isolate. Joyeux Noël.

FRIDAY 18 DECEMBER

Boris has reluctantly caved to the inevitable and agreed to cancel Christmas. We've not announced it yet. Clearly the existing system isn't holding things in check – the R is now officially above 1 – and I finally won the argument about introducing an extra tier. Short of a full national lockdown, making people in the worst hotspots stay at home is all we've got left. In Tier 4, people will need a reasonable excuse to leave home, and non-essential retail has to close. London and most of the south-east and east of England will go straight into this category. The whole 'Christmas bubbles' idea is cancelled in these areas. For everyone else, Christmas bubbles will only be allowed on Christmas Day. That's it. Frankly, we would have been far better off saying it will be a Zoom Christmas from the start. I'm kicking myself. I deliberately stayed out of the whole Christmas debate and now I think I should have been more proactive. Raising expectations only to dash them at the last minute was a mistake and by not engaging I played my part.

The MHRA has finally – somewhat grudgingly – approved lateral flow tests for home use. This is going to be transformative. On the flip side, Dido messaged tonight warning me of problems with lab capacity heading into the weekend. She says they are 'going to need to take some action to manage demand', which sounds ominous. She's hopeful it's just a blip. 'It never rains but it pours!' was her cheerful sign off. More of a monsoon from where I'm sitting.

As always, Damon messaged me about tomorrow's front pages. Both *The Times* and the *Telegraph* are splashing on Covid-related stories based on leaks. *The Times* claims – wrongly – that the MHRA are blocking plans for home testing by mailshot, criticising me for not 'sorting out' regulatory issues. They're going to look a bit daft, because I've literally just unblocked it, but I'm still annoyed. The *Telegraph* splash is exactly what I told the PM in front of No. 10 comms colleagues yesterday, namely that the Oxford jab should get the green light before New Year. I really thought this inveterate leaking would stop when Cummings left. As I told Simon Case, sharing sensitive information about the vaccine programme becomes exceptionally difficult if it immediately appears in a national newspaper.

'Fucking unbelievable,' I told Simon – who is going to instigate yet another leak inquiry. I think he thinks it's come from Boris direct.

I was interested to read that Austria is going to test its entire population for Covid, starting on Boxing Day. I sent Dido a link to an article about it in the *Daily Mail*.

'The curse of Slovakia is alive and well!' she replied.

SATURDAY 19 DECEMBER

There's no good time for Test and Trace to crumble, but this is literally the worst. Dido tells me there's a critical shortage of pipette tips – showing the level of detail we have to go into to make this operation work. Our failure to get hold of these little bits of plastic has led to a backlog of 182,000 tests. Though the scale of the problem isn't public, there's no hiding it, not least because part of the Test and Trace website has crashed.

After an angsty call with Dido's team, a gloomy Damon reported that they regaled him with 'all sorts of constraints', which is Whitehall speak for 'reasons they can't deliver'.

'Testing falling over just at the time a new strain arrives is extremely dangerous territory,' he observed helpfully, as if I hadn't already figured that one out myself.

Meanwhile various people, including deputy chairman of the 1922 Committee Charles Walker, are calling for my head over the Christmas farce. Boris announced the changes to howls of dismay in what will surely go down as one of the messiest political U-turns in modern history. In his public statement, he rightly blamed the Kent variant, which new data suggests could be 70 per cent more transmissible. Walker seems to hold me personally responsible and thinks we deliberately delayed the announcement until Parliament went into recess so we didn't have to manage the fallout. It's an irony, because I wasn't involved in the Christmas decision at all. Maybe I should have come in and played hardball over it right from the start – but I can't be Mr Miseryguts on everything.

Actually, the reason we couldn't announce it all before Parliament rose was the Treasury holding things up. Time and again, HMT's institutional view of how to respond to this crisis has been wrong. They've played a blinder on furlough and support for businesses. But their attitude to lockdown has been entirely static. It's just like how they refuse to acknowledge the dynamic effects of tax cuts: you cut the right taxes at the right time and economic activity and revenue go up. In this case, it's the dynamic effect of the virus: you let it get going and it grows exponentially until eventually you have to have a tougher lockdown. In this case, there isn't even an economic reason to keep things open – but there is an immense emotional and very human reason to.

Jamie tried to make me feel better by saying the Christmas bubble policy was 'always mental ... a catastrophe waiting to happen'. He's right that while the U-turn is rough, sticking to the flawed policy would have been much worse. 'Even if we hadn't had this new strain, it would have been political suicide. Every death that happened in January would have been blamed on government allowing people to mix at Christmas,' he said.

He reports that his girlfriend is fuming and 'thinks everyone should be sacked'. Right now, I suspect most of the nation shares her view.

In response to our Tier 4 announcement, Sturgeon unveiled a travel ban with the rest of the UK. I'm sure she's been yearning to do that all her life.

SUNDAY 20 DECEMBER

We're an international pariah. Germany, France, Italy, the Netherlands, Canada, Belgium, Turkey, Iran and even Ireland have stopped flights to and from the UK. France has also halted ferry traffic for forty-eight hours and the Port of Dover is closed. It's a desperate attempt to avoid the Kent variant. I don't blame anyone for shutting us out: I've done the same to other countries in the past few months. Still, it's profoundly depressing. Jens called, perhaps feeling sorry for me. Looking for a bit of cheer, I picked up. He apologised for having to suspend air travel to the UK but was sure I'd understand. He asked me how many people we've vaccinated and I told him that we're aiming for half a million by tonight. He said how envious he was and I thanked him for the German technology behind the vaccine. He's under huge pressure on jabs but has to wait for EU supplies. He expects Brussels regulators to approve what he calls 'the BioNTech vaccine' in days. 'At least I have someone to blame for the delay,' he said wearily.

What I didn't tell him is we're having another panic about our own supply. The closure of Dover has created logistical issues. I spent the evening talking to the team, trying to figure out a way round it. Nadhim messaged this morning to say we have 700,000 doses en route by lorry from Belgium escorted by police and private security. The journey seems to be going smoothly. 'The vehicle does not need to return through France so no issue,' he added, promising to let me know when it's here. He says we can expect two to three more consignments before New Year, which will come via the Hook of Holland. We have planes on standby in case of any problem. We've checked with the regulators, who are rightly very cautious about transport, and they're happy with these routes. The vaccine has only been tested with a small amount of the kind of shaking and bumping that is unavoidable in transit. It also needs to be kept at −60 degrees. Imagine the consequences if we accidentally neutralised it by jostling it around.

What this means is that I have to restrain my normal bullish attitude: we can't afford to be injecting a vaccine that doesn't work. Nadhim is clearly relishing this whole challenge, and I think we make a good team. 'We will do this and people will see what you have done is truly a massive thing,' he said encouragingly. Nice of him, but I'm acutely aware that public expectations are very high. Unlike Jens, who can point the finger at the EU, I've got no one to blame if this goes wrong: it's on me. As the Christmas thing shows, I even get blamed when it's not my fault. I warned him that we will now come under HUGE pressure to go faster and need to be totally across the delivery schedule. Stephen Metcalfe, Tory MP for South Basildon and East Thurrock, messaged flagging up a problem with the rollout in his area. We're not aware of it. Metcalfe says it's a terrible Labour council, so cock-ups are to be expected.

Damon alerted me to a shit-stirring article in tomorrow's papers claiming we're considering vaccinating secondary school pupils following advice from SAGE. It's nonsense.

'Vallance needs to grip SAGE. Their briefing is out of control,' he said.

'Hit it very hard,' I replied.

I messaged Patrick, saying that stories like this are extremely unhelpful in this very difficult situation.

'Grateful if you could tell SAGE they have no role in the vaccination rollout. If I want their advice, I will ask you and Chris for it. Thanks,' I said, a bit brusquely.

Damon put out a line making it clear that SAGE has no locus in these decisions, which are for ministers advised by the JCVI. No such idea has been put to ministers and we have no plans to vaccinate children yet. The tricky thing is I don't want to rule it out, but if we go there, it will require months of highly sensitive preparation.

Later Patrick checked the minutes of the latest SAGE meeting, which note that the JCVI want SPI-M – their modelling sub-committee – to model the effects of immunisation in schools. It was a request from JCVI to see what would happen if vaccines have a very significant impact on transmission and whether that would alter their thinking on jabbing younger people. This confirms it was a JCVI request – not a SAGE request – relating to potential future scenarios. Slightly messy, but we've batted it away for now.

MONDAY 21 DECEMBER

Damon says Boris is 'slightly aggrieved' that we've described the virus as 'out of control' and that I've suggested things won't be back to normal until at least March. Well, it's the truth! I don't know why he's upset. Last night, I almost called him to tell him we're unlikely to get schools back in January and there is no way out of this until the vaccine is rolled out. Surely we're best being straight with people? I suspect he's still feeling resentful about the whole festive season situation. Nobody, least of all Boris, wants to be the man who cancelled Christmas.

More than forty countries have now suspended flights to the UK. Patrick has been on the radio saying he expects the Kent variant to spread across the whole country. The logic of his argument is for a national lockdown. That's what I've been fighting to avoid all autumn, but it's the obvious endpoint. On the plus side, we've hit half a million vaccines. We'll even be vaccinating on Christmas Day. Meanwhile the EU has finally approved the Pfizer/BioNTech vaccine. I sent Jens a text congratulating him and he replied that he was worried they don't have enough doses. 'German media are panicking,' he said. He asked me how much we have.

I felt a teensy bit smug replying, '340 million doses,' but as he knows, we have no idea how long it will take for them all to be delivered.

TUESDAY 22 DECEMBER

Uğur Şahin, chief executive of BioNTech, says the vaccine does work against the Kent variant. It's a massive relief. Pascal has also been in contact to say AstraZeneca thinks its vaccine will too. I asked both companies to get the news out ASAP. Hopefully it will calm everyone down a bit.

In another positive development, Macron has agreed that lorry drivers and EU citizens can continue to travel to and from France subject to a recent negative Covid test. Ben Wallace messaged this morning to say he has a battalion on standby to help at the border. Grant Shapps is fuming because the French won't accept lateral flows – of which we have millions – and are insisting on PCRs, which take much longer and are considerably more expensive. Still, it's progress, and given that supermarkets are beginning to run low on basics because cross-Channel transport has seized up, we've got to get on with it.

At lunchtime I attended the last G7 call hosted by Alex Azar, my US opposite number. He's leaving when Biden is inaugurated, and I'm taking the chair for 2021. He ended by saying he's going back into the private sector and if any of us needs a job, to give him a call. I'd rather stay where I am!

I chased JVT re. the possibility of delaying the second dose. If we're going to go for it, the sooner we announce it the better, as there will be a backlash. JVT says the MHRA are still looking at it but promised to try to move things along. Later JVT, the Prof and I went to see the PM to talk him through the idea. Rishi was also there. Boris was worried about disappointing elderly people who were expecting their second dose sooner. I said I backed it wholeheartedly, and Rishi also agreed, so in the end it was an easy decision for the PM.

Then, sitting in my office doing my box, my phone pinged with a message from Tony Blair. Unbelievably, he's got wind of our proposal and, like an over-enthusiastic junior minister, is calling for it before it happens! This is annoying, but much worse is that he's written an article saying we should focus our vaccine efforts on the individuals most likely to spread the disease, like students. This is bonkers: why vaccinate people who are at less at risk from the disease ahead of those for whom it's life-threatening?

Taking a deep breath, I stayed calm and messaged him suggesting we talk. 'Interesting piece on vaccines,' I began chirpily (I want to keep him onside). Then, some flattery: 'I think some of what you say is very wise.' Then: 'But other parts not quite right – would it be helpful to have a briefing, as I'm keen to ensure your excellent interventions are well informed?' I signed off with my very best wishes. Hopefully he'll catch my drift.

I was just about to collapse into bed when there was a new blow: confirmation via private office that the South African variant is here. I got straight onto the phone to Nadhim, who swore and asked whether it is resistant to the vaccines.

'We don't know, but more likely to be,' I replied gloomily.

We will now have to do to South Africa what everyone else has just done to us. Painful.

WEDNESDAY 23 DECEMBER

Blair got back to me before dawn, thanking me for my offer of a briefing. He said he's around all week (isn't everyone?) and mentioned that he was doing a radio interview this afternoon.

'If there is anything you think shouldn't be said, happy to take on board,' he offered. Very good of him. I've arranged a clinician to call him – the Prof or JVT – to try to talk him down from the vaccinating students position. We've done the work and are highly confident not only will it save fewer lives but it will also lead to a longer lockdown as it would take jabs away from protecting the most vulnerable.

The spread of the Kent variant is incessant. We've not even made it to the official review date, yet I've had to put Suffolk into Tier 4, along with whole swathes of England. I've also had to reverse the Herefordshire decision. Rates there have jumped, which is probably no surprise given that, according to Jesse, the pubs have been 'heaving'.

In better news, AstraZeneca has submitted its full data package for the Oxford vaccine to the MHRA. JVT phoned me to say it's in good shape but it will take them a couple of days to process. Sign-off would be the best possible Christmas present.

And we've finally started vaccinating care home residents. Hot on the heels of identifying someone called William Shakespeare to become the second person in the world to get the Pfizer jab, Simon Enright has pulled it off again, finding a nurse called Pippa Nightingale to vaccinate Chelsea Pensioners. We're paying GPs double the rate they get to deliver jabs in standard walk-in clinics to vaccinate elderly people in these settings. It works out at £25 per resident, which is pretty nice money for something that only takes a few minutes.

While officials in the department were working out how to get GPs to play ball, they made a remarkable discovery: there is absolutely nothing in law requiring us to negotiate payments for doctors with the BMA.

For the best part of two decades, Health Secretaries have been letting the BMA push them around over GP contracts, on the assumption that they were legally obliged to negotiate with the union. In fact, we could have just consulted publicly, like government does on everything else. Following this happy discovery, we were able to fix payment for vaccinations in care homes at the stroke of a pen, and I resolved that in future we won't be led a merry dance by the doctors' union.

THURSDAY 24 DECEMBER

Boris has been on TV saying we've done almost 800,000 jabs so far, when the actual figure is 745,000. He got the number from Nadhim. He's been fretting that America has now jabbed more people than we have. I had to explain last night that as a proportion that means we're six times ahead – and they're jabbing anyone, including Congresswoman AOC (Alexandria Ocasio-Cortez), who is still in her early thirties. Now he's latched onto an inflated figure, it will only get worse.

I listened to the PM get it wrong with a sinking feeling, knowing it will swiftly rebound. Messaging Nadhim, I warned that we'll get into 'serious trouble' if we use any more unconfirmed figures. 'We have to stop,' I said.

My view is that part of the problem is that the statistics regulator Sir David Norgrove seems to hate Boris. I strongly suspect he's never forgiven the PM for his notorious '£350 million more for the NHS' claim during the Brexit referendum campaign and is primed to pounce on any hint of misrepresentation. What this means is that I am frequently bollocked for these sorts of mistakes. I really resent being caught in the crossfire, because I've fought hard to maintain the accuracy of statistics, and have a background in it myself, so I feel my professional integrity is being called into question. I even passed an Act through Parliament giving the ONS powers to use modern data techniques.

'We both have to stop giving him figures,' I told Nadhim firmly. 'I'm not getting bollocked again.'

'Who dares bollock you?' Nadhim teased, with a thumbs-up emoji.

Unfortunately, plenty of people.

The latest ONS data, published early because it's Christmas tomorrow, shows that one in eighty-five people currently has Covid, with the Kent variant accounting for 38 per cent of cases. Very unhelpfully, there's a major outbreak at the largest testing lab in the country, in Milton Keynes, adding to the backlog.

We do, however, have a Brexit deal with the EU. It was never really in any doubt, despite both sides whipping it up, but nor were Brussels ever going to make it easy. At least that's done for now.

FRIDAY 25 DECEMBER

Today is my first real day off since summer. I told my family I'd do no work at all on Christmas Day, and I kept my promise. All the urgent things – the US banning flights, Ireland seeing the Kent variant for the first time – can wait.

Instead, we had a very small Christmas and watched the Queen tell people struggling without friends and family on Christmas Day that they 'are not alone', before praising the British people for 'rising magnificently to the challenges of the year'. She is wonderful.

SATURDAY 26 DECEMBER

As a consequence of yesterday's day off, Boxing Day was no holiday. I was back at my desk at 7 a.m., feeling a bit guilty about all the emails I ignored yesterday. The team have been working so hard. The NHS always works on Christmas Day, of course, and the Prof was on ward rounds, but so much of the civil service team and so many of my advisers were working too.

Almost everywhere in England is now in Tier 4 and it's obvious we're heading for another lockdown. We keep being told to wait for the data to settle after Christmas – but I don't think we've got time to do that. The new variant has changed all the old calibrations of what level of restrictions keeps R below 1.

The big question is whether kids can go back to school in January. Unfortunately, Gavin and I do not see eye to eye on this one. He is adamant we should keep schools open, which I suppose is his job, whereas I think it's nuts, which I suppose is mine. I just don't see how we can control this new strain with schools remaining open. Damon tells me Gavin's people are busy briefing about how worried he is about the damage to kids' education if they don't go back, so that the media knows he's put up a fight. Of course the damage of locking down to education – and mental health – would be significant, but the damage to life if we do not would be catastrophic.

SUNDAY 27 DECEMBER

Pascal Soriot has told the *Sunday Times* they've found a 'winning formula' with the Oxford/AstraZeneca vaccine. It should be approved for use in the UK in the next few days. Michael Gove agrees with me that we have to go into another lockdown. It's time to face facts.

MONDAY 28 DECEMBER

The beauty of Zoom meetings is that if you're clever with the camera – or just switch it off – it's perfectly possible to have a parallel dialogue with one or more participants. This is a very useful way of strategising if things aren't going well, and so it was that several of us were trying to figure out how to handle Gavin as he went batshit over the potential closure of all schools. He has compromised on the need to keep some closed, in Tier 4 areas, but that will just lead to more closures as the virus spreads. Of course I really, really want to keep schools open, but looking at the figures, I just can't see how we can get R below 1 unless they close. There are now 20,426 people in hospital with the virus – more than at the peak of the first wave – and we've had over 40,000 cases in just twenty-four hours. I don't need more data to know we have to lock down or we will overwhelm the NHS, and hundreds of thousands more people will die. We are in a worse place than we were in the spring. Gavin doesn't have an answer to how we stop that happening. What he does have is a lot of passion and energy, and in this meeting to discuss what to do about next term he was going absolutely gangbusters, insisting that there must be a reopening of schools.

Michael Gove, Emma Dean and I watched his performance open-mouthed, surreptitiously WhatsApping.

'What is Gavin going on about?' Michael asked, awestruck at the passion the Education Secretary was displaying.

I have no idea, I thought, but it is quite something to behold.

'I think he sees the whole thing through the lens of political competition, not policy,' I said eventually. This was probably unfair: he was, after all, standing up for the millions of children whose education will suffer if they can't go back. Then again, we are teetering on a precipice. People will die. What happens with schools is totally tied in with how we get out of this mess. Ever diplomatic, the Prof was struggling to maintain his usual neutral expression as Gavin continued his diatribe.

'Chris Whitty's face is a picture,' Michael said.

'PM doesn't seem to be buying it,' Emma observed.

Perhaps sensing the PM's scepticism, Gavin upped the ante, becoming so shouty that I had to turn the volume down.

'He's freaking out. You can just tell he isn't being entirely rational,' Emma said, sounding genuinely worried.

'Are you coming in to rescue this?' I asked Michael, because we really needed someone other than me to counter the onslaught. My own view is that shutting schools till February except for pupils in exam years would be best, but I doubt we'll get there.

Michael did his best to inject some cool rationality into the debate, pointing out that we can shorten Easter and summer holidays to make up for lost classroom time. But none of us were a match for Gavin, and the meeting broke up with no decision to close schools – i.e. for the time being, he's won. There's no way this will hold.

I switched off Zoom and put my head in my hands.

'The next U-turn is born,' I said wearily.

Emma asked if I wanted her to set up a call with Test and Trace later to go over the plan for school testing.

'No, I want to find a way – Gavin having won the day – of actually preventing a policy car-crash when the kids spread the disease in January,' I replied. 'And for that we must now fight a rear-guard action for a rational policy.'

No surprise that within hours, several journalists were chasing the story, details of Gavin's robust defence of the nation's schoolchildren having mysteriously leaked. The strict instruction from No. 10 was not to engage, and so we left it to Gavin's over-enthusiastic outriders to do their worst. Accordingly, tomorrow's *Mail* has a screaming headline imploring the government not to 'betray our children'.

No. 10 may be glad we stayed out of it, but I'm marooned in the middle, as shots are fired all around. This is the conundrum when someone briefs against you.

Apparently the PM is cross, but not as cross as I am. I messaged Boris direct, saying I can't believe the meeting leaked.

'You had so effectively stopped all that crap,' I said.

That was my polite version. The more direct version, to Dan Rosenfield, made it clear that I was 'pretty fucking appalled'.

'This is hard enough without that sort of behaviour,' I said.

Amid the mayhem, late tonight Michael messaged me saying he thinks we 'CAN' get to a better place on schools, 'BUT we need to show No. 10 we are busting every gut on vaccine/testing'.

Well, we are! What would be ridiculous would be to reopen schools in some parts of the country and not others. This one isn't over.

TUESDAY 29 DECEMBER

Dan Rosenfield messaged early doors to say the PM is 'furious' about the leak and instigating yet another inquiry.

'Good,' I replied. 'We also need to settle the policy.' I care far more about that.

Yesterday Gavin suggested some concessions, but since then, DfE has been rowing back. As I told Dan, my spirit of communal love and compromise is somewhat waning. This morning the DfE SpAd was onto Emma, saying they want to rule out testing of primary school kids and are pushing for teachers to be prioritised for vaccination – neither of which I am going to agree to.

'This is backtracking on all the things Gavin floated in the meeting,' I said.

'It was a very strange call,' Emma agreed.

Later she and Gavin had a discussion about what to do re. universities, during which he indicated that he would be very happy to agree to a staggered return over eight weeks 'provided the position on schools remains unchanged'. Seriously?! A) there is no agreed position, and b) as I pointed out to Emma, you can't negotiate with the virus.

'That's been their attitude,' she replied. Well, time for what Jim would call an 'attitude adjustment'. Dido says they have never seen such high rates at local authority level as they are seeing in London and Essex now and messaged offering to show Gavin the figures.

'Yes please,' I replied. Maybe it will help.

Overall figures are record breaking anyway: 53,135 new cases as the figures catch up with data that went unreported over Christmas. When I saw the data, I tried to reach the Prof. He texted back to say he's been out of contact as he's been back on the Covid wards. The figures are so bad that everywhere needs to be in Tier 4, a national lockdown in all but name. Ben Wallace messaged, annoyed that part of his Lancashire constituency is bouncing from Tier 2 to Tier 4, when it's 80 per cent rural. I told him that the figures are very high nonetheless.

'It's fucking depressing,' I conceded.

He says Cumbria had one of the earliest outbreaks of coronavirus, which he puts down to 'lots of travellers and skiers', though he also mentioned a North Yorkshire choir which travels the world and 'came back from China at the end of 2019'. The mind boggles.

As we lurch inevitably towards another lockdown, Boris is surprisingly sanguine – the data has done the talking. However, he is still digging in on schools. I will have to go into battle again tomorrow.

Happily, the MHRA have finally approved the Oxford vaccine. It's with Jim again for the technical sign-off. This time we don't need a formal meeting with the Prime Minister. We're going to announce tomorrow morning. I'm impatient to start the rollout – after all, this one comes from Wrexham, not Belgium – but Simon Stevens thinks we need the bank holiday to prepare, and the Scots want to wait till 4 January anyway. I reluctantly agreed: though it would have been nice to get it started in 2020, it's still within a year of our first meeting and a few extra days will allow for a smoother start.

Before I had time to tell Jens, he messaged asking if we can expect Oxford approval soon. They're keen to have the vaccine in Germany as quickly as possible. I dropped a very heavy hint in the affirmative. It's great that the Germans are asking for it; just such a pity Jens and I haven't been able to work on it together like we did in the summer.

Finally, the papers are reporting that hundreds of Brits did a midnight flit from Verbier after Switzerland imposed a retrospective ten-day quarantine on anyone from the UK due to the Kent variant. A bunch of skiers bust out of their resorts and hotfooted it to the Swiss border and thence to Paris, where they were able to get the last Eurostar home, making it back just in time for Christmas.

Top marks for chutzpah – though obviously I disapprove.

WEDNESDAY 30 DECEMBER

Words fail on the schools front. Gavin's still insisting that kids go back, with the exception of those living in the worst hotspots. Someone has come up with a figure of 22 per cent for the proportion of primary schools that can close. The result? We are fiddling around with random quotas and poring over maps of the outbreak to put in place a ridiculously complicated policy I know for certain will not hold.

'Why are we going for an arbitrary figure rather than what's needed to have a shot at protecting the NHS?' I asked Dan Rosenfield, exasperated. 'Seriously, in the state of the pandemic right now, I think we are under-gunning this. We know that the scientific advice is that with schools open, we can't hold this thing.'

I hate this horse trading: what we should be having is a proper public policy discussion. For now, though, no joy: Downing Street is siding with DfE, and DfE continues to lead us all a merry dance.

This morning I agreed the 4 January start date for the Oxford/AZ rollout with the devolved administrations. I still can't believe that two of our portfolio vaccines have come off so fast and that both are now being manufactured at scale. Poor Jens is now seriously fed up with the glacial pace of progress in the EU. He messaged congratulating me on the Oxford approval and asking when the UK will get to the immunity threshold. I thanked him and said that I hoped we'd be there by spring.

'And I need to wait for Europe again,' he replied gloomily.

'Dexit – you can get a really good deal,' I suggested jauntily, feeling that a bit of gentle teasing wouldn't go amiss.

His reply was just a zipped mouth emoji.

Later this morning, we announced the plan to extend the interval between the first and second doses of the jab. Lo and behold, who should pop up to claim credit but none other than Tony Blair! I let it pass. If he can help us land it, great.

One mercy is that most – though not all – of our anti-lockdown MPs are calming down. A new set of Covid regulations passed at an emergency recalled Commons today without a vote as support was near unanimous. Helen, who was keeping an eye on proceedings, says those opposing restrictions who are in denial about the data 'just look ever more out of touch'. There is a lot of justifiable unhappiness about the messy compromise over schools, which involves reopening some but not others.

'The announcement today is frankly a total shambles. Best we keep well clear of that,' I advised.

'Agreed,' she replied, adding that it's very hard to explain to Kent MPs why east Kent schools are still due to open when we are busy helicoptering patients from the area to Bristol because hospitals are overrun. Quite.

THURSDAY 31 DECEMBER

As predicted, the schools 'policy' is already blowing up.

'Glad you're not running DfE?' I asked Wormald mischievously.

I now have Tory MPs in Harrow complaining they're not in the area where schools will remain open, and the editor of *The Sun* on my back because one of the many geographic anomalies affects her family. Meanwhile everyone is trying to pretend this is all really well thought through.

'I'm just ducking,' I told Wormald.

Predictably, the BMA is kicking off about the second dose interval. The debate must not become political, so I kept well out of it. Instead, all four UK chief medical officers put out a response explaining that you get more protection by vaccinating a greater number of people with the first dose than by treating a smaller number of people with both.

This evening I was able to tell the PM that we have done more than a million vaccines in England: 1,004,740 to be precise. We have been debating what target to set for the rest of the rollout. He wants to go as fast as possible, obviously, but whatever we announce needs to be achievable. I'm not being set up for a fall, and neither should he be.

It's a very tricky judgement, as we're not in control of supply. I've told the supply team their job is to get in so much the NHS can't deliver it, and the NHS their job is always to be able to deliver whatever the supply team can get their hands on. So far, supply has always been the rate-limiting factor. That's how it should be: that we get it into arms as soon as it's available.

For now, Boris and I have agreed a vague pledge to 'offer' a vaccine to the most vulnerable people by mid-February. The point about the target being to 'offer', not to 'inject', is Simon Stevens's key ask: he's up for pushing the NHS hard, but if people don't come forward, you can't blame the NHS for that. Underlining my point about the uncertainty of supply, the companies aren't telling us about all their stock, only what they expect to be able to deliver – which is itself uncertain.

Sir John Bell messaged to say he thinks AstraZeneca has a secret stash in Gaithersburg, Maryland.

'We must get our hands on this now. Fly it over!' I told Nadhim excitedly. He says he's on it.

Less cheerfully, Geordie Greig has been in touch with a long list of what he calls (in capital letters) 'NAGGING QUESTIONS'. He wants to know why volunteers eager to help deliver jabs are being 'frustrated by excessive red tape' (good question); why we promised to deliver 30 million doses of the vaccine by September when far fewer are available (we never made that promise); and why we've increased the gap between the first and second doses of Pfizer when the manufacturer's research does not support this (see clinical advice).

So, we deliver the first vaccine in the world, with the fastest roll-out anywhere except Israel, and still the media is grumpy. I think it was Margaret Thatcher who said if you want approval, go into show business.

JANUARY 2021

FRIDAY 1 JANUARY

New Year's Day but no rest for the wicked. The boss wants to know why we can't boost our vaccine supply by getting it made in India. We should have pursued this more actively months ago, and it's partly my fault. The Serum Institute of India, AstraZeneca's Indian production partner, reached out to me back in October offering to help. I told the civil service to follow up, but nothing came of it.

I've told the PM that Indian production isn't regulated to our standards and we don't have any kind of mutual recognition arrangements in place. The Vaccine Taskforce say it will take longer to work our way through all the red tape than it will to scale up production elsewhere. I checked with Nadhim today and he confirmed that the MHRA would have had to visit every single factory producing the vaccine, which would take months, so it's a no-go.

Sensing the PM is on the warpath about the pace of the rollout, I reminded him that we're doing better than almost anywhere else. 'We have the earliest, and per head of population the biggest, supply of any major country. Except for minnows (e.g. Bahrain, Israel) countries would give their eye teeth to be where we are. We should always be pushing the VTF to go faster – as they have with Pfizer, securing another 3 million doses yesterday – but that's the reason for the current schedule,' I said.

The reason this wasn't followed up properly in October is that I didn't chase it personally. I have a rule with private office that I should only have to ask for something once: it's their job to make it happen. This works 99 per cent of the time, and I couldn't do the job if I had to keep a list of everything that needs chasing, but the system isn't infallible. I'm annoyed I didn't push this one.

I strongly suspect that fretting about vaccine supply is displacement activity for the PM, because he's worried about what will happen when we inevitably go for a full-blown lockdown. It's quite clear that the tier system isn't doing enough. He's due on *Marr* on Sunday and will need to be very well briefed.

Gavin is gradually conceding on schools. He's now agreed that London schools will stay shut. I've done my best to be collegiate and he's been gracious, cheerfully telling me after yet another difficult meeting today that he felt like he'd been 'mugged by a polite and friendly mugger'. He knows how stupid we'll look if we announce one thing then almost immediately have to change it.

I told Helen Whately that he'd been generous, having had to swallow a fair bit of humble pie.

'How long until he's ready for seconds?' she asked mischievously.

SATURDAY 2 JANUARY

The situation with the Serum Institute of India is getting more awkward. They are now actively pushing to sell us more doses and Downing Street is stressing. The last thing we want is a row with either the SII or AstraZeneca, and we can't risk a diplomatic spat with India by implying that their manufacturing systems aren't good enough. Then again, we don't want headlines about ministers desperately resorting to 'unregulated' vaccines. Damon suggested that Kate call the PM direct to calm him down, but I wasn't convinced this would work, as she's been unenthusiastic about these doses throughout. We dug out the minutes of the meeting when the VTF decided not to buy from the SII and thrashed out a substantial response to Downing Street, making it clear to them that our supply chain has to be assessed by a world-renowned regulator to ensure safety. The question is whether we can say this publicly without offending India. I told the team it was up to No. 10 to make the call on the balance between diplomacy and vax defence. Damon reports they're wary of being seen to criticise India's regulatory process but will do so if they're really feeling the heat.

'Yes, we may have to pull that emergency valve,' I agreed.

Meanwhile the Cabinet Office is stressing about NHS capacity. 'I am getting various noises that we are in dire straits now and will be in an apocalyptic position by end January/early Feb,' Simon Case told me. He asked if they're right.

'No. But it is tight and right to question,' I replied. We'll give Downing Street and the Cabinet Office the lowdown on Monday.

As the pressure mounts, Ben Wallace is once again feeling a bit used and abused re. requests for military help. 'We aren't the magic porridge pot!' he said grumpily.

He's been bombarded with requests, the latest of which is for combat medics to help with the vaccine rollout at the Nightingales and in Essex. All 111 army doctors available are already deployed in the NHS. Unfortunately, it's a pretty finite resource. He has asked his planners to find a solution that isn't robbing Peter to pay Paul.

'Understood,' I said. 'You have been a wonderful porridge pot but not a magical one!'

I am getting quite hacked off with what feels like relentless media negativity right now. Simon Case sent me a link to an outrageous story in the *New York Times* claiming the UK is opening the door to what they label 'mix and match vaccines', which they claim is 'worrying experts'. It's absurd – any suggestion we give people doses from different vaccines is obviously something that would be based on advice from our experts, who are world class. I agree with him that the piece is grossly irresponsible and that we need to hit back hard. Tomorrow's papers are also a bloodbath: there are claims of a 'postcode lottery', criticisms of a 'patchwork rollout' and claims people are being forced to drive ten miles for a jab. The driving ten miles bit is nonsense. As for some areas getting the vaccine faster than others, that's a fair cop, and as I told Damon (in stressed-out all caps) ABSOLUTELY THE RIGHT THING TO DO. Our initial sites are located according to where we can reach the greatest number of vulnerable patients. I told Damon not to stand for it. We can't let this false narrative gain any momentum.

Is it any wonder we are cautious about putting facts into the public domain when the papers act like this?

'Literally can't win,' Damon agreed resignedly. 'They are psychos.'

SUNDAY 3 JANUARY

The boss was fine on *Marr* – his usual showman act – but by this evening it was ancient history. The latest Covid figures are truly shocking and it's patently obvious we can't avoid a national lockdown. I messaged Boris this evening setting out how bad things are. I sent him the latest data and graphs, all of which point to one thing: the whole country needs the strongest possible measures.

I sent him a long list of steps we need to take, including closing takeaway alcohol outlets and click and collect services. I also want to end the boozy 'work lunches' and 'work dinners'. I know people are abusing the system.

'No consumption of alcohol at work meetings. 10 p.m. curfew. Very strong stay-at-home messages in all circumstances, with very limited reasonable excuses,' I said. I have made sure that everyone in my own department gets this message: I am banning alcohol on the premises.

I think secondary school non-exam years are going to have to switch to online learning until at least half-term. As for primary schools, they'll need to shut entirely.

We're going to have to be straight with people: this is going to last weeks.

Boris rang me back straight away and we talked it over. I left him in no doubt that unless we do this, the NHS will be overwhelmed. He was resigned and receptive. It doesn't matter how much you hate lockdown; this is increasing exponentially and we know where it will end up unless we act.

Later Tedros called to say Barbados is having a shocker and needs urgent help. Having previously been virtually Covid-free, they're now having a huge outbreak and are desperate for vaccines. Tedros says they're looking for 10,000–20,000 doses of AstraZeneca. I demurred, because I know other countries have made similar requests of the Foreign Office. We can't fulfil all the requests and the FCDO doesn't want any favouritism. Tedros linked me with the Prime Minister of Barbados, so after I finished my box I called her on her mobile and we spent an hour talking over the phone. Barbados hadn't really had a first wave, so this was her first real experience of the misery. I said I would do everything I could. The whole thing turned into more of a mutual counselling session than a business call about vaccines.

MONDAY 4 JANUARY

Millions of children returned to school today, only to be told schools are closing again tomorrow. After sleeping on it, Boris agreed that we have no choice but to go for another national lockdown, so all that to-ing and fro-ing with Gavin was indeed a waste of time.

When I arrived at the morning meeting to go through the data, he was there, standing, gripping the back of his chair. 'We're going to have to do it,' he said. My phone call had obviously had the desired effect. We went through the latest grim figures, and the conclusion was obvious. There was a consensus that we had to act, despite the painful consequences. I'd won, but it didn't feel like a victory.

A Cabinet call was arranged for 6 p.m., and nobody was opposed. We spent the rest of the day hammering out the detail. I wanted to make taking exercise easier than it was during the previous lockdown. This time, people will be allowed to exercise with one other person outside. The PM announced it all at 8 p.m. He looked tired but was very clear.

It gives me no pleasure that I've been warning about this since September. If only we could have got the vaccine out before this wave, but there was just no way of going any faster.

I was up early to witness 82-year-old Brian Pinker become the first person to get the Oxford AstraZeneca vaccine. I had tried to get a Union Jack on the label (Ben Wallace's idea!) or even the box, but regulators said no – apparently packaging is tightly controlled. The best we could do was use it on social media. Very annoying: I'm sure if it were French, it would be plastered in the tricolore.

In between all this, we firmed up the new vaccine target: 13 million doses by mid-February, covering all the priority groups. Once the vulnerable are jabbed – as I told *The Spectator* in an interview today – it's 'Cry Freedom'.

I had hoped to keep the mid-February target slightly vague, but at the last minute Dan Rosenfield changed 'mid' to '15' February in the announcement, so now we'll have to work to that specific date.

Nadhim's already under massive pressure, so I cheered him up by telling him that the boss was singing his praises in Cabinet. Nadhim was delighted and started going on about how much he loves working with me, how it's really refreshing, the only good thing about his job etc.

'The only good thing? What about saving the country?' I teased.

He replied that as an Iraqi Kurd who fled Saddam Hussein's regime to find sanctuary in the UK, he feels this country has given him and his family everything.

Tony Blair is still being a pain on the vaccine rollout, arguing for a different approach. Trying not to sound too passive aggressive, I offered to help bring him up to speed on our policy.

'Hi Tony, I'm very worried you've not been well briefed on the vaccine rollout. Your points this morning were not all correct. I've asked the department to organise a briefing – but maybe we should talk in the interim,' I suggested.

He replied promptly, saying he was happy to do that.

Someone has got wind of the difficult exchange I had with Ben Wallace yesterday over the use of combat medics and has briefed a garbled version to Times Radio's Tom Newton Dunn. TND is now claiming that I originally 'refused to accept any MoD help', whereas now I am taking it, which Tom claims is a 'sign of the pressure I'm now under'. Untrue and annoying! I messaged Ben saying I had no idea where it's come from since it's total rubbish. Ben says he'll do what he can to kill it. Incredibly tedious.

TUESDAY 5 JANUARY

An early morning panic after Downing Street unilaterally decided we should announce vaccination figures at the daily press conference. The media is pushing for it – this morning, the *i*, *The Times* and *The Sun* all called on the government to start publishing daily data, complaining that our limited figures won't do – and the PM is clearly feeling the heat.

The problem is that we only have numbers for England, and extracting daily updates from the devolveds will be a nightmare. Damon says he's trying to talk No. 10 out of it.

'Tell them it's not agreed,' I instructed.

'They can't announce something that's undeliverable,' Emma said. Unfortunately, bitter experience suggests otherwise!

I then had to deal with a farce over security vetting for volunteers at vaccine centres.

When we launched the programme, officials rightly stressed that we need to make sure that everyone who registers to help is kosher. I signed off on it, assuming they'd do some basic checks to make sure we don't unwittingly hire convicted criminals/other undesirables. In a classic example of Whitehall gold-plating, the civil service took this to mean that I wanted everyone involved to be fully vetted. I can just imagine the instruction from some blank-faced bureaucrat: 'The Secretary of State has said everyone needs to be properly vetted.' Then the securocrats would have got a hold of it, and they like nothing better than a lengthy clearance process. The result: logjam. Apparently they've been running around trying to figure out how to deliver on my 'instruction' without the whole system collapsing. Thankfully Emma got wind of it, and I explained that I meant basic checks, not a full-blown security vetting.

No sooner had I put out this fire than I got a very grumpy message from Jonathan Gullis, the Conservative MP for Stoke-on-Trent North, saying that clinics and care homes in his constituency were all set to jab a load of people this weekend, only to be told, at the last minute, that their scheduled vaccine delivery has been 'pulled'. Apparently hundreds of people have had their appointments summarily cancelled. Gullis described the situation as 'mayhem'. He says the clinical director of Newcastle North Primary Care Network is furious and busy claiming that the delay is 'impacting on the mental health' of the vaccination team. In what is becoming a familiar refrain, I told him I'd get Nadhim onto it.

Jim has been doing more groundwork on the potential for vaccine passports. He says he's 'nudging along thoughtful and sensible ideas' but is running into headwinds. He reports that a submission on the Israeli green pass scheme was not well received by ministerial colleagues ('had a very bad vibe', as he put it). Wheeling out one of his favourite phrases, he says there needs to be some 'attitude adjustment' on the part of sceptical colleagues. He describes the response to the sub as 'gratuitously risk-averse, back-covering and emotionally negative'.

Slightly awkwardly, Nadhim suggested we definitely weren't going to go down the vaccine passport route when he was asked about it in the Commons in December – or rather, he said we have 'absolutely no plans' to do so. In Whitehall speak, that does not mean we absolutely won't do it, but it does make it more awkward. Jim thinks Nadhim needs to be 'inducted' into what he describes as the 'medium-term inevitability' of some sort of documentation – for example, when other countries require it for travel.

For all my moaning about the media, the *Telegraph* has run a nice comment piece praising the vaccine programme. Alex Phillips writes that 'when it comes to vaccinations, our little island is blazing quite the trail'. There are only a few days to go to hit our first target of vaccinating 1.5 million people by Monday. Emily Lawson, who is heading up the vaccine deployment programme, has scheduled what she's calling a 'no holds barred' team meeting about how we get this done. Nadhim is affronted not to have been invited. When he asked her why, she told him he 'scares the team'. Hard to imagine, as he's such a charmer.

WEDNESDAY 6 JANUARY

Boris has been lying awake at night worrying that other countries are overtaking us on the vaccine. 'I woke up at 3 a.m. in a cold sweat about all this', he told me this morning.

I pictured him tossing and turning, fretting that Britain is trailing in the international league tables that are starting to appear.

I sent him a link to the *Telegraph* piece and he replied slightly testily that European countries are now ahead of us.

'No, they're not', I protested. 'What makes you say that?'

'Denmark?' he replied.

'Behind us', I replied briskly.

He wasn't satisfied and asked for more comparisons, which I'm happy to provide, as they will show us doing well.

'Now you've set our huge target, what the team need are motivation and accountability', I said, for which read: we're already busting a gut and it gets a bit demoralising if we're only criticised for not going faster. Last year we funded Our World in Data, run by Oxford University, so the comparisons are all in the public domain.

It turns out the ridiculous gold-plating of security clearance for vaccine volunteers has been repeated in training sessions. Andrew Murrison – who's a public health doctor as well as an MP – went for his induction and rang me afterwards to tell me what's been going on.

'You won't believe what they're asking me to do!' he said.

Unfortunately, I entirely believed it, and I had to unravel it all again. My instruction that people should be 'trained properly' did not mean they needed to complete every conceivable module: counter-terror training, lifting and shifting training, safeguarding training etc. Seriously?! My fault, but I didn't think I'd have to spell it out – I just don't have the time. A complete lack of common sense at the other end. I've now asked to see every training module myself and have said it should be the absolute minimum required.

Extraordinary scenes in Washington this afternoon as a mob of disaffected Trump supporters stormed Capitol Hill. They were trying to interrupt the final counting of electoral college votes, which will confirm Biden's victory. Unbelievable that Trump has let this happen.

THURSDAY 7 JANUARY

An SOS from Isle of Wight MP Bob Seely, whose local NHS is in crisis. He fears what he described as a 'perfect storm': small hospital, rising infections, an ageing population and a slower vaccination process than parts of the mainland. His message was polite and constructive, and I took his point. Frankly, the Isle of Wight NHS struggles to cope at the best of times. I've promised to look into it. Why does it face so many challenges?

On the *Today* programme, Chris Hopson set hares running by suggesting that the NHS is discharging patients to care homes because hospitals are full. Helen Whately says it's true. We are both alarmed – the last thing we can afford is a repeat of the issues around discharges to care homes in the first wave – even though the analysis shows that infection was mostly thanks to staff working in more than one care home, moving between them, not discharges. It makes sense to use care homes for Covid-negative overflow, but we need to be incredibly careful.

Meanwhile I want to solve something that's been bugging me for weeks: we're not doing nearly enough to make the most of the UK's vaccine success to boost 'Brand Britain'. I have made clear that in all comms we should refer to the AstraZeneca jab as 'the Oxford vaccine' or 'the Oxford AstraZeneca vaccine'. We've got to get the point across. I know Jens is irritated that Pfizer get all the kudos for what is actually a German vaccine. BioNTech barely get a look-in. Both are massive international collaborations, but we've got Oxford and should own it. 'It should be seen as a Mini. Made in Oxford. A brilliant piece of British engineering. Accessible to everyone. Ready to change the world,' I told Nadhim enthusiastically. He agrees.

Uptake is going well so far. The Queen has had her jab and the

Palace will quietly make it known. They are such pros. I'm still worried about vaccine hesitancy, especially among younger care workers. Also, we still don't know whether the vaccine works against the South Africa variant. Apparently scientists at Porton Down don't yet have what they need to do this research. I messaged JVT asking him to push things along and also make sure we're doing clinical trials in South Africa. JVT promised to speak to Porton again. He thinks they're under-promising but will over-deliver. I hope he's right. He says the World Health Organization also needs to get better at coordinating the global response to new variants. He's going to talk to them.

JVT has told the Faculty of Travel Medicine that he thinks Covid vaccines will become required travel vaccines.

'No vaccine, no Benidorm,' he told me robustly. 'All self-respecting young Brits will be vaccinated!' I hope so.

Finally we have movement on getting the MHRA to be much quicker at signing off consignments of the vaccine. They've been taking up to twenty days to rubber-stamp new loads, which was not helpful, and are now indicating they could do it in five. In a sign of their confidence, they've briefed the *Daily Mail*. Obviously I'm delighted. I have been pushing for this change for two months.

This morning Jim signed official approval for the Moderna vaccine. It comes with specific interval dates for the first and second dose. If we alter these intervals, we'll have to go 'off label', meaning we'd be using the drug in a way that does not precisely match its licence. For now, we don't have any stocks, so it's not an issue.

Jim says the MHRA are moving to authorise the vaccine for children with serious health issues like cerebral palsy. He rightly notes that giving the jab to kids is highly contentious, so we will need to be careful about how any new policy is presented.

FRIDAY 8 JANUARY

There's a fake NHS video doing the rounds purporting to be a public service announcement to 'Covid hoaxers, mask deniers and general conspiracy theory nutcakes'. To a sombre soundtrack, a funereal voice instructs these people to 'shut the fuck up, mask the fuck up, grow the fuck up'.

'Follow these guidelines to stop being an arsehole,' it concludes.

It is dark perfection and I really, really wanted to tweet it. Indeed, I came within a whisker of doing so. In the end I restrained myself, but I enjoyed the fleeting fantasy.

All week I've been fretting about whether the measures we're taking will be enough. The reality is that we have no more levers to pull. Hospitals are now at breaking point – much fuller than in the first wave – and I am left with a sense of powerlessness. It's the most nervous I've been since the same point in the first wave – watching and waiting for the worm to turn. When I wake up in the night, I tell myself it's too early to hope for the data to move. I'm desperate for a sign that what we're doing is paying off, but nothing yet.

The thing I dread more than anything – that continually hangs over me – is having to issue directions on which critically ill patients to prioritise. Should we put old people first, because they're more vulnerable, or young people, because they have longer to live? Government is often about taking the least-worst decision. In this case, choosing who should live and who should die is the worst 'least-worst' decision I can imagine.

The Prof is equally worried. He says any such awful decisions should be taken as locally as possible. My fear is that the BMA leadership – ever eager to pile pressure on governments – are gearing up to call for some kind of central direction on this dreadful question. We must avoid that at all costs.

Blair is again trying to be helpful and has been privately attempting to secure additional vaccines from Johnson & Johnson. He says he's working hard behind the scenes and has further calls lined up over the weekend. He wonders whether there is any additional AstraZeneca supply lurking somewhere outside the UK that we could access earlier. He says pharma companies that have stock squirrelled away will be very reluctant to commit to anything for fear they can't deliver, but that he will suss out the real room for manoeuvre and let me know. Worth a try...

SATURDAY 9 JANUARY

The Palace announcement has worked wonders. They did it so artfully: quietly letting it be known that Her Majesty waited for her turn and then simply confirming she's had it without the hullabaloo of doing it in public. It's great for take-up – if it's good enough for the Queen etc...

Less encouragingly, Lord Darzi, the eminent surgeon, caught Covid despite being jabbed. He told me he had the vaccine in December and then helped with the rollout. He then caught Covid from a patient after Christmas. He says he's fine, but it doesn't seem to be a one-off. In fact, he told me it's quite a common story. I mentioned it to the Prof because it could create a little media anxiety. The reality is that it takes a while for immunity to build, so we should not be surprised this is happening.

I asked the Prof where we are up to on the system for monitoring events after rollout. We have two parts to what's called the pharmacovigilance system: one to register all adverse events to check they're not worryingly regular and another to check if anyone gets Covid afterwards.

'I was told that we were doing it, but I worry that the details will be shonky,' I said.

The Prof replied that the system is 'reasonable' but needs to get better. We agreed a meeting with the team to go through where we're up to and how we can step it up.

The boss has been asking me whether the MoD could be doing more to help the rollout. As I told Ben Wallace, what's holding us back right now is vaccine supply: we have enough vaccinators and good logistics. All the same, I asked Ben to keep me informed about what assets he has available. He replied that he needs more information about supply so that he can anticipate what support we'll need and allocate resources.

'I don't want to offer the PM delivery capability that's ahead of stock, which would only raise expectations,' he said reasonably.

I told him that supply is still uncertain due to the realities of production challenges. 'On the current schedule – unless we get seriously good news on availability – we shouldn't need much more [help],' I said. Where we will need MoD support is within the NHS, where capacity is going to get tighter and tighter over the next two to three weeks.

Ben has been totally brilliant throughout this, for which I thanked him again.

'You and I both have an interest in managing everybody's expectations,' he replied.

'Exactly – including the boss!' I replied.

Pressure on hospitals is being exacerbated by the reluctance of care homes to accept patients who've been discharged from wards, even if they've clearly tested negative. Operators are worried about being sued. We've been working on an indemnity scheme, which is now urgent. Helen Whately is gripping it. I messaged her warning that hospitals are now in serious trouble.

'We need to do everything we can on discharge,' I said.

Jim says there are various Covid outbreaks at vaccine manufacturing facilities. 'The people making the vaccine at AZ need some vaccine themselves, I gather,' he reported.

Not vaccinating the individuals required to keep making the stuff – meaning they get sick and can't keep coming to work – is clearly daft. I tell the team we should define them as healthcare workers.

SUNDAY 10 JANUARY

I am very worried about funeral and mortuary capacity. Apparently funeral directors are struggling for staff. I messaged Michael Gove to say we'll need to prioritise them for the jab, alongside healthcare workers. 'A problem in the mortuary space would be terrible. Can we fix it together?' I asked.

Meanwhile I've inadvertently upset Downing Street over schooling for children of key workers by reiterating our official policy on TV today: namely, that if only one parent is a key worker, if at all possible, their children should stay at home like everyone else. Kids are only automatically eligible to keep going to school if both parents have frontline jobs. I was barely off air when Damon got an angsty message from James Slack, the Downing Street comms director.

'This is not government policy. Where the hell has this come from?!' James demanded. He was very wound up, suggesting my hardline approach on this will 'take out' the security services, the National Crime Agency etc. 'We can't freelance on stuff like this,' he said angrily, telling Damon we have to row back.

'It's the actual policy,' I pointed out, feeling aggrieved. I was bewildered as to why No. 10 seemed so het up. It turns out that it's the Cabinet Office. Apparently they're being inundated with complaints from NHS leaders, police and intelligence agency chiefs etc. saying their staff are being told kids can't go in. As a result, critical services are not running. Meanwhile lawyers who aren't even in court are sending their kids in. They're trying to avoid a situation in which conscientious public servants are struggling to do their jobs with their kids at home while commercial lawyers abuse the system. I agree and did my best to clarify during the rest of the media round. Later Dom Raab, who'd been watching me on the media round, messaged to say I'd been very 'clear and reassuring'.

'Aiming not to be too reassuring!' I replied.

The PM – usually so reluctant to impose measures – now wants to go even further than I do with restrictions. He is pushing to ditch the provision allowing two people to meet up for outdoor exercise together. I don't want to budge – the ability to exercise with someone else is really important for both physical and mental health. The Prof says it's a double-edged sword, because the system is being abused but if people are determined to meet up, it's better for them to do it outside than in. Personally I really want to be able to keep doing this. Last year I did almost no exercise all year. I'm losing fitness and know I need to do something about it. Since Christmas I've been running part of the way into work with my brother Chris. I take my government car as far as his flat, going through my work boxes en route, then leave the vehicle and run with him through Hyde Park, Green Park and St James's Park to work. It's a real joy. Chris and I haven't seen much of each other for several years as we've both been so busy; the half-hour jog is a great way to catch up. I know millions of people feel the same – I don't think we should take this away from them. I warned Simon Case that if the PM tries to push this, it could have serious implications for people's ability to stick to the lockdown and could also drive socialising indoors, which is much more dangerous.

Simon suggests that in the first instance we announce that we know people are flouting the rules and warn that if they don't stop, we'll have to kill it off for everyone. Perhaps this will generate a bit of social pressure.

MONDAY 11 JANUARY

I'm keen to keep all the former Prime Ministers onside, so I've been trying to get them all together for a Zoom briefing, which finally took place today. Given my impossible schedule and their complicated diaries, it was a nightmare to organise. The only time that worked for everybody was while I was visiting Epsom Racecourse vaccination centre, so this lunchtime I found myself in a cavernous reception room, surrounded by empty bookmakers' stalls, talking to four former British premiers. The four quarters of my screen consisted of Gordon Brown, Tony Blair, Theresa May and David Cameron. The only one who couldn't attend was John Major.

I sat at a tiny table, staring at my laptop as these extraordinary figures from history stared back at me. I explained the vaccination rollout plan and asked them to support it. The funny thing was that all four played directly to their public personae. Cameron was charming and asked a very sensible policy question. Blair asked a question to which he already knew the answer. Ever the diligent constituency MP, Theresa asked about the rollout in Maidenhead. Gordon was very quiet. Finally he made an incredibly incisive point about how best to demonstrate the value of the union by stressing that all this is a joint effort: UK and Scottish institutions working together, vaccines bought and developed by UK government, rollout done by local Scottish NHS, and all supported by the British Army.

On my way back to the office, I received a message from a friend tipping me off that straight-talking cricket legend Sir Geoffrey Boycott is very unhappy about the delay in the second dose. He's a childhood hero of mine, so I volunteered to call him personally to explain. I rang him from my car as we whizzed past, believe it or not, the Oval. Flattery got me nowhere: he gave me such an earful I felt like I'd run him out at Lord's. I made the case as well as I could, but it was clear he was far from persuaded.

Sadiq Khan is on manoeuvres, complaining that Londoners are being let down over the vaccine rollout. It's true that rates are much lower in the capital than elsewhere. While we try to establish why, we need to square him off. I asked Nadhim to organise a summit with him and other London leaders to bind him in. Sadiq is mercifully predictable and easy to deal with. He really cares about being respected and taken seriously. If you include him in the process, he's usually quite reasonable. He's a complete contrast to Andy Burnham, who will play any process for the politics.

Meanwhile I'm starting to be bombarded with messages from MPs about problems with the rollout in their constituencies. Feedback from colleagues shows the scale of the challenge we face. I've had a long list of complaints, including: elderly and vulnerable constituents receiving letters telling them to travel very long distances to get vaccinated; vaccination centres not having enough warning of when vaccines will arrive, so they can't plan; difficulty of vaccinating in rural areas; some clinical commissioning groups being very slow to set up hubs; GPs not stepping up; and some CCGs playing politics with the doctors. One colleague thinks his local NHS are 'not interested in the Prime Minister's timetable' (or, perhaps, would quite like him to fail?) and that the PM 'will become the fall guy for their lethargy'.

'All part of the Rolls-Royce service,' I replied breezily, as my heart sank.

TUESDAY 12 JANUARY

Not only is Boycott in the press having a go at me; now Betty Boothroyd is kicking off as well. Given that I personally ensured she got her first jab fast, it feels a bit rich. The delayed second dose policy is fully justified, but it's a classic case of winners and losers in politics: those who lose from a decision shout much louder than those who win, and the people whose lives are saved aren't identifiable so don't have a voice at all. As a result, an excellent policy gets a pasting. It's particularly miserable being criticised by people I've grown up admiring and went out of my way to help, but welcome to the life of a politician.

Emma messaged this evening saying that a bunch of GPs are refusing to go into care homes where there are Covid cases. Apparently there are cases in about a third of care homes, meaning many residents aren't getting vaccinated.

'Seriously?' I replied, shocked.

'Yep,' she confirmed.

Evidently I was naive to think £25 a jab would be enough of an incentive. Once again, we may have to use the army to fill the gap.

The *Telegraph* has run a story claiming that we're funding a trial of vaccine passports. I had no idea. It turns out to be a tiny grant (just £75,000) from the government's science and research funding agency. Nadhim says the Covid Recovery Group are going nuts. He's already had Steve Baker on the phone but has managed to calm him down.

Case numbers are just starting to flatten out. They were under 50,000 yesterday and today. It's very hard to look day by day, because they're always higher on a Tuesday as more people test on a Monday. But you can reliably compare to a week ago, and these are down. I have a spreadsheet that tracks the daily figures and compares to a week ago. I also have a brilliant daily data feed from my private office, where I've embedded a data scientist called Adam Langron, who has invented a new way of presenting the daily data to make sense of it. The result of all this: tentative signs that the new lockdown is working. A massive sense of relief.

WEDNESDAY 13 JANUARY

The Joint Biosecurity Centre is going to recommend all travel corridors are closed. Jim, who's been liaising with them on this issue, says he encouraged them to be bold.

'This may be the "Ming vase moment" that makes people realise we're facing a different level of threat,' he mused. I know the Prof agrees and told Jim we should back the JBC on this one. Given how relaxed the Prof has been on travel, this is telling.

I finally made my statement to Parliament on mental health reforms, something I've been wanting to do for weeks. There have been awful abuses in residential mental health settings and it's time to drag the law into the twenty-first century. I tried to keep it as uncontroversial as possible and Jonathan Ashworth was wonderfully supportive. It has been a long haul on an issue that doesn't excite the media, but the plans will be life-changing for some very vulnerable people.

New data from Israel suggests the vaccine is halving infections from fourteen days post-jab. Very encouraging.

THURSDAY 14 JANUARY

We've done 3 million vaccines! We're on track to hit the PM's target next month and might even do it with a day or two to spare.

Priti Patel wants to introduce a requirement for people flying into the UK to have negative tests. I am fully supportive and think they should be mandatory. I told my team to support the Home Office, and that my view is there should be no entry to the UK without a negative test and a properly filled in passenger locator form, and if you lie or give your name as 'Mickey Mouse', you should face serious consequences.

I've recommended that for the next month we bar all foreign arrivals; require all British citizens flying into the UK to quarantine for ten days; and introduce a strict testing regime for anyone transporting freight. I think we need much stronger enforcement and a much tougher testing system for any international travel.

Later I took part in a Commons debate on Vitamin D as a

preventative treatment for Covid. It's something David Davis, the Tory MP and former Brexit Secretary, and Labour MP Rupa Huq are now pushing. The theory is that high doses may provide some protection. Doctors say it's unproven, but DD rightly argues that this is because we haven't really tried. I'm keen. Vitamin D is harmless except in huge doses, so let's give it a crack. Unfortunately, however, because Vitamin D is generic, the pharma companies don't make any money out of it, so the clinical trials required to see whether it's effective just don't happen. I'm no socialist, but I do think there's a gap in medicine which leads to a bias towards in-patent pharmaceuticals. It's the same with social prescribing. Cheap or free solutions like exercise or music just don't get the research investment that a new drug gets, and so don't get the weight of evidence; therefore they aren't prescribed. Unusually, the Prof and I disagree on this one. He says there's no clinical evidence yet on Vitamin D. But my view is that when the lack of clinical evidence is down to a market failure like this, the state has a duty to step in.

FRIDAY 15 JANUARY

An extraordinary row with Pfizer bosses, who are trying to divert some of our vaccine supply to the EU! The first I heard of it was a message from Natasha saying I needed to get over to No. 10 right away. I called Ben Osborn, who heads up Pfizer UK, to try to find out what was going on, but he didn't pick up.

By the time I got to Downing Street I was on top of the basics: Pfizer production is behind schedule and they're under massive pressure from EU leaders, who don't like daily headlines about how far they've fallen behind the UK, so now they're trying to reduce our supply to appease Brussels.

When I got to the Cabinet Room the PM practically had smoke coming out of his ears. He was in full bull-in-a-china-shop mode, pacing round the room growling. What really riled him was the fact that only last night he was speaking to Pfizer CEO Albert Bourla, and Bourla made no mention of it!

JVT is also seething and thinks Bourla has been totally disingenuous.

'Claims not to know. Really, the MD of the UK business??' he spluttered over WhatsApp.

'I know,' I replied. 'Not just the MD of the UK business but the global CEO! We are using this to put serious pressure on them.'

'Good!!!' JVT replied.

Either Bourla didn't know and should have or did know and didn't say anything. Neither is good.

Watching Boris huffing and puffing, I knew he was also nervous about the potential blowback on him. He was the one who tightened the target for the rollout, putting a specific date on it to put more pressure on me to deliver. If we miss it, he can't blame me.

Nevertheless, I was wary: when the PM is in this mood, he can really lash out. I've seen it before and knew I'd need to be as diplomatic as possible if I wanted to avoid getting caught in the crossfire.

As Boris was steaming about it, Osborn rang me back and I darted out of the Cabinet Room to take the call. I went into the little study overlooking the garden so we could talk privately.

'Listen, Ben, we've always been straight with each other,' I said, dispensing with small talk. 'Your global CEO spoke to the PM last night and didn't mention a word of this, and now we are likely to miss our target. Either he's being disingenuous or he doesn't know what's going on in his own company. Which is it?'

Ben was mortified and gave me some bluster about challenges with production lines etc., but I could tell he knew it wouldn't fly.

'You cannot behave like this,' I said firmly. 'We gave you the gold-standard world-first approval, and now you're dumping all over us like this? The public will want to know why our delivery has slowed down, and we will have to explain what happened.' In other words: your reputation is on the line. As head of Pfizer UK, he isn't the final decision maker. I knew he would need plenty of ammunition to take to the company's global board.

Hanging up, I went back to the Cabinet Room and gave the PM a diplomatic version of our exchange. Thankfully he seemed to have calmed down. He asked for another call with Bourla, and my team was tasked with finding a Plan B. As we wrapped up, I seized the opportunity to make a tentative point about the importance of wriggle room.

'We should always under-promise and over-deliver,' I said, trying not to sound too 'told you so'.

Still recovering from this drama, I checked in with JVT about the human challenge studies, which involve inoculating volunteers and then infecting them with the virus, to test the efficacy of the jab. He told me the trial is finally up and running. It's taken a year! At least we've now got the system going: in future, it's got to be much quicker. Next time, if we're able to infect volunteers as part of Phase 2 trials (after initial safety has been tested), it could take months off the time to develop a vaccine. As long as the volunteers are fully aware of the potential risks and have fully consented, I think the ethics are straightforward.

SATURDAY 16 JANUARY

Good news and bad news: the PM has accepted my hardline travel restriction recommendations, but it's up to me to deliver them. That was the deal I had to do to get the plan through No. 10. So I'm now chairing a new cross-government committee on border arrangements with Grant and Priti. Frankly, borders policy has always been a total muddle: there are just too many different authorities. Ports and airports are run by private operators under DfT regulations, Border Force reports to the Home Office, and now Covid rules are set by the Department of Health. The aim is to pull it all together. Whether a new Whitehall committee can sort it out God only knows, but we'll give it our best shot.

This afternoon I took the boys to the park to play some rugby. We messed around chucking the ball and did some tackling. They like the rough and tumble. Later I was astonished to find myself at the top of a news website for a perfectly legal – in fact encouraged – bit of outdoor exercise. Damon tried to get them to change the copy, which was ridiculously accusatory in tone, but they wouldn't shift. They did at least pixelate the children's faces. Since when is park rugby with the kids front-page news?!

SUNDAY 17 JANUARY

Bad news in a call from the Prof. They have found a number of new variants, including one in Liverpool, for which the vaccine may be less effective. We're waiting for more information, but there are suggestions that neither Pfizer nor Moderna may work as well against some of the new strains emerging. Very worrying, but at least we've caught these ones early.

Someone has briefed the *Sunday Telegraph* that all over-eighteens could have the jab by the end of June. It just isn't true and raises unrealistic expectations. Damon asked me to speak to Nadhim to 'do a bit of course correction'.

MONDAY 18 JANUARY

I've been pinged by my own app! There I was, working on my boxes in my office, and ding! Up pops a very unwelcome message of the sort that other people all over the country have been getting, saying I have to self-isolate. What a pain. It means I'll have to join Cabinet remotely tomorrow morning, and everything else for that matter. Very annoying, but I can hardly make an exception for myself.

On the upside, Pfizer has relented. Following a robust exchange between Bourla and the PM, lo and behold, they've located an 'emergency supply', which is now heading our way.

They've clearly calculated exactly how much we need to meet our public commitments and are going to pony up. What a relief.

Meanwhile the numbers are definitely starting to turn. After an excellent presentation at the No. 10 dashboard meeting, it was clear that cases are finally falling. We will know for sure on Wednesday when we get the first cut of figures being published on Friday – but I'm encouraged.

We've been shown a draft design for a gallantry medal for healthcare workers who risked their lives to treat patients at the beginning of the pandemic. I quite liked it, until Ed Argar messaged with what he called a 'note of caution'. He fears it bears rather too much resemblance to the Kaiser's highest gallantry medal in Imperial Germany during the First World War. That's the end of that one then.

TUESDAY 19 JANUARY

Jim has been doing battle to push through my travel regs. After a meeting with various key players today he reports there's still a lot of 'Old Think'. He says he 'didn't go full "Fortress Britain"' but wants colleagues to change the way they're thinking about this disease. His view is that we should be aiming to eliminate this thing.

'We should be walking steadily towards zero Covid,' he says. I'm all for tough measures at the border to stop variants that could skewer the protection from the vaccine, but we'll never get to zero Covid – and it would be wrong to try.

WEDNESDAY 20 JANUARY

Not content with attempting to swipe some of our Pfizer supply, Brussels is plotting to ban vaccine exports from the EU. Wow! This would be a direct attack on our vaccine flow. Their target seems to be the small proportion of the Oxford jab that AstraZeneca make at Halix in the Netherlands. Don't they realise they could have had access to these vaccines too, if they'd got their act together like we did?

Just because the manufacturing site is in the EU doesn't mean it belongs to the EU! If they are mad enough to go ahead, there will be a major diplomatic row. I'm seeking urgent advice on how to respond and have called Raab and our ambassador to the EU, Tim Barrow. This one will need all arms of government to get the response right.

Worryingly, there are growing questions over the efficacy of the vaccines against the South African variant. Sir John Bell has been in touch saying early research is not encouraging. We urgently need to accelerate plans to tweak it. Meanwhile we must keep borders closed.

I called Patrick. He agrees it's a real concern, and the VTF are already on it. They are going to come up with a proposal by Friday.

At today's dashboard meeting we went through the data again. Definitely trending down. Crucially, the ONS figures are clearly lower. They still have two more days' data to put in before publication, so it's cautious optimism, but the rate looks to be dropping faster than in the first lockdown. This is the vaccine effect: not only lockdown but vaccines are bringing case numbers down. It's a great chart.

THURSDAY 21 JANUARY

We've hit 5 million Covid vaccine doses. That's almost one in ten adults, including JVT's mum! The range of places we're using as vaccine sites is expanding and now includes cinemas, mosques and the Blackpool Winter Gardens.

Infuriatingly, someone's leaked the discussions we've been having over possible one-off government payments for people who are forced to self-isolate. The proposal is contentious and we've been trying to thrash it out behind the scenes without a big public debate. My money's on HMT, who have never liked the policy. I messaged Dan Rosenfield, who is also hopping mad.

'The leak of this self-isolation payment paper is a fucking nightmare,' I said. 'We've been discussing this policy bilaterally with HMT for months. As soon as it goes in a Covid-O paper it leaks.'

'Am furious. Talking to Simon. Totally shit,' he replied.

Evidently we need to massively tighten the whole Covid-O structure. People complain when they're not in the key debates, but this sort of thing is why No. 10 restricts the number of people in meetings.

In other 'challenges', aka nightmares, ITV is preparing to run a very negative piece about the suffering of care home residents because of visiting restrictions. Helen Whately wants to find a way of allowing indoor visits again. I'm hardline on this: we cannot have Covid taking off in care homes again.

'For now, save lives,' I instructed.

Jim had what sounds to have been a difficult meeting of the new committee on travel restrictions. He says not everyone is entirely onside with some of our proposed measures. Apparently some aren't convinced the South African variant will take off in a major way, and even if it does, they're optimistic it may not be too serious. Jim described this attitude as 'fatalistic'.

'I made our case, and emphasised that even if the vaccine-escaping-high-transmission-mutant scenario was low-probability, it was so severe we needed a plan to deal with it by addressing border management with hotels, pre-registration etc. But his set-up did undermine things a lot,' Jim reported.

However, he says Grant was very helpful and that the devolveds are 'totally onside' with enhanced border measures and a joint approach. As for the Home Office, Jim worries that they're talking the talk but not walking the walk. He says they made no material comments during the meeting whatsoever. Strange, given they're meant to be responsible for the borders.

FRIDAY 22 JANUARY

Just as I feared, the £500 self-isolation payment proposal is blowing up. Politico says it could be 'dead on arrival' because the Treasury 'had no idea it existed until it appeared in the press'. They quote a source saying HMT was 'flummoxed' by the idea and that they think it's 'mad'. Utter tripe. We've been talking to them about it for months!

Boris agrees this has to be HMT trying to kill off the policy. I've messaged Rishi to see what he has to say.

Meanwhile someone has secretly recorded me talking about the South African variant on a confidential Zoom with business leaders the other day. Charmingly, they've leaked it to the *Mirror*. The angle is me saying the South African variant could make vaccines 50 per cent less effective. In what is becoming a tedious ritual, Damon alerted me to the story and we wasted a bit more time wondering who was responsible.

Peter Westmacott, former ambassador to Turkey, came back through Heathrow Terminal 2 this afternoon and immigration was jam-packed. He tweeted a dreadful photo of the queues.

'T2 Heathrow Friday afternoon. No ventilation. Long delays. Super-spreading,' he declared. Presumably everyone is trying to get home before we impose mandatory quarantine. It's a terrible look. Sam Coates, deputy political editor at Sky, retweeted the image accompanied by the words 'Borders... open.'

When I saw the picture, I exploded. This makes a total nonsense of everything we're doing. I shared the images with Dan Rosenfield. I hope the boss gives the Home Office a rocket.

I've told Downing Street we should not be satisfied until we have 100 per cent compliance with travel-related Covid restrictions and zero imported new variant cases. In an internal briefing note, I've said that if a traveller arrives in the UK without proof of a negative Covid test, they should be barred from entry and sent back where they came from. If they're a UK citizen, they should be arrested and quarantined for public protection. I just don't think fines go far enough. We need to emphasise that it's currently ILLEGAL for people to be travelling abroad, except in extremely limited circumstances. I also think we need to create a 'red list' of countries that are completely off limits. There should be no entry to the UK at all for non-UK nationals travelling from these countries. No exemptions. As for returning UK nationals, they should all be forced to quarantine, with daily physical checks to make sure they're doing it. I've recommended huge fines for breaking quarantine. No exceptions! Seriously – there is no point messing around.

SATURDAY 23 JANUARY

The boss texted asking us to do everything we can to identify the leaker of the £500 payments story. He suggested the culprit might actually be in our department, not HMT. Not likely – it's not in our interest – but we'll go through the motions.

SUNDAY 24 JANUARY

The teaching unions are still pushing for their members to jump the vaccine queue. They claim it would help accelerate the reopening of schools. This is an old canard and we've debated it ad nauseam. It's a terrible idea. I messaged Boris to make sure he holds firm. We've got to keep vaccinating according to who is most likely to die: that's the fastest route to freedom. Three quarters of over-eighties have now had their first jab. We couldn't have done that if we'd put teachers at the front of the queue, and we couldn't have done it if we'd given second doses at three weeks, not twelve. For all the brickbats and abuse, this really is life-saving work.

On *Marr*, I was very firm about celebrities going abroad on holiday. I can't believe so-called social media 'influencers' are swanning around in Dubai. Why would you do that in a national emergency? I am beginning to think we may have to introduce some kind of forced hotel quarantine, like they have in Australia and Singapore. Damon agrees and wonders if we could go even further.

'Like what?' I asked.

He suggested we expand the red list on the basis of precautionary principle and introduce a system for quickly triggering additions to the list. I agree.

MONDAY 25 JANUARY

No smoke without fire: the EU really was plotting to hamper our vaccine supply. Stella Kyriakides, EU health commissioner, has tweeted that 'in the future' any company that produces vaccines in the EU will have to provide 'early notification' if they want to sell it to a third-party country. In other words, they'll need permission. Totally desperate stuff! They're doing it purely because they screwed up procurement. This is no way to behave. We should all be pulling together, not trying to deprive other countries of their share. Thank God I insisted on domestic production. At the time, I insisted on exclusivity clauses because I was worried about Donald Trump. Looks like I should have been more worried about Ursula von der Leyen.

I ask Jens whether he thinks all this is just rhetoric from Brussels or whether it's real. I always knew there would be geopolitics, but this is taking it too far.

He called me and said it wasn't about blocking, just 'transparency'. Yeah, right.

Luckily the EU threat only raises a question mark over 5 per cent of our Oxford AZ supply, but it's enough to derail our 15 February target. If they come after our Pfizer supply – which is all from Belgium – it will be a complete disaster.

All the same, I don't want to wind things up any further than need be. Nadhim's on the media round tomorrow and it's vital he gets the tone right. I told him to resist any temptation to point score with the EU.

'Remember you are talking to worried grannies,' I said.

His lines to take are: yes, we are confident of our partners delivering the vaccine; no, we do not think that this will have any effect on vaccine delivery; yes, we are working to build up domestic capacity; and no, we will not be retaliating.

'We beat the EU by being the grown-ups,' I advised.

'Totally my instinct,' he agreed.

Later Emma Dean took a call from one of the Home Office SpAds, who says Priti is going to call for a full travel ban. Over time, she wants it to morph into a hotel quarantine system.

The Home Office wants our support to make it a UK-wide system and is looking at the best legislative route. It tallies with what I've been pushing and I'll throw my weight behind it.

Late at night, I opened my spreadsheet again and studied Adam Langron's charts. Today's cases are just 22,195 – they're falling far faster than in the first wave and are definitely on a sharp downward trend. So now we know: lockdown is working, the vaccine is working and we're on the way out.

TUESDAY 26 JANUARY

The Germans are going tonto. They're now putting it about that our jabs don't work. Today's *Bild* carries a totally inaccurate report claiming the Oxford vaccine is only 8 per cent effective.

I texted Jens at 8 a.m. asking him what was going on. I told him the 8 per cent figure is totally wrong and asked him to inject some objectivity into the debate. He replied that it shows how heated the whole situation is getting. Uh, yes – but it's his department briefing it?! As diplomatically as I could, I pointed out that some of the constituent parts of the Pfizer vaccine are made in the UK. The last thing we want is a trade war over this. While I know Jens gets it, I'm not sure the most political parts of the EU machine do at all. They are so ideological, even in a health emergency. Evidently it's all about 'the EU project' for them.

The Cabinet Office asked if I could get the MHRA to talk to the European Medicines Agency about the *Bild* story. They want it knocked down authoritatively and think the regulator is best placed. I told them I'd already asked Jens to deal with it. 'He is being helpful but clearly finding it difficult,' I said.

Nadhim was awesome on the morning bulletins, managing not to pour fuel on the fire.

While the 8 per cent figure in *Bild* is outrageous, I am worried about early efficacy data from the JCVI that was brought into my office in between meetings this morning. It's totally contradictory and unclear. The question is how to explain it to the PM without him freaking out and deciding we might as well give up on restrictions altogether because the vaccines 'don't work'. I asked the Prof his thoughts.

'I'm about to wrap a metaphorical towel round my head and try to understand the figures,' he said.

I told him my single biggest fear is the PM doing a complete flip. The Prof replied that the figures show that the Pfizer vaccine has what he called a 'non-trivial effect'.

'I am pretty doubtful we can say much more than this with these data,' he added.

For now, we're best fudging it with the PM. We'll tell him truthfully that it will take a few more weeks for an accurate picture.

Today we reached a really grim milestone in the pandemic: more than 100,000 deaths in this country. I study the numbers every single night but I've never become inured to what they represent: so many people grieving; so much loss. I gathered the team to talk about the data. Everyone is affected by the number of deaths. The Prof, ever the professional, told the team that with the lockdown and the vaccine both working, it will never be this bad again.

WEDNESDAY 27 JANUARY
A humiliating climbdown from the EU, who clearly realised their 'export ban' wouldn't end well. It followed frantic diplomacy on our side, with the PM calling Ursula; Dom Raab calling EU trade commissioner Valdis Dombrovskis; and me speaking to Stella. Meanwhile our lawyers worked flat out to figure out what legal basis Brussels might have for their threat. I know our contracts with AstraZeneca and Pfizer are pretty watertight and – based on what we know of the EU contracts – our lawyers confirmed that they wouldn't have been able to block our supply anyway. Once the EU were hit with that cold, hard dose of reality, hey presto! They retreated. Just after 5 p.m., Dombrovskis issued a waffling clarification, saying they were 'not planning to impose an export ban or export restrictions'. The statement claimed it was all about introducing an export transparency mechanism 'to bring clarity on production capacity of manufacturers, numbers of doses produced, at which production centres, how many doses sold to which countries'.

'This is backing off!' I told the team jubilantly. Crisis over, but what a ridiculous waste of time and energy.

A new poll suggests 80 per cent of people support the lockdown. I sent a screenshot to Gove. 'There is no public clamour to start lifting measures,' I told him, adding that the survey could be useful next time anyone says the public are straining against lockdown. 'They aren't. They want us to keep people safe,' I said.

'Yup,' he replied.

Tonight I'm doing a nightshift at Basildon Hospital. Frontline staff are still under horrendous pressure. I hear a lot about this, but the best way for me to understand is to see it for myself. People really tell it to you straight at 2 a.m.

THURSDAY 28 JANUARY

The night shift was incredible but has left me completely drained. I don't know how they do it day in and day out: heroic.

My first stop was the hospital's vaccination centre, where several staff confided that they were nervous about having the jab. They explained they'd been persuaded despite what social media has been telling them. I did my best to sound sympathetic, but it's frustrating that people are still being influenced by anti-vax rubbish. I then headed to the Covid wards to help in any way I could through the night.

As a Secretary of State, it's hard to strip away the layers of formality, so I donned full PPE, which is very anonymising, and got stuck in, helping to turn patients and fetch and carry. In intensive care, I watched a man consent to being intubated because his blood oxygen levels were dropping and weren't sustainable. He spoke to the doctor, who said, 'We want to put a tube in, because we don't think you'll make it unless we do that.' His chances of waking up were 50:50. He knew that. It was an unbelievably awful moment: you could tell he really didn't want go under, and who could blame him, knowing there was such a significant chance he would never wake up? Worry etched on his face, he asked the doctor if this was really needed, to which the doctor said yes. He reluctantly agreed, and within a minute he was flat out on the ventilator. The doctor next to me said, 'I don't think we'll see him again.' It was extraordinarily sobering and left me very reflective about what these doctors are doing every day, putting people to sleep knowing there's only a 50:50 chance they'll open their eyes again.

When my shift was over, I went down to the rest area, where a mental health hub had been set up to support staff. One of the registrars followed me down and we had a chat. He told me he'd just had to phone the wife of the patient to say he'd been intubated.

'We're doing this, we all know it's our duty, we're coping with a second wave – but we can't have a third,' he said. Then he burst into tears.

Back in the office this morning I felt completely wrung out. I don't think I'll ever forget the experience. It's important that I had a glimpse of the harrowing reality: for patients, their relatives and frontline staff. I couldn't stop thinking about the man who had been intubated.

My mood was slightly boosted by some brilliant Test and Trace stats: over 90 per cent of test results returned the next day, and more than nine in ten contacts reached and required to self-isolate. Also, the Novavax results came through: 89.3 per cent effective! Another one comes off! And it's going to be made in Teesside, a particular relief after all that EU sabre rattling. This is such an emotional rollercoaster.

FRIDAY 29 JANUARY

Helen has alerted me to scandalous behaviour by certain care home operators, who are unscrupulously using staff with Covid. She messaged me this morning to say that Care Quality Commission inspectors have identified no fewer than forty places where this is happening. Wow. I am shocked. How could management do this, knowing how vulnerable their residents are? It underlines why we need to make jabs mandatory for people working in social care. The PM supports me on this. There will be howls of protest, but we need to make it happen.

The European Medicines Agency has finally approved the Oxford vaccine. Just as well – EU member states are going to need it.

SATURDAY 30 JANUARY

Mum has been jabbed! She sent me a pic from a vaccination centre in Cheshire where she and Bob, my stepdad, both got it today. Hooray.

Helen is pushing for some relaxation to visiting restrictions in care homes again. She worries that isolated residents may lose the will to live. She thinks old people may start 'just giving up'.

'Yes on visiting but only after a few weeks,' I replied firmly. It's still too risky.

SUNDAY 31 JANUARY

Sad to hear that Captain Sir Tom Moore has been admitted to hospital with Covid. He's been such a hero of the pandemic. It would be heartbreaking if he became another victim of this awful disease. Yesterday we set a new record, jabbing almost 600,000 people in one day. Incredible! Now the EU have backed off, we're on track for 15 February, and we're on track to get out of this pandemic soon.

FEBRUARY 2021

MONDAY 1 FEBRUARY

Do I want Bill and Melinda Gates making an appearance at the G7 health summit I'm chairing? Well, yes and no. Normally, who wouldn't want the world's greatest living philanthropists? At the moment, however, it would completely undermine the message we're trying to get across. There's a reason we're holding it in Oxford. The Oxford jab is doing more than anything else to vaccinate the world – because I stopped it being sold to Merck and together with AstraZeneca we're delivering global at-cost distribution. The push to vaccinate the world is about getting manufacturing going as widely as possible – but the debate Bill and Melinda are spearheading is all about donating doses, having a go at us in the process. Sure, let's do that too, but it's tiny compared to what we've done already. Teach a man to fish, I say.

Unfortunately, the Cabinet Office didn't bother asking my view and just steamed ahead, setting up a vaccines discussion between Bill and Melinda and Boris. I think they were just attracted to the big name. The meeting was all nicey-nicey and 'Why don't you do a turn at the summit?' Now we're going to have to row back. I complained to Rosenfield that it might be best if mandarins don't give the PM ideas without asking me first. According to Natasha, the diplomat responsible 'wasn't aware of the steer on Melinda'.

'He won't know about the steer on lots of things if he doesn't ask. He has screwed up here and needs to get back in his box,' I replied crossly.

In better news, a YouGov poll suggests 70 per cent of Britons think the government is handling the vaccine rollout well, while 23 per cent think we're doing badly. Feeling more cheerful, I forwarded it to Simon Stevens.

'Who the heck are the 23 per cent, for goodness sake!!' he replied.

I don't know. Maybe the same 20 per cent of people who believe UFOs have landed on Earth? Or the 5 million Brits who think the Apollo moon landings were faked?

Allan messaged late to say that Andrew Bowie, Tory MP for West Aberdeenshire & Kincardine and an all-round good guy, is 'bored and looking for something to do'. Allan suggested getting him involved in our efforts to show the value of the union when it comes to vaccination.

'Yes, yes, yes!' I replied enthusiastically.

The work to stop Scottish separatism needs such sensitivity. Bowie is first-rate on that. The campaign has to be cross-party too. Scottish Labour types are very tribal, but Allan's due to talk to the old Scottish Blairite Jim Murphy this week. I want all unionists to help make the case that Scots wouldn't be getting their jabs so fast without the union.

TUESDAY 2 FEBRUARY

Captain Sir Tom Moore has died. I knew he was ill so it's not exactly a shock, but it's still incredibly sad. He was a great British hero and showed the best of this country. People tend to focus on the £33 million he raised for the NHS, but to me his contribution was so much more than that. Not only did he raise a staggering amount of money; he brought the whole country together at a time when we really needed it. We will have to find the right way to commemorate him. There are suggestions of a statue. It would certainly be fitting given all he's done and the huge sum he's raised for the NHS.

Not public yet, but things are not looking good re. the Oxford vaccine and the South Africa variant. It underlines the urgency of border controls. Simon Case messaged this morning warning that the pressure to speed up hotel quarantine is going to become 'overwhelming'. I went through the plans with the team last night and the main problem is technology. Officials say the earliest we can get this up and running is 15 February. I'm demanding it goes live next week.

Simon agrees, with the caveat that we frame the first week of the scheme as a pilot. That would give us some room to make – and rectify – mistakes.

'And let's face it, if the customer journey is crap, that will just be more of a deterrent for those who want to come!!!' Simon said.

Downing Street wants us to write to the Scottish government offering to help with their vaccine rollout. Damon says No. 10 is keen 'to subtly highlight' how slow they've been. Allan has told them to tread carefully. Say what you like about Sturgeon, but she's not stupid. If we're too clunky, it will rebound on us.

Some ignorant lout verbally abused the Prof as he was waiting to get his lunch from a street stall in Westminster today. The video footage is shocking. Poor Chris just stood there calmly while this rude boy laid into him, labelling him a 'liar'. This stuff really makes me angry. The Prof is not only an eminent scientist but also one of the most selfless individuals I have ever met. He does not deserve this abuse.

Very encouraging news from Oxford on the delayed second dose policy: lengthening the gap between doses appears to make the vaccine even more effective than the original approach. Not all the risks we've taken have paid off, but I'm banking this one.

Jim is working very hard on hotel quarantine, his restless brain whirring with creative schemes at all times of day and night. One of the things I like most about him is his boundless energy and enthusiasm, though it does result in some wild ideas.

This evening he messaged saying that Taiwanese citizens who do what they're told get a small cash reward from their government. This got him thinking about sticks and carrots. He wondered whether we could offer people a free jab in return for doing the right thing.

'A nice incentive,' he mused.

Off he trotted to run this by a small focus group, aka his family, before returning to his phone twenty minutes later with an update. In short: scrap that.

'We'd be flooded by rich people of the world trying to get the vaccine. Daft idea. Goodnight.'

WEDNESDAY 3 FEBRUARY

Having landed me with responsibility for hotel quarantine – a mission I readily accepted – some genius in the Cabinet Office has decided the buck actually stops with Michael Gove. I very much doubt that Michael has any idea, but he's not exactly going to be thrilled to find officialdom proposing he carries the can. There is every prospect that it will go wrong, and he will not want to be in the firing line.

For my part, I can't make this work unless I'm formally in charge. That's just how it is in Whitehall. Unless you are officially responsible for a particular task, the machine just doesn't respond. I messaged Simon Case telling him that the appointment letter has been bungled and that I'm not doing this without the levers.

'If you want Gove to run it, he can run it,' I told Simon huffily.

Simon, who knows better than anyone how the system works, says he will try to sort.

Shortly after I got into the office, Helen messaged flagging up some awful statistics about the mortality rate from Covid among people with severe learning disabilities. For those aged eighteen to thirty-four, the risk of dying from the disease is thirty times the risk for others in that age group. She has been pushing for these very vulnerable individuals to be prioritised for the jab. I told her I'd see what I can do. Meanwhile Jim has been doing some work on long Covid. He warned me that we're going to be hearing a lot more about it. So far, it looks as if as many as 160,000 people are going to need some sort of NHS support for ongoing symptoms, and that's before this latest wave. Evidently it's going to be a serious healthcare demand and he worries we're not doing enough. I agree. He says care for these patients is currently 'very weak' and is drafting a pitch to HMT for big money to put into it.

'It's shone a light on NHS failures on "rehab" generally and this is a key "levelling up" issue,' he said. He thinks we'll need some kind of national plan.

Tomorrow's World Cancer Day. Despite the stress the pandemic is putting on the NHS, people need to know that diagnosing and treating cancer remains a top priority. I'll be going to the Royal Marsden Hospital in Chelsea to make the point.

THURSDAY 4 FEBRUARY

Tobias Ellwood thinks GPs are deliberately discouraging patients from using vaccination centres so they get their jabs in surgeries instead. I'm sure he's right that this happens. That way, the GPs make more money. Top marks for enterprise, but no points for public spirit. In some vaccination centres, the result is a lot of people hanging around doing nothing. This is what's happening in Tobias's Bournemouth East constituency, apparently, where there are hundreds of vaccinators and other volunteers but not enough punters.

'Apparently one in three vaccination lanes has no queue. The facility has a maximum capacity of 1,600 jabs a day and is doing less than 400. GPs are discouraging the hub's use. Why? Because they're getting paid £20 a jab!' he reported.

He's not quite right about the figures – they are paid £12.50 a jab in clinics, though it's more in care homes – but he makes a point.

We intentionally set up the pharmacists and GPs to compete to vaccinate people. It's the secret grit in the oyster that's made such a success of the rollout so far. In most areas, they've risen above the pure financial incentive and worked alongside each other – competing, sure, but not aggressively. But in others there's clearly some over-enthusiasm.

But this problem is worth having because the NHS has consistently delivered all the supply we can get. The carefully thought-through incentive structure has worked wonders. Empty lanes or not, we are on track to hit the 15 February target. Yesterday we confirmed we'd reached 10 million jabs. Today we passed the threshold of one in five of the population jabbed. Now the boss is demanding we set a target date for the over-fifties. After the Albert Bourla near-miss, he's learned his lesson about over-promising/under-delivering and has given us a decent lead-in time. We have set on May.

The biggest risk to this timetable is Brussels restarting its futile vaccine war. Apparently Olaf Scholz, Merkel's deputy, thinks the EU Commission's vaccine strategy is 'richtig scheisse gelaufen', which the *Financial Times* translates as 'a total shit show'. I don't disagree: they've reached just 3.5 per cent of the population, while we've hit 20 per cent.

Earlier we had an unusually constructive meeting with the PM about the rollout, testing etc. The only bit I didn't like was a suggestion that we could reopen non-essential shops on 8 March.

Afterwards, I told Dan Rosenfield that this is a very bad idea.

'I think we should go for 1 March and overachieve,' he replied.

I wasn't sure whether he was winding me up.

'Overachieve the return of the virus?' I replied.

FRIDAY 5 FEBRUARY

Sky News claims chaos and confusion over the hotel quarantine scheme is 'making Whitehall look like *The Thick of It*'. Damon is going berserk, but they've got a point.

I spent much of the day at Gatwick, nobody's idea of a pleasure at the best of times. The place was deserted, but somehow, it's still a shambles. The extraordinary thing is that nobody in government is in charge of our borders 'end to end'. Different departments are responsible for different bits, with the inevitable weak/non-existent coordination, buck passing and other systemic failure.

Simon Case seemed to be in a good mood, so when he asked me how I got on, I was quite blunt, telling him that it's high time that a specific department – or at the very least a Transport or Home Office Minister – has overall responsibility for our borders.

'Exactly,' Simon agreed. 'It is mad... I have said to PM that this needs fixing.'

To make matters worse, the airlines and airports are totally offside.

They just don't see it as their job to support Covid restrictions and have no interest in helping us enforce hotel quarantine.

'Completely unhelpful. Don't get that there's a war on. And of course, very hard for them as they're going bust,' I told Simon.

At least Priti and Grant are playing ball and HMT is being uncharacteristically efficient signing off the finances. So, as I reassured Simon, we can make this work.

'Don't make it look too good or else people will think it's OK to travel!' Simon replied.

I told him that this isn't about making hotel quarantine look inviting; it's about making the system look competent.

'Ha ha! That would be good!' he agreed. I told him we're making a point of giving big families all the suites and putting pop stars in the box rooms. The thought of the expressions on the faces of people coming out of First Class and into a Premier Inn shoebox amused us both.

Later I messaged the excellent civil servant I've put in charge of the hotel quarantine programme, listing key action points. I told her Border Force is worried about how it will cope if passenger numbers rise. There's a real risk of people trying to give us the slip.

I was also struck by the total absence of Covid-related signs at the airport this morning – nothing on Covid anywhere and no instructions to self-isolate. 'Very, very weak,' I told her.

Unconnected to the pandemic, I've been working on moving the NHS back under the control of the Department of Health. It's long overdue. Andrew Lansley's reforms from the early Cameron years – which devolved power to the NHS chief executive and a long list of quangos – just haven't worked. The buck needs to stop with the Health Secretary, who is accountable to Parliament and to voters. There's a risk that Lansley, who had a very rough time getting the changes through in the first place, will take this personally. Jim has been trying to square him off. When the pair of them discussed it today Lansley regaled him with a long list of reasons why we're making a big mistake, but he promised to stick to the policy debate so long as we did too. If we're too critical of what he did, he will go ballistic, Jim says. Fair enough! I certainly wouldn't be rude about him – he should know that's not my style. I messaged Ed Argar, who's been talking to the BMA etc., saying we're going to need some supporting fire. He says Chaand Nagpaul and Chris Hopson 'weren't unhelpful'. Better than the reverse, I suppose.

SUNDAY 7 FEBRUARY

We need to get our ducks in a row on vaccine passports. On *Marr* this morning Nadhim labelled the idea 'discriminatory' – but didn't draw the distinction between domestic and international use. We can't control what other countries do and some kind of certification is inevitable to go abroad. Test and Trace has been developing the data system that is pretty much ready to go, including on the NHS app.

MONDAY 8 FEBRUARY

I've finally, finally got my way on making vaccines mandatory for people who work in care homes. It's a simple duty of care to use medical science to protect the very vulnerable people being cared for. These jabs are safe – so what possible reason is there to refuse? If the NHS isn't built on medical science, we might as well pack up and go home. Boris has been very supportive throughout, but the system is emphatically opposed – without good reason. So I've first got the care worker policy over the line – that's the most urgent. Next, the NHS, and once that's agreed, I want to add flu jabs to the list. One step at a time.

We've now vaccinated more than 12.2 million people. That's almost a quarter of all adults in the UK! So far, take-up has been way better than we thought. We expected around 75 per cent, but it's coming in at more than 90 per cent. One week to go till the 15 February target.

There's been heavy snow and JVT had an epic journey from Lincolnshire to London for today's press conference. He ploughed on and made it on time, despite five inches of the stuff in some parts of the country. It seems nothing will stop that man getting to a press conference.

According to Damon, tomorrow's *Times* 'Red Box' features Ipsos MORI polling of MPs naming me as the 'second most impressive parliamentarian'. Crikey. No need to ask who comes first.

TUESDAY 9 FEBRUARY

Taking something of a leap of faith, I announced the hotel quarantine plans in the Commons. It's another example of breaking the Whitehall convention of only announcing things when you're certain they'll work. We don't have time for that, given the need to keep new variants out. I think I looked suitably grim faced as I spelled out the dreadful consequences for anyone who tries to dodge it (up to ten years in jail), but the truth is I'm not certain this will be a finely oiled machine. Heathrow seems almost as riven by tribal divisions as Westminster, with no love lost between Border Force and the company that runs the airport.

Later I had a long chat with my counterpart in South Africa, Dr Zweli Mkhize. We commiserated each other about the damage the Kent and South African variants have caused our countries. The blame game feels unfair: there's every likelihood these variants began elsewhere, and we have been penalised for identifying them.

Annoyingly, the very early Pfizer efficacy data has leaked to SAGE, meaning it will probably leak everywhere. As the Prof told Boris last month, it's way too early to draw any conclusions. What we don't want is the anti-vax nutters getting their hands on it and spinning it into something it isn't. Damon messaged this evening in something of a panic, his head full of imaginary headlines, but relaxed when I told him No. 10 has known about it for ages.

'It shows Pfizer works, but we don't know exactly how much... The numbers are not credible – CMO doesn't think there's enough data to be meaningful,' I explained. If it gets out, we'll have to play it down as statistically unreliable data and get the verified figures, which hopefully look a whole lot better, out as soon as we can.

WEDNESDAY 10 FEBRUARY

Meg Hillier, who chairs the Public Accounts Committee, has started an infuriating campaign accusing 'Tory ministers' of running a 'chumocracy' over PPE contracts. How pitifully low. I'm incandescent. The PAC is meant to be an august body for challenging the value for money we get for taxpayers' money. She's proposing to turn it into another arm of the conspiracy drive. What Meg fails to acknowledge is that when the pandemic began, of course we had to use the emergency procedure for buying, which allows officials to move fast and not tender everything for months. And when people got in contact after we went public with the need for PPE, of course we forwarded on the proposals for civil servants to look at. Even the Labour Party were getting involved, and I thank them for that – it was a national crisis and these leads have proved invaluable. Rachel Reeves, Michael Gove's shadow, wrote to him at the time, complaining that a series of offers weren't being taken up. Officials looked into her proposals too.

I'm even more offended because I served with Meg on the PAC and I used to respect her. It is so offensive for a supposedly grown-up politician to bend the truth in this way. So many good people worked so hard ensuring that as a country we never actually ran out of PPE. It would be perfectly reasonable to have an inquiry into how we can speed up purchasing in the next emergency, or into what worked and what didn't. But this is just insulting.

By contrast, I was hugely cheered up that Prince Charles and Camilla have announced they have had their jabs, a month after the Queen and Prince Philip had theirs. They're both in their seventies and setting a fine example. It's almost a year since the Prince of Wales got Covid.

Boris has said people shouldn't pin their hopes on a summer holiday this year, even in the UK. After a bad day, this did nothing to improve my mood. My God, we all need something to look forward to! I seriously hope the PM is being unduly negative. My hope is we'll have a great British summer. I don't think we should be raising any expectations of a foreign trip, but I'm already dreaming of Cornwall.

THURSDAY 11 FEBRUARY

So here we are, in the depths of the bleakest lockdown, with the virus still picking off hundreds of victims every week, and Test and Trace officials have been having secret talks about scaling back. Unbelievable! I told them there was no way they should stand down any lab capacity, but according to Jim, who has a meeting with them later, 'they are getting a very different signal from the Treasury'. What do you recommend, he asked?

'They made a massive error talking to the Treasury before talking to me. They need to sort this. I'm frankly furious about it,' I replied.

Sensing that if I try to sort this out personally, I may well lose my rag, Jim has offered to 'politely admonish' the relevant people and act as 'ministerial shield' between Dido and the Treasury.

'I will confirm that I am the Minister for Testing and they need to run things through me,' he offered.

FRIDAY 12 FEBRUARY

The left never ceases to amaze. The bleeding hearts who run North West London CCG (one of many health quangos nobody will miss when they're abolished) have taken it upon themselves to prioritise vaccinating asylum seekers. Damon messaged me this afternoon revealing that they have fast-tracked no fewer than 317 such individuals – 'predominantly males in their twenties and thirties'.

'They've WHAT?' I replied, in disbelief.

So, while older British citizens quietly wait their turn, we are fast-tracking people who aren't in high-risk categories and may not even have any right to be here? Unbelievable.

Tentative talks are under way about how we begin to unlock, with an initial meeting in the Cabinet Room this morning. The Prof's main ask is that there should be five weeks between every step, so we can assess the effect of the previous lifting. That makes sense. My main objective is a plan that is irreversible. Going backwards would be a disaster and people wouldn't forgive us. The boss agrees. Understandably, Rishi's priority is to reopen everything as fast as possible, but even he accepts that reversing would be awful. Essentially we're all agreed on strategy – it's just a judgement call about pace.

The draconian jail sentences I announced for people who lie to the authorities to avoid hotel quarantine have caused a bit of a storm. Someone is putting it about that Solicitor General Michael Ellis thinks it's over the top. Cue front-pagers based on 'Whitehall sources' complaining that the punishments don't fit the crime and are disproportionate. I told *The Times* that I make no apology. After all the sacrifices people have made, we can't have a handful of irresponsible travellers jeopardising our progress.

This afternoon I went out to Heathrow to talk to the various people involved about how it's going to work. Frankly I was horrified: it's worse than Gatwick. The inability of different parts of the airport – the company, Border Force, G4S security personnel, health officials – to work together beggars belief. They all seem to hate each other. They wouldn't even meet me together, so I had to do a series of individual meetings. During these one-on-ones, they all spent most of their time telling me how awful the others are. Even worse, they all report to different people – different departments or shareholders – so there's not even any single person to sort it out. It will be a miracle if we can pull this off.

From Heathrow I headed to Stoke Mandeville Stadium, which is now a huge vaccination centre. What a contrast! I watched in wonder as a beautifully efficient flow of patients arrived for appointments, waited no more than a few minutes to be seen and left shortly after; job done. It was magnificent to observe. If only the NHS always worked like that – and our borders, for that matter. It helps that we set up a modern, well-thought-through data architecture right at the start, so everyone's working off the same information.

Less wonderful was the discovery that some of our vaccine supply has met an untimely end. I had just reached the end of a particularly tricky meeting when a sheepish-looking official knocked on my office door. I could tell by his expression that he was not bearing good news, and sure enough, he had been dispatched to inform me that half a million doses of the active ingredient that makes up the vaccine have quite literally gone down the drain. Details of the incident are sketchy, and I haven't had a written report, but what I've been told doesn't sound complicated: some poor lab technician literally dropped a bag of the vaccine on the floor. Half a million doses in one dropped bag! I can only imagine the collective horror as the precious liquid formed a sorry little puddle around his or her feet. My eyes bulged slightly as I fleetingly wondered whether anyone had been tempted to try to salvage it. I pictured the panicked culprit rushing round trying to find some kind of pipette to suction it up. But of course not: the moment it hit the deck, that was that.

I decided not to calculate how much Butter Fingers has cost us, or to make anyone feel worse about the half a million people who will now have to wait a little longer for their jab. Doubtless they already feel terrible. Bad things happen, and I am only grateful that the accident wasn't a few weeks ago, when we were in more of a panic about supply. There's no point issuing reprimands now. Mistakes happen and so long as it doesn't happen again that's the end of it for me. It's amazing you can get half a million doses of active ingredient in one bag – and just goes to show quite how precious this stuff is.

Con Home have run a gushing profile of Nadhim, describing him as a 'rising star who also knows what it is like to fail'. They included a quote from Robert Halfon, the Harlow MP, who told them Zahawi would 'get you mangoes in the Antarctic and Brussels sprouts in the desert'. Back in the 1980s, Nadhim worked for Jeffrey Archer, who's described him as a 'born organiser'.

'If you said to him, I need six taxis, three aeroplanes and a double-decker bus all in thirty minutes, he went ahead and did it,' Archer said.

Sounds like pretty good training for what he's doing now.

I've given an interview to the *Telegraph* reiterating what I said to *The Spectator* last month: vaccines and treatments mean Covid-19 will become an illness we can live with, like flu, by the end of the year. That's where we need to get to over the next few months.

SATURDAY 13 FEBRUARY

Gavin says Michael Ellis hasn't been briefing against my hotel quarantine punishments and is really upset that I might suspect he has.

'I'm certain it wasn't him, if only on the basis that I know he was defending you. He's also one of your biggest fans and was really gutted that you may have thought he was causing you grief,' Gavin said.

Actually, I never thought it was him, but I knew he was worried about it because he called me himself. I thanked Gavin for alerting me and reassured him that all is well. I like Ellis and he has been nothing but supportive. 'He's such a legend and has been amazing during the crisis – finding ways to make all sorts of stuff legal,' I said.

The army has produced some amazing footage showing how they're supporting the vaccine rollout in Scotland. I messaged Ben to thank him.

'Your Scottish Army vaccine video has EVERYTHING,' I told him gratefully.

'Your vaccine programme has been your success. We should all be grateful. In the end the public will only remember the beginning and end of this pandemic,' he replied.

'Very kind of you to say. Big team effort. Totally agree re. beginning & end – we must drive this thing home,' I said.

Helen is increasingly anxious about people with learning disabilities getting the jab. She says she keeps seeing notes that only those with 'severe' learning disabilities can be prioritised. Apparently that data about the mortality rate from Covid being thirty times higher in these groups was not limited to those with severe conditions and MENCAP are seeing more deaths in this second wave.

'I have yet to see a clinical rationale for the current position and don't see how we can stick with it,' she told me anxiously.

I replied that I've signed off a more expansive definition which should cover everyone who needs it fast. 'We can't have "all LDs" as that's huge – it includes me!' I pointed out. Clearly my dyslexia does not justify an early jab, but when you start to drill down into it, drawing these sorts of boundaries within groups can be exceptionally tricky.

Steve Baker's crew have written to the PM saying there's no justification for legislative restrictions beyond the end of April. Let's see.
I don't want this dragging on any longer than necessary either – but
what we absolutely must not do is backslide.

SUNDAY 14 FEBRUARY

We've hit the target: more than 15 million people have now had their
first jab. I woke to a congratulatory text from Pascal. 'Dear Matt: I
hope you are doing well. Looks like the vaccination strategy is working, you will be the winner of this debate!' he said.

Maybe, but it's way too early for any backslapping. I'm particularly
worried about what's going on in the north. The virus is falling right
across the country except in Bradford and some other parts of West
Yorkshire. It's exactly the same problem we had last summer: tight-knit
communities, often of Asian descent, often with several generations
of the same family living under the same roof and not necessarily as
able to follow social distancing rules. They've been going gangbusters
on vaccines, so it's definitely not that. The Prof and I discussed it and
agree that the PM needs to know, otherwise he'll see the overall infection figures (which are good) and take that as the green light to ease
restrictions, when we still have this major hotspot.

Jim has been having more meetings with Border Force officials.
They're very keen to brush off any problems at Heathrow as 'Heathrow's problems', but the reality is that they're shared issues. As Jim says,
long queues at passport control matter, 'even if Border Force thinks its
secondary to their staff rotas and strange ways of doing things'. We
need to sort all this out, because we might be living with red-list management and quarantine hotels for months to come. The truth is that
Border Force needs reform. The Home Office has never gripped it. It's
one of the last bastions of old-school strike-threat unionism – like the
railways. This is the imperative we need to get it sorted. For now, the
Home Office and DfT seem OK with us playing in this pool, but No.
10 may get resentful about remit-spread – and it's not a remit I want.
What it really needs is a Minister for Borders who takes responsibility

for all border-related issues from all parts of government that are affected – Transport, Home Office, HMRC, DEFRA, Health etc.

MONDAY 15 FEBRUARY

The kids are off for half-term, though the so-called break is meaningless since there's nowhere to go and nothing to do. I feel sorry for them and miss them so much. I just don't have time to do any Dad stuff. They don't complain, but I am conscious of how quickly childhood goes and know I won't get this time with them again.

To that point, the PM has decided to set out a roadmap for lifting restrictions a week today. The Cabinet Office proposes five steps, starting with schools, then shops and hospitality, each one a progressive relaxation. In classic Whitehall fashion, there will be four tests for each step, each clear enough to be meaningful but loose enough for discretion. They are:

1. The vaccine deployment programme continues successfully;
2. Evidence shows vaccines are sufficiently effective in reducing hospitalisations and deaths in those vaccinated;
3. Infection rates do not risk a surge in hospitalisations that would put unsustainable pressure on the NHS;
4. Our assessment of the risks is not fundamentally changed by new variants of concern.

Sounds good to me.

Boris is getting impatient: he can see a glimpse of light at the end of the tunnel and is wondering whether we can hurtle towards it any faster. I've been batting him off quite well, because we are already at full stretch, but he is still on my back.

'Look, Prime Minister, we've got to have a target we can hit. I've got some back pocket here, but we might need it,' I said, trying not to sound exasperated. I know it's his job to push, push, push, but I'm doing exactly the same.

Gavin and I have agreed a plan for mass testing to keep schools open when kids finally go back. Relations between our respective departments weren't exactly sweetness and light a few weeks ago, but he doesn't seem to hold grudges, and neither do I.

'A pleasure doing business with you,' I said, after we'd thrashed it out.

'And with you. I think it will work rather well. We will aim to be your golden child of testing!!!' he replied cheerfully.

Hotel quarantine has started. So far we've done deals with sixteen hotels, providing 4,963 rooms. A further 58,000 are on standby. We've changed the law to give powers to Border Force, built a new IT system and done our level best to get all the different stakeholders in the airports to work together. Deep breath!

Politico has run an annoying little story suggesting that government Covid doctors are unhappy about 'science by press release'. It's based on a brief, leaked email exchange between various figures at PHE, including Susan Hopkins, in December when we announced the Kent variant. She messaged me saying she's 'extremely annoyed' by the 'divisive' story and making clear she has no problem with the way the announcement was handled.

'Science by press release has occurred all year... for exactly the reason that information needs to get out fast to the public,' she said. Precisely!

Following last week's 'jabs for asylum seekers' shocker, I've been tipped off about another queue-jumping outrage: nannies. This afternoon a friend discovered that her daughter's nanny 'and all her nanny friends' have been getting vaccinated on the grounds that they are 'carers'.

'Apparently they're all at it,' my friend said.

Head in hands. At least they're enthusiastic.

TUESDAY 16 FEBRUARY

Simon Case messaged to ask how many people we locked up in hotels yesterday. 'None,' I replied. One hundred and forty-nine people chose to enter the country and are now, of their own free will, in residential quarantine, having elected to pay a four-figure sum for the privilege.

Simon laughed.

I can't imagine it's remotely funny for the individuals concerned. They could easily have avoided it all by spending a couple of happy weeks at their liberty in a country that isn't on our red list before entering the UK – or better still, stayed away – but that's their lookout.

The latest vaccine efficacy data, which I received today, is a bit messy. Overall, it appears goodish, but there's a worrying uptick in Pfizer cases after Day 35. Does this mean the vaccine effectiveness wanes that quickly? I asked the Prof whether he is concerned about the dosing schedule.

'Not yet,' he replied. He says the efficacy is unlikely to go down rapidly: the main risk is that it does not go up enough. I've recommended that we do not circulate the information at this stage.

WEDNESDAY 17 FEBRUARY

I visited the Queen Elizabeth Hospital in Birmingham with the Prince of Wales and the Duchess of Cornwall, their first public engagement this year. I met HRH and Camilla at the entrance. Prince Charles quipped that he would have come sooner but he was waiting his turn to be vaccinated – a joke news camera crews picked up on their mics. They were both a class act, talking to as many staff and volunteers as possible and showing real interest in the work.

Other royals are making congratulatory calls to some of our busiest vaccine centres. Among those who have been invited to a virtual audience with the Queen are Emily Lawson and the national vaccine rollout team. I am thrilled for them: they completely deserve it.

Emma is worried about long Covid. She says the default for GPs is just to sign people off work so they can unpick suspected long Covid symptoms from the general stresses of life. We don't yet know the numbers, but they could be very significant. As Jim has been privately warning, it could have huge implications for the NHS and the economy. We need to keep pushing for proper funding from HMT.

THURSDAY 18 FEBRUARY

Just as we finally land the extra vaccine doses from the Serum Institute of India, the VTF have kicked off and another senior member is threatening to resign. It transpires that he and Kate have a fundamental problem with us buying vaccines from India, and he's let it be known that if we do so, he'll quit.

All this explains why we didn't get the Indian doses last year: he and Kate were working against it, and completely ignoring ministerial steers. I suddenly feel less guilty about failing to drive it through: clearly no amount of chasing would have made any difference. No wonder I never got anywhere and then had to deal with an inquest by No. 10.

'*That's* why we kept getting bullshit excuses,' I told Boris.

All this would be water under the bridge, save that we still want the doses. The VTF are refusing to engage, so I'm going to have to sort it out personally.

It's unreal. The government of India has told the SII that it has no problem, and the UK government wants to buy the doses. Yet the VTF have blocked it from the start and are threatening to resign if they don't get their way. What's infuriating is that the reason the Indians are so supportive is that they know that without Oxford and AZ giving them the rights to make this stuff for free, there'd be no vaccines for India at all – and nor for most of the rest of the developing world. It's a great deal for India, and my duty as the UK Health Secretary is to get the UK vaccinated. Still, at least now we've identified the blockage, and I've tasked Nadhim with getting the vaccines physically here.

As and when lockdown ends, home testing is going to be crucial. After winning the battle to get it signed off, Jim is worried that Test and Trace have taken their eyes off the ball.

'I have real foreboding about this,' he said, warning that unless we get a better system in place, home testing will 'work out v badly and will ultimately fail'. It's a useful warning – and it has taken an age – but last time I checked in, their plans were well advanced. I put it on the agenda for my weekly meeting with Dido and will check she's across it. Often just putting something like that on the Secretary of State's meeting agenda has the desired effect.

FRIDAY 19 FEBRUARY

The Times front page claims there is 'hope for holidays overseas' this summer. I doubt it!

We are MILES from being able to open internationally.

'Kill it,' I told Damon.

'Apparently it's better than it was going to be,' Damon replied gloomily. He says No. 10 tried very hard to hose it down.

I'm doing the Sunday media round and have suggested making the key message 'the vaccine is working'. Weirdly, No. 10 is against.

'Why?' I asked Damon.

'They worry it raises expectations too much,' he replied. I've told him to push hard: we need to reassure people that we are getting there and encourage them to keep coming forward for jabs.

Amid some secrecy, the Cabinet Office has been fine-tuning the roadmap to easing restrictions. Everyone is paranoid about leaks, so the draft document is in very limited circulation. Officials are being given numbered copies to look through in a supervised reading room, so nothing can be snuck out or reproduced. The reading room is actually just an office in the Cabinet Office – comically numbered Room 101 – used for these purposes. The Prof is increasingly optimistic about the direction of travel, so we're starting to get into the detail. While the PM obsesses about what will and won't be allowed in private gardens in each step, I am more concerned about what we say on international travel. I've been pressing for a very cautious tone. I am terrified of what Jim calls a 'vaccine-eating variant'.

Separately, a High Court judge has ruled that the department – and therefore I – 'acted unlawfully' by failing to publish Covid procurement contracts within the thirty-day period required by law. Jolyon Maugham, the pompous leftie barrister who brought the case, is crowing. He's been telling anyone who'll listen that he 'wishes there were no need' for his so-called Good Law Project – all the while pursuing questionable cases that seem designed for media attention. Hard as I find it to take him seriously – this is, after all, a man who bludgeoned a fox to death while wearing a silk kimono – it's very frustrating. We defend these judicial reviews as if they are substantive, whereas they strike me as largely political and aimed at generating media coverage, with him putting his own spin on the judgments. It's a massive waste of time. After all, who the hell would have acted differently: in the heat of the crisis, should my civil servants have prioritised the paperwork over buying PPE? The question answers itself.

We finally managed to secure almost 10 million extra doses from India. In the end, the MHRA only took a few weeks to inspect the SII production facilities. I'm trying not to think about the fact that we could have had these doses in December, had Kate and her allies not been working behind the scenes to block it.

All day I resisted the urge to engage with her, hoping the whole row would simmer down. Sure enough, this evening Nadhim messaged to say no one is going to resign.

'Triumph!' he declared jubilantly. Hmm. Let's get the doses here first.

SUNDAY 21 FEBRUARY

Here we are in the midst of the gravest health crisis in modern history, and the NHS has no idea what its budget is going to be in five weeks' time. This year's allocation runs out at the end of March. Who knows how much money we'll have after that? I certainly don't, and nor does Simon Stevens, because neither HMT officials nor Downing Street seem remotely interested in agreeing a figure until the last possible minute, which makes forward planning more than a little bit difficult. My solution was to insert a line about NHS funding into the roadmap, but as I perused the latest draft this morning, I realised to my intense annoyance that some scoundrel has deleted it, leaving us no further forward. I got straight onto Dan Rosenfield and asked for it to be reinstated. I told him that leaving the NHS with no budget at all from the end of March is nuts. An hour or so later he still hadn't replied, so I took it up with Simon instead.

'What happened to NHS funding in the document? It's only five weeks to the new financial year and they don't have a budget!' I protested.

He had no idea but promised to look into it. A few minutes later he came back to say that the funding line had 'gone into square brackets' and then been taken out after HMT objected on the grounds that it requires a separate discussion. Well, yes, it does – but nobody in the Treasury seems to want that discussion, and the clock is ticking.

I told Simon I'll take HMT's lack of engagement as an assumption that we'll roll over the current – elevated – budget to next year. There is no credible alternative.

By lunchtime Dan still hadn't replied, so I messaged him saying I wanted to register how frustrating it is to be left high and dry.

'Let's come back to the NHS point,' he replied dismissively. I know he's busy, but this nonchalance really frustrated me.

'It can't wait to Budget. It's nuts! I have an NHS to run,' I protested.

Luckily none of this came up when I appeared on *Marr* this morning. I was able to announce that we'll offer a vaccine to everybody in categories 1 to 9 by 15 April and all adults by the end of July – which puts a real end-date on this whole thing.

I thought my appearance had gone quite well but was quickly disabused of that notion in the car home when I received a message from Helen saying that I've upset Edel Harris, CEO of Mencap. She's not happy that I said people with learning disabilities are now getting their jabs.

'They are!' I retorted.

'No, that's been the whole battle. It's only those identified as "severe" or in residential settings,' Helen replied patiently.

'That's what Marr asked about!' I replied, genuinely confused. I thought I'd said all the right things during the show. Andrew and I had discussed radio presenter Jo Whiley's campaign to draw attention to this issue. Her severely disabled younger sister Frances almost died of Covid.

'Tell Mencap to talk to the JCVI,' I said firmly. We have to follow their advice.

Unfortunately, Helen does not think this will pacify Mencap at all. She says Edel is 'very angry' and has 'volunteered she has time to speak later today/tomorrow with you'.

Hmmm. Not appealing!

'If you're willing to talk to her, I think it would be v worthwhile. This is not going to go away,' Helen said.

Fine – I'll do it if it will calm things down, but we can't budge from the scientific advice from the JCVI. We have to be guided by the science, or the whole queue concept will break down.

MONDAY 22 FEBRUARY

Piers Morgan is thrilled that the government has had a rap over the knuckles over Covid contracts and thinks I should be 'locked up' for 'breaking the law'. The comedian Jim Davidson was clearly listening to *Good Morning Britain* while he was getting dressed and was so incensed by this comment that he rushed straight into his recording studio to fire back.

Clad only in a fluffy grey dressing gown, he rounded on Piers: 'What is the matter with you?' he demanded. 'It should be you locked up... in a nut house. Why are you so angry with everybody? We've had the most successful vaccine thing in the whole of Europe! Why is it not good enough for you? You want to lock Matt Hancock up now and do you know why? Because he went out and bought a load of PPE stuff instead of sending it out to a thousand different firms to get a thousand different quotes. He needed it and he needed it now! And do you know why? There was a shortage!'

Davidson was so annoyed that his dressing gown was in grave danger of coming undone. He told Piers that he should be braced for a shortage of 'anti-gravity boots', because in a year's time 'the earth's going to lose its gravity and we're all going to float off, and I hope you go first'.

It was a spectacular rant. The video is getting hundreds of views, mostly from Nadhim, who's a massive Jim Davidson fan. Never in a million years had I expected to take such joy from a partially dressed Jim Davidson, but this pandemic is unprecedented in so many ways.

'Love it!!' I said. 'And by the way, I didn't "break the law". Government action was deemed "unlawful". There's a big difference.' It's not like we went out of our way to do something illegal – it's that a court has looked at what happened afterwards and found the paperwork wanting. It's always frustrated me that, by antiquated precedent, these legal cases are made out in the name of the Secretary of State, rather than the name of the department, which gives a completely misleading impression. I know I sound defensive, but this contract stuff does my head in and so does Piers, with his endless negativity.

Now there's been enough time for a proper assessment of the Pfizer jab's efficacy, the results are looking good. The latest data suggests a single shot of the vaccine cuts the chance of hospital admission and death by more than 75 per cent. It also significantly reduces the risk of infection. It confirms that we were right to wait before releasing the figures: as the Prof always said, earlier data was pretty meaningless.

Later Boris published the roadmap, making clear that the decision on each stage will be based on data, not dates. Not a word of dissent at Cabinet. There was a minor drama later when an unnamed source told journalists that you 'cannot vaccinate your way out of this', which is literally the opposite of our policy. You absolutely can vaccinate your way out of this and that is precisely what we are doing.

'Who the fuck is saying this?' I asked Damon.

He initially thought it might be someone in No. 10, but they denied all knowledge. I told him to keep a very close eye on it and hit it hard if journalists ask.

'This is very, very damaging if it gets going,' I said.

After a bit more digging, Damon thinks he's tracked down the source: a well-meaning official whose words were taken out of context. Fortunately, it seems to have fizzled.

With something of a heavy heart, I kept my word to Helen and spoke to Edel at Mencap. To my surprise, it was an extremely useful discussion.

'How did it go?' Helen asked afterwards.

'Superb. She was so reasonable and very persuasive,' I replied enthusiastically. I told Edel I couldn't move from the science on this, but she was so thoughtful she convinced me to ask the JCVI to re-examine the issue. Helen is delighted. Well done her for pushing.

TUESDAY 23 FEBRUARY

Sounds to me like JVT has been winding up the Germans. He messaged me this afternoon warning me that Jens might call, after he was slightly less diplomatic than they might have expected about their attitude to the AstraZeneca jab. Not only have they cast aspersions over its safety in elderly patients; they've also been very sniffy about the delayed second dose policy. During a meeting about the pandemic with German ministers today, JVT threw caution to the wind and told them bluntly that people will have died as a result of their attitude.

'I think I may have put the cat among the pigeons,' he told me, sounding slightly sheepish.

'As in you told them what we are doing is right?' I asked.

'100 per cent pulled no punches,' he confirmed.

'Legend,' I replied. I'm glad he said it as it is.

On the morning media round, I caused a bit of a furore by arguing that there was never a national shortage of PPE. It was a close-run thing – we certainly had distribution issues and there were shortages in particular places – but overall, we never actually ran out. Naturally, Labour is squealing with righteous indignation, but it's the truth.

I was equally robust about 'contracts for cronies'. The notion that nobody who knows anybody in government should be allowed to have

a contract for anything is patently absurd. If we'd ruled out every potential PPE supplier with any connection to any parliamentarian, we'd
have missed out on a lot of life-saving kit. For that, we would rightly
have been crucified. Of course there are plenty of things I could have
done better, but delivering PPE in the teeth of a pandemic when the
whole world was desperate for it wasn't easy.

Jim is anxious about vaccine passports. He describes work on certification as 'quite low-energy' and thinks people are waiting for Simon
Stevens to grip it. The real issue is that the concept is fundamentally
unconservative. Whatever the justification on health grounds, many
of our natural supporters will hate it.

WEDNESDAY 24 FEBRUARY

I'm still getting an absolute battering over PPE contracts. It's beginning
to get to me. Jamie sent a long and sympathetic series of messages,
joking that at least I've now got a really good answer when people ask
what I wish I'd done differently during the pandemic.

'You could say, "I wish we'd moved people off the PPE procurement
team and into the DHSC audit team so we could buy less PPE but do
all the paperwork faster. Because at the time we assumed that the lives
of doctors and nurses who needed life-saving PPE gear was more important than prioritising technical paperwork, but clearly we got that
wrong,"' he suggested sarcastically.

'Utterly ridiculous' is his view of the whole thing, which it is. The
question is how to take the sting out of the relentless political attacks,
which are such a debilitating distraction – especially when the battle
isn't over.

Jamie had multiple constructive suggestions. Trying to pass the
buck won't do me any favours, but if I'm really feeling the heat, Jamie
thinks people should know that Cummings was the one who shouted at officials to cut the bureaucratic crap and just buy whatever we
needed. 'I was in the meeting when he lost his shit over ventilators
and was furious that officials were trying to build a business case for
it,' he said. Indeed, at the time, No. 10 made a virtue out of cutting red

tape to get things done fast. The way I see it, the key point I need to get over relates to values: we were working every hour to keep nurses safe. Meanwhile Labour just busies itself with endless political attacks.

Nadine is also backing me up. 'We were facing the unknown. It all could have been so, so much worse. You did good,' she said kindly. Apparently Downing Street focus groups are very supportive of us on this one. People are glad we refused to get bogged down in a legal quagmire and just got on with the job.

'Exactly, because that's how rational humans see it! It's common sense to grab what you can to fill the gap. Remember, everything shifted every day, and dramatically so,' Nadine said.

My political woes are considerably less important than the life-or-death threat to people in developing countries who have no access to vaccines. Today Ghana became the first beneficiary of the COVAX initiative. A delivery of 600,000 doses of the Oxford vaccine – manufactured in India – arrived in Accra on Wednesday. It's the start of a plan to deliver over 2 billion vaccine doses globally by the end of the year – all organised by the UK government and paid for by taxpayers. I love this work.

THURSDAY 25 FEBRUARY

Woke up to *Bild* – the biggest-selling paper in Germany – congratulating us on the vaccine rollout. 'Dear Britain, we envy you!' said the headline. The accompanying article notes that more than 17.7 million people have received a jab in the UK compared to 3.4 million in Germany. They're yet more furious that the gap is growing, as we vaccinate nearly three times as many people as they do each day.

I'm acutely conscious that we could yet be knocked off course by a horror mutation. I messaged Nadhim asking where we are up to on the roadmap to variant vaccines. He says we should have a document setting out a timeframe in 'about a week', which is Whitehall speak for 'in about a fortnight, if you're lucky'. Nadhim doesn't yet have years of experience of civil service inertia. To make this happen he'll need to shake the system.

'Drive it hard. Take no prisoners. Remove any barriers on the critical path. Then repeat,' I said. He replied with six emojis: three bicep curls, and three thank-yous. Or are they prayers?

We were due to attend a No. 10/Cabinet Office meeting this evening on what to do about France, which is a hotbed of variants of concern. Some are pushing the case for putting it on the red list, but that would create huge import/export issues for both countries and is politically incendiary. At the last minute, Downing Street bumped us off the cast and limited it to the PM's team only, I suspect because Boris didn't want to come under huge pressure. I messaged him direct, warning him that this could jeopardise everything we've achieved.

'France has 5 per cent of cases from the South Africa new variant. This is the killer fact. We simply don't know how effective the vaccines are against them. Holidays are already banned until 17 May, so the cost of action is already limited until then,' I argued. By 17 May we'll know far more. If the vaccine *does* work enough against new variants, we are fine and won't have lost much. If it doesn't work, we will have to keep restrictions until we have something that does, and we'll be very glad we took this action now.

'It's very diff,' Boris replied, clearly torn. 'Economic downside big and we don't know whether it would really make any difference.' True.

FRIDAY 26 FEBRUARY

Boris decided not to put France on the red list. We've got a problem in another quarter, though, as behavioural scientists are complaining that we included provisional dates in the roadmap. They seem to think it's 'dangerous'. According to Professor Stephen Reicher, a member of the SAGE subcommittee on behavioural science, the Prime Minister is undermining his own message about reopening being guided by 'data, not dates'. Reicher says people are already seizing on the rough time-frames we've given to book holidays, and events like the Reading and Leeds Festivals are now expected to go ahead – when there's a danger it might all have to be cancelled again.

'It gives hope if you can stick to those dates; if you don't, it brings despair,' Reicher opined gloomily.

I'd argue the exact opposite. If we don't give people any idea of what's happening and when, they'll simply give up. That's just human nature.

On a positive note, I've managed to get us out of something we really didn't want to do, just by picking up the phone to Rishi. It's a great example of how the machine sometimes conspires. The Treasury has been pushing very hard for an independent review on vaccine procurement. There may well be a time for that, but right now it's too soon: we still need total focus on the task at hand. Yet HMT officials have been refusing to let it go. Cue lots of agonised Whitehall exchanges about terms of reference etc. I said I was against it happening now but was open-minded about a 'lessons learned' exercise afterwards – after all, you've got to learn lessons from successes as well as failures. When Emma checked in with HMT this morning, she was told that they'd 'decided at official level that we are too far apart' and 'have advised Chx [the Chancellor] to drop the idea for now'. I rang Rishi to make sure he wasn't too sore about it, and to my amazement, he was completely unaware of the proposal. He didn't agree with the idea either and was quite taken aback when I explained that his department has been on our backs about it for ages. We joked about how we are both generally against independent reviews in principle – if we want to act, we should act. Looks like someone in HMT was keen on the idea and pushed it in Rishi's name, without taking the trouble to check. Shows the importance of ministers actually talking to each other.

SATURDAY 27 FEBRUARY

Oh, to be part of the international jet set. It seems Covid is just a minor inconvenience for them. In fact, I reckon they quite enjoy the challenge of finding ever-more imaginative ways to maintain their usual lifestyles. Take Sir Philip Green. Now he's a tax exile in Monaco, he's not subject to UK restrictions, so he's swept his daughter Chloe off the Maldives to celebrate her thirtieth birthday with 'around twenty-five of her best friends'. According to the *Daily Mail*, they're currently luxuriating at the £1,000-a-night Four Seasons Hotel for what Sir Philip is characterising as a low-key celebration. This behaviour is just so spectacularly insensitive. It makes everybody who is stuck at home doing their bit feel even worse. Annoyingly, Priti has confirmed there's nothing we can do. 'He lives in Monaco and any trip to the Maldives would need to be questioned by Monaco authorities if breaking their rules (including curfew) rather than the UK,' she told me.

If he comes back here on return from Monaco, he'll have to submit a PLF and self-isolate at a private property, but Monaco isn't on the red list, so sadly he would not have to suffer the humiliation of a fortnight at the Heathrow Premier Inn. Border Force officials are going to check aviation records just to be sure there hasn't been any funny business, but I think our hands are tied.

'Always thought it is strange politically that our side has sat back and not been critical of his overall biz and tax conduct,' Priti said wearily.

'Totally agree,' I replied. I've had one brush with him in which he was incredibly abusive to one of my junior aides and I have refused to have anything to do with him ever since.

Despite the utter wretchedness of this lockdown, we have our biggest poll lead over Labour since last summer. Benefiting from a vaccine bounce.

SUNDAY 28 FEBRUARY

A potentially dangerous new variant has been identified in the UK, but we can't find Patient Zero. We know someone in Britain has it, but whoever it is failed to provide the correct contact details when they took their Covid test, so we don't know who or where they are.

Cue a frantic search for the so-called 'orphan' – the funny term epidemiologists use for lost cases – which we're going to have to escalate into a public appeal.

Annoyingly, No. 10 failed to brief Rishi properly before he went on *Marr*, as a result of which he inadvertently declared that there's 'no evidence of new variants spreading in the UK'. At that very moment, we were mid-panic about the orphan, which we think originated in Brazil, and trying to work out when to tell people.

'What Rishi said is *technically* correct,' Damon observed, pointing out that there's no evidence – yet – of the Brazil thing spreading. All the same, it jars. Meanwhile PHE is still trying to work out how dangerous the variant is.

According to their risk assessment, there are 'a lot of unknown unknowns', which doesn't really help us any. The task is made harder by the poor quality of data from Brazil. So far, it looks similar to the South Africa variant, which is not encouraging.

Damon says Test and Trace think it may have been a DIY test, rather than someone going to a Covid testing centre. If so, I'll be relieved.

'Much, much easier to explain,' I said. 'The idea someone sent back a home test without filling in the paperwork is less of an operational screw-up and more that the person just didn't do the paperwork.'

If the idiot failed to provide his or her contact details, Test and Trace is off the hook: it's hardly Dido's fault.

Meanwhile Italian researchers have found that the Pfizer/BioN-Tech vaccine may be less effective in people who are very overweight. Data suggests obese healthcare workers only produce around half the number of antibodies in response to a second dose of the jab compared with people with a healthy BMI. I can't say I'm surprised: previous research has suggested that obesity increases the risk of dying of Covid-19 by nearly 50 per cent, as well as more than doubling the risk of ending up in hospital. One to keep an eye on, in case there's something we can do in terms of giving those who are overweight extra booster jabs.

MARCH 2021

MONDAY 1 MARCH

'How is the hunt for our man from Brazil?' Boris asked anxiously. It was 8.17 a.m. and despite a nationwide search, the orphan had been neither identified nor located. What to say? Actually, a remarkable triangulation operation was under way. When a lab technician first spotted the new variant, we didn't even know which part of the country the positive test had come from. Since then, thanks to some fancy sequencing and a high-quality data system, we've been able to identify the batch of home test kits involved, through which we've narrowed it down from the whole of England to just 379 possible households in the southeast. We are now contacting every single one of them, so very soon we should know who our mystery patient is. The PM was obviously too busy for this detail, so I just told him that we're on it.

TUESDAY 2 MARCH

The net's closing. We now know that the PCR test was processed at 00.18hrs on Valentine's Day and went to the lab via a mailing centre in Croydon. The search is narrowing to south-west London.

The *Daily Mail* has got wind of our plan to mandate jabs for NHS staff. The unions will object, but I'm relaxed. The story quotes a 'Cabinet Office' source.

'Best not to deny', I told Damon.

Sturgeon is on the rack over her handling of sexual harassment allegations against her predecessor Alex Salmond and could be forced out within twenty-four hours. I'm supposed to be heading up to Scotland later this week to look round their vaccination and testing centres – all part of low-key efforts to shore up the union. Now I'm having my doubts about the trip.

'Are we SURE I should be going? On the grounds of "don't interrupt your enemy when they're making a mistake"?' I asked Allan apprehensively.

'I think it's fine on the basis that we don't get sucked into it all. So it looks like while the SNP is imploding there's still one government that's cracking on delivering for the people of Scotland,' Allan replied.

Apparently the Scottish Tories still want me to go up. Good. Let's see how things look tomorrow.

WEDNESDAY 3 MARCH

The boss has been reading a book about cancer called *The Emperor of All Maladies*, written by an American oncologist. The *New York Times* described the book as 'a history of eureka moments and decades of despair'. I have no idea how he has time for this kind of reading, but he sent me a nice message at the crack of dawn praising the vaccine effort and talking about what's next. Before the pandemic nightmare, he and I talked about a 'cancer Moonshot' – to turn cancer into a survivable disease, not just for the lucky few but for everyone. When this is all over, he thinks I should get back onto it.

'Next big thing for you. Not for now and not until the backlog is cleared etc., but worth setting as a goal,' he enthused.

'Love to,' I replied.

Sturgeon is still in post – just. I'm heading up to Glasgow by sleeper tonight.

Meanwhile Test and Trace think they may have found the orphan. Public health officials are on their way to interview him or her. No confirmation as yet.

THURSDAY 4 MARCH

Not much sleep as we thundered north on the train. I lay in my narrow little berth worrying about the mystery Brazilian and wondering what else we can do in this 'Where's Wally?' operation if we haven't got the right person. Shortly after 5 a.m. I gave up trying to shut out the rat-a-tat-tat of the wheels on the track as we sped up the west coast and messaged Allan in the next-door berth. He was awake too but hadn't heard anything. Then: a breakthrough. They've found him!

'Do we definitely have Wally?' I asked Dido.

'Yes, we do,' she confirmed. She didn't have any more details about how he was infected but is sure we have our man. Dido says that he was on the shortlist of 379 households and that officials tried to reach him by phone, leaving various messages. He eventually returned their calls at 4 p.m. yesterday. Apparently he tried to register his test but got the details wrong 'which is why he was orphaned'.

We know his name and age (thirty-eight) and that he has been very ill. 'He called an ambulance but didn't go to hospital,' Dido said. He claims not to have left his house for eighteen days. This is extremely good news: assuming he's telling the truth, he has not been out and about super-spreading.

'He's located in Croydon, almost exactly where our search led us,' she said.

'Well done, team!' I replied. What amazing detective work. Apparently he doesn't realise he triggered a massive manhunt, so we'll have to be careful to protect his anonymity. We agreed to wait until we've checked out his story about not leaving the house for three weeks before declaring victory.

Piling off the train into spectacular dawn sunshine in a deserted Glasgow Station, we jumped into a huge convoy of taxis. To abide by social distancing, we're only allowed one official per taxi, so snaked through Glasgow bumper to bumper to the Lighthouse testing lab – run by the incomparable Anna Dominiczak – to see their test processing in action. Their ability to spot variants is amazing. We then moved on to a vaccine centre run by NHS Scotland, manned by British Army soldiers alongside the local council. A brilliant example of the union in action.

Later we went to Edinburgh University to see their scientific contribution, and I took half an hour out to clamber up Arthur's Seat. I love the hills outside Edinburgh, but I think I surprised some of the other hikers who were not expecting to bump into me. It was a glorious spring day as Allan and I, along with Oliver, my private secretary, climbed up high over Edinburgh and the Firth of Forth in our work garb, lockdown-length hair flying in the wind. On the way down, we got chatting to two local hikers, who asked politely why we were there. I explained that as UK Health Secretary I'd come to see Scotland's work on testing and vaccination. 'No,' she said, somewhat bemused by my rather formal answer: 'What on earth are you doing halfway up a mountain in your suit?'

While I was heading back from Scotland, Jim updated me on the mood among Cabinet colleagues on vaccine passports. Overall, he reckons there's broad support for some form of certification for international travel but not much love for anything domestic. 'Basically went very well, with green light for the thrusters and arse-covering for the certificate-sceptics,' he concluded colourfully.

Later Simon Case texted to congratulate us on 'capturing' the Brazilian. 'Incredible he stayed at home – restores a bit of faith in humanity!' he said cheerfully. I told him Dido and Susan Hopkins did a great job. They deserve the credit, not me.

Meanwhile the bollocking JVT gave the Germans seems to have worked. They've belatedly accepted that the Oxford vaccine is perfectly safe for the over-65s – let's hope the damage isn't done. It's so reckless. Perhaps we should dispatch JVT to talk some sense into the Italian government? They've just blocked the export of 250,000 doses of AstraZeneca to Australia. JVT messaged to tell me that they're using the EU's new regulation (the one they claimed was just about 'transparency') to stop the shipment, on the basis that the pharmaceutical company hasn't sent Italy as many doses as promised. Not much we can do about this one – but Pascal, who is a naturalised Australian, will be very upset.

FRIDAY 5 MARCH

Another Friday in the office when I should be in Suffolk, preparing for another press conference on the vaccine rollout. In the midst of preparations, pacing around my office with the draft script on the big screen, editing away, I received a curious message from Chipping Barnet MP Theresa Villiers alerting me to a potentially serious blunder on the passenger locator page of the government website. Apparently we've upset British Cypriots by including the 'Turkish Republic of Northern Cyprus' in the list of countries of origin from which passengers can select.

'The UK government has never recognised TRNC,' Theresa told me.

I'm no expert in that particular territorial dispute, but I can quite see that a lot of people will be very unhappy indeed if decades of foreign policy is inadvertently overturned by the gov.uk website. Apparently the correct terminology for that part of the world – at least as far as the FCDO is concerned – is simply 'the north of Cyprus'. In a classic case of Whitehall buck passing, Theresa says she raised it with Grant's department, who referred her to the Home Office, who told her it's a Department of Health and Social Care project and they're just implementing it. Very much hoping nobody in the FCDO has noticed, I reassured her that we will get onto this before it causes a diplomatic blow-up and asked Allan to fix it forthwith.

We have now vaccinated over 21 million people – almost two fifths of the entire adult population of the UK – and Covid deaths have nearly halved within a week. Mortality is falling faster than it was last month. The vaccine is clearly saving lives.

'Incredible, and something we need to protect with border measures,' Damon said. Agreed. Unfortunately, we're coming under increasing pressure to bring back international travel, even though it could put the whole thing at risk. I hope we don't all come to regret it.

SATURDAY 6 MARCH

We've now vaccinated three quarters of the over-sixties and are ready to move on to the over-55s. Gavin's on the media round tomorrow, so I offered him a bunch of positive statistics to wheel out. In line with the roadmap, schools are reopening tomorrow. It's not long till the end of term, but anything is better than nothing.

MONDAY 8 MARCH

Schools are back. Naturally the teaching unions are bleating about it all being too risky, but we had to get on with it. I was very nervous. Would schools actually open? Would the unions win? By the end of the day, it was clear the vast majority did open, testing went down well and the message about ventilation seems to have got through. Great excitement at home as the children got to see their friends again, although I did detect some grumbling that all the windows were open while it's still early March.

In other good news, the first batch of SII doses have finally arrived: 5 million! Better late than never.

TUESDAY 9 MARCH

Piers Morgan has stormed off his *GMB* show after a dramatic on-screen row with a colleague over Meghan Markle. I can understand why his co-presenter Alex Beresford finally snapped during yet another of his rants about 'Princess Pinocchio'. He flounced out, huffing and puffing about it being 'his show', and it's not at all clear he'll be back.

An interesting update from Porton Down on the accuracy of lateral flow tests versus PCRs. Surprisingly, the cheap tests seem more reliable than the so-called gold standard option, at least when it comes to false positives. Previously, they thought the false positive rate was one in 1,000. They now think it's more like one in 3,000. That's a lower rate of false positives than you get with PCRs, which Jim (who's been liaising with the scientists) says can be distorted by shards of old virus. Lateral flows can miss some virus but essentially detect transmissibility, and people are now getting much better at swabbing themselves, reducing that problem. The only real issue with these cheap DIY tests is that some people still don't know how to read them, mistakenly thinking that one stripe means the test is positive, when in fact it's two.

Sir John Bell still doesn't think we're doing enough to make the most of the 'Oxford vaccine' brand around the world. He says he took a call from Simon Case, who made the same point. As Jim says, the FCDO should lead on this, but the whole government needs to think about it. Jim also suggests we incorporate it into our G7 health summit plans.

'100,000 per cent agree,' I enthused.

Hospitalisations for Covid are now so low that we've decided to stand down the Nightingale hospitals. Another step on the road to normality. I wouldn't do this unless I was confident we won't be going back. Let's hope I'm right.

Helen has suggested we celebrate Piers's departure at our team meeting tomorrow. Perfect. Since I banned alcohol in the department, we can't toast the news, but we can mark it. The junior ministers in particular are relieved. He has a huge amount of talent, but simply shouting at politicians is not enlightening and doesn't hold anyone to account. I think British politics is better off without him.

WEDNESDAY 10 MARCH

Can you imagine if we hadn't bothered to set up a contact tracing system? And if we'd decided it was all too difficult and expensive to do mass testing? How much grief would we have got had we not raced against the clock to build a formidable machine to identify anyone who might have come into contact with a positive case and ask them to self-isolate? Would we ever have been forgiven if we'd failed to establish a system for identifying clusters of cases or new variants? No – and rightly so.

Yet a cross-party committee of MPs has come to the conclusion that Test and Trace was basically a gigantic waste of time and money. According to the Public Accounts Committee, it's unclear whether its contribution to reducing infection levels can justify its 'unimaginable' cost. Skimming their press release last night, I felt the red mist descend. It is beyond unreasonable.

I knew it was going to be a rough day when I looked out of the window and saw a camera crew hanging around on the doorstep. It was a little after 7 a.m., the sun was barely up, and I was in no mood to apologise for anything.

'TV crew on the doorstep!' I told Damon, trying to WhatsApp while wolfing down some breakfast.

'That's outrageous,' he replied.

'How to handle?' I asked, telling him I wasn't going to be remotely defensive. Yesterday we did 1.5 million tests – in a single day! No other European country has built such a capability.

Of course I'm not going to pretend that the system is perfect or that it hasn't had lots of problems. And yes, it's expensive – though most of the cost is on the free tests now very widely available. Overall, though, I think Dido and her team have done a fantastic job, under exceptionally difficult circumstances and immense pressure.

Outside, my ministerial car was waiting.

'My suggestion is to put your suit on and get in the car and if you really want to say something for them, go with "Test and Trace is doing a phenomenal job helping stop transmission and protecting people. We did 1.5 million tests yesterday. The team are doing an amazing job,"' Damon advised. Precisely.

Damon has put in a formal complaint to the broadcaster, as has No. 10. I never mind answering questions, but I don't think this select committee report justifies hanging around outside my family home at 7 a.m. It's horrible for the kids.

THURSDAY 11 MARCH

The Test and Trace row is rumbling on, as is a ridiculous story about me supposedly helping a guy who used to be the landlord of my local pub in Suffolk land a multi-million-pound Covid contract. As I've said ad nauseam, I've not had anything to do with awarding Covid contracts.

I know Alex Bourne, having met him when he bought the pub in the village where I was living. When that didn't take off, he instead turned his entrepreneurial spirit to a plastics factory and, when the call came, turned that to making the little plastic pots you put your swab into. We needed millions of them and it was better to be making them here than in China. But here's the rub: he never got, nor applied for, a contract from either the government or the NHS. He was a sub-contractor – making the accusation even more ridiculous.

I find these attacks on my integrity incredibly hurtful. Yet there's a problem in how to respond. Put out a robust statement and you only inflame the story, giving it extra legs. Ignore it and it looks like you're guilty. The departmental advice is to be very cautious, issuing only the blandest of statements that 'all contracts are awarded in the proper way'. But that's what the journalists call a 'non-denial denial' and they treat it as virtually an admission of guilt. So far I've tried to rise above the hostile reporting, which is mostly confined to *The Guardian*. But I wonder if I'm making a mistake. Maybe I should fight harder to ensure people know the truth.

FRIDAY 12 MARCH

After thinking long and hard, No. 10's finest creative minds have settled on a name for Public Health England's successor body. I was quite excited to hear their big idea, having charged them with coming up with something that encapsulates the new organisation's identity as public health warriors battling tirelessly for the health and wellbeing of the nation. I've given it the working title of the National Institute for Health Protection, which fits with international norms but doesn't exactly roll off the tongue. I waited impatiently for signs of white smoke from No. 10, where the final deliberations were being made. Then, at 8.32 a.m., came news via a WhatsApp from Dan Rosenfield that they had made their choice. My heart beat slightly faster in anticipation. What was it to be?

'United Kingdom Health Security Agency,' Dan announced proudly. I blinked at the screen, wondering if I'd read it correctly. Was it some autocorrect horror? How had they managed to make it sound both boring and creepy at the same time?

'Terrible,' I said. Which bright spark thought it would be cool to draw inspiration from Orwell's *1984*?

'Is awesome. PM's choice,' Dan replied breezily.

'Not without discussion,' I snapped. Another hour, another battle...

Oh well, at least Geoffrey Boycott is happy. He texted me to say he'd got his second dose. I'm very pleased and he seems genuinely grateful. I resisted the temptation to tell him that good things come to those who wait. We now know that he'll be even better protected than he would have been when he made all that fuss.

SATURDAY 13 MARCH

JVT sent me a picture of a vaccine certificate from 1859. It was issued to the parents of a four-month-old baby called Caroline, from Sheffield, who received a smallpox jab under the Vaccination Act of 1853, which made vaccination compulsory for children. He was sent it by an amateur historian.

'Absolutely fantastic. Turns out compulsory vaccination is a fine British tradition!' I replied cheerfully.

SUNDAY 14 MARCH

Jens messaged alerting me to what he described as a growing issue with thrombosis in young and early middle-aged women, linked to the AZ jab. I sent him back the safety data we routinely publish, which does not show any cause for concern.

MONDAY 15 MARCH

I went for a run with Dan Rosenfield, although we had to have a little walk in the middle while he caught his breath. I didn't rub it in – a few months ago, that would have been me huffing and puffing. My brother has done wonders for my health and fitness. We talked about what life will be like after the pandemic, something I've hardly dared to do till now. He says that No. 10 can't wait to get on with everything an eighty-seat majority allows you to do.

Germany is not the only country worried about the AZ jab. Today the Irish authorities announced they're suspending the vaccine while they look into blood clots. Several EU countries are following suit. We'll do what we've always done and stick with the science.

Our big task tomorrow is to work out how to explain the vaccine rollout slowdown. The second batch of 5 million more SII doses is behind schedule. We're still just about on track to cover all over-fifties by our mid-April target, but I very much doubt we're going to do any better than that. Damon has started managing expectations.

'It's our biggest win at risk. We can't blame the Indians. And so far the EU hasn't blocked anything,' I said anxiously.

'Provided we hit our targets we will be OK,' Damon replied. I told him that Jeane Freeman is extremely worried about whether they will pull it off in Scotland. If they fail, Sturgeon will doubtless find a way to blame us. It's going to be a tricky weekly vaccine meeting with the boss on Wednesday.

Officials tell me that Steve Barclay is still messing around on the Budget. I asked Dan to tell Rishi's SpAds they need to settle it NOW. Speaking of Steve, Jim tells me he's declined to sign off a very large lateral flow test order. Test and Trace's purchasing strategy may not be perfect, but we can't stick to the roadmap if we don't have these kits. As Jim says, it's wishful thinking to imagine that the virus will somehow evaporate. Plus, we'll be clobbered by the supplier for failing to honour the contract. These are false economies.

'Turn the tables on HMT,' I told Jim. Cancelling these orders is poor value for money.

TUESDAY 16 MARCH

To my astonishment, and eternal gratitude to Shona Dunn and her excellent officials who have done the hard graft, hotel quarantine is working. There's a weird new variant from the Philippines, but the two cases we've identified have gone no further than their airport hotel rooms. Both were detected in a hotel at Heathrow, both patients having travelled from Johannesburg to London via Doha, arriving on 21 February. The individuals concerned weren't on the same flight and followed quarantine rules to the letter. The team are checking what contact they may have had with anyone else in the airport or in transit to the hotel, but it all looks good. It was an opportunity to thank the team and remind them that what they're doing is so important for the country. Until we know a variant can't knock out the vaccine, or until people have been boosted so much they're protected against variants, we've got to maintain this routine.

My Indian opposite number has invited me to a UK–India health summit when the PM travels to the subcontinent next month. I've told No. 10 I'm keen to go.

I've written a piece for *The Sun* reassuring people that the Oxford jab is safe. More than 10 million people have now had it in the UK. Adverse side effects are vanishingly rare.

WEDNESDAY 17 MARCH

It's exactly 100 days since Margaret Keenan became the first person in the world to get the first Covid jab, but no victory laps for me. Instead I spent the day dealing with a spectacular row over vaccine supplies, trying to appear calm while feeling anything but.

Last night Simon Stevens asked me to approve a letter to the NHS warning of a significant reduction in the number of doses available from the end of this month. I didn't like the draft and specifically told him not to send it. It was badly written and very obviously designed to direct any flak away from the NHS. To my astonishment, half an hour before I was due to lead this evening's Downing Street press conference, he released it anyway, catching me completely off guard.

I was quietly seething about this and wondering how best to manage the fallout when – in a desperate attempt to save face over the EU's shambolic vaccine rollout – Ursula von der Leyen suddenly declared that Brussels will block vaccine exports to countries with higher vaccination rates than they have – i.e. us. It was clearly designed to be inflammatory and make it look as if Brussels is doing something, *anything*, to get a grip of their vaccine programme.

I couldn't believe my luck: just as I was about to have to explain why we're in danger of falling behind schedule, the EU provided the perfect excuse. What Ursula clearly doesn't realise is that a) our exclusive and expertly agreed contracts with AZ protect us from this kind of skulduggery and b) now everyone will think any supply problems are their fault. After all, Brussels is a tastier target for the media than the Department of Health or the NHS.

None of this made me any less annoyed about Simon's behaviour. He clearly knew he'd done wrong because he kept ignoring my calls. He didn't dare blank Boris, though, and got an earful when he took the call. Dan messaged me mid-bollocking, updating me on who was saying what.

'What's he saying?' I asked. 'It's a total outrage.'

'PM saying letter totally bonkers and blindsided. Didn't need to go now. Simon arguing had no choice,' Dan replied.

'Simon sent it AGAINST my advice,' I said, before correcting myself. 'Not advice – *instruction*.' True: much to Simon's annoyance, at the beginning of the pandemic I introduced a rule that he had to run all major NHS circulars past me before sending them out, to make sure we were always aligned. God knows what other unhelpful freelancing he and his team would have done if I hadn't made that change.

Earlier, Cummings popped up in front of the Science and Technology Select Committee to give evidence about a new research agency he championed. Naturally he couldn't resist the opportunity to characterise everyone except himself as stupid and incompetent. In his usual ludicrously over-the-top style, he labelled PPE contracts an 'absolute, total disaster' and claimed the scramble for protective gear left the Department of Health a 'smoking ruin'. Lest anyone fail to get the message about his own brilliance versus the rest of the world's uselessness, he suggested that I personally could not be trusted to lead the vaccine programme, so someone else had to be put in charge. Given that I was the one who drafted in Kate Bingham, and that I spent a great deal of time battling to protect the vaccine rollout from his interference while he continually briefed that I was 'too obsessed' by the quest for a vaccine, his narrative beggared belief.

Watching the whole thing from afar, Jamie was outraged. 'You went out and backed him over Barnard Castle and he responds by briefing against you relentlessly, in private and now in public,' he messaged indignantly. 'He's a fucking psychotherapist,' he added, pressing send before noticing the funny autocorrect.

'*psychopath,' he clarified. I think he means sociopath.

'We are rising above it,' I declared loftily.

'Also, you had people briefing against you in October saying you were the "only person in government who thought there would be a vaccine",' Jamie pointed out.

'Quite. Worth saying that Dom wasn't anywhere near vaccines, at all,' I replied.

'He was briefing against you over testing; then started to try to paint himself as the mass testing guy. He was briefing against you on vaccines; now is trying to take credit for vaccines,' Jamie recalled, adding that Cummings originally wanted to let the virus rip.

I absolutely can't get into a slanging match, but it's frustrating not being able to respond.

'Why should we take this crap lying down?' I complained.

'I suppose because until six months ago he could get you sacked,' Jamie pointed out reasonably.

Well, he can't now.

La vendetta è un piatto che va servito freddo, as Don Corleone put it.

For now, I shall content myself with pointing out that I don't recall Cummings making any of these arguments while I was defending him over his little trip to Barnard Castle.

Damon messaged this evening to say that *The Times* has got wind of the row with Simon over the letter. Apparently they're running something tomorrow.

'What angle will they take?' I asked Damon.

'I think that the letter as drafted came as a surprise.'

Fine. It did. Tomorrow I'm formally going to direct the NHS that no announcements go from them without our sign-off.

'They did this in the MoD about eight years ago and it was transformational. This is the moment,' I told Damon – meaning, this is the moment Andrew Lansley's unfortunate 2012 experiment with the so-called independence of the NHS is unceremoniously laid to rest.

Today was my son's birthday. His second of the pandemic. Another special occasion missed. We had breakfast together, but there was no way I could join the birthday tea with family. I hope to make it up to him – to all of them – when all this is over.

THURSDAY 18 MARCH

Paris is back in lockdown and Jim fears we've taken our eye off the ball on international travel. He describes controls at Heathrow and other entry points as 'OK but frayed'. There are 'wobbly operational bits', he says, and the official in charge of hotel quarantine spends her time 'whack-a-mole problem solving'. That pretty much sums up the usual state of government. The big picture is that DfT is eager to get overseas travel moving again, just at a time when the EU's vaccine strategy has stalled and there are nasty variants stalking the continent.

'I have a strong sense we're walking into March 2020 2.0,' Jim summarised gloomily. He is scathing about Border Force, for whom everything seems too difficult, and thinks No. 10 spends too much time worrying about 'the *Daily Mail* and Saga vote'. Worryingly, JVT says that global vaccine manufacturing will be too busy fulfilling pre-paid backorders this winter to have any capacity for orders of vaccines designed for variants. We could be stuck with border controls for some time.

After yesterday's drama, I made a statement in the Commons setting out the situation with vaccine supplies. I've never known the House so united in its view on Brussels. Suddenly the European Commission, which ardent pro-Europeans see as a bastion of progressive values and the rule of law, has been exposed for what it is: a highly politically driven operation, prepared to do anything to cover its back.

FRIDAY 19 MARCH

An emotional day for Jim as he got his Covid jab, and an emotional day for the rest of us as we were treated to the sight of his naked torso. Quite what came over him when the moment arrived for him to have his vaccine I don't know, but he seemed to feel the need to strip off and treat us all to a vision of his bare chest. Standard procedure for blokes involves a manly rolling up of the shirt sleeve, a stoic smile when they say 'sharp scratch coming', then over and out. Not for Jim, who videoed his semi-striptease and posted it on social media. To give him his due, he's in excellent shape, but that is not a body that has seen sunlight for a while.

What we don't need is the rest of the population mistakenly thinking they have to follow suit, or vaccine centres across the land will be swarming with semi-naked bodies. Much as I love him, I won't be retweeting that one.

JVT has discovered that the USA is loaning 1.5 million doses of AZ to Canada. They get it next week.

'Why not us?' he enquired. We're working on it.

Natasha tells me Nadhim Zahawi also got his jab today. Here's hoping he kept his kit on.

SATURDAY 20 MARCH

Priti agrees that we can't afford to relax on borders. I spoke to her last night and she said we need to do much more on hauliers, the red list etc. I've told the team to liaise with the Home Office to make the case.

After all the rumpus about the vaccination slowdown, yesterday we hit a record number: 711,156. To date we've vaccinated over half of all adults. Bloody good going.

SUNDAY 21 MARCH

The EU is now in a panic and is upping the ante in the vaccine war.

'I think we all need to calm down,' the EU's financial services commissioner declared on *Marr* this morning, after a series of provocations she knew would have precisely the opposite effect. Mairead McGuinness knows Brussels has screwed up and admits European citizens 'are growing angry and upset'.

'Frankly none of us have had a great Covid,' she told the BBC this morning, and then added to the EU's long list of misjudgements by once again refusing to rule out an export ban. She claims it's fair enough for them to go down this route because we have a long list of medicines that we don't send them. (True, but that has nothing to do with vaccines.)

Dom Raab got straight onto me after the show, saying we need to push back hard. I agree.

Later Simon Case messaged to say that the PM had 'a couple of tough calls' with Macron and Merkel. For now, Downing Street thinks the less said the better and is keeping that quiet.

'Summary of conclusion is that we will try to talk to them to avoid export bans. It will be tough going, though,' Simon said. Tim Barrow is heading to Brussels to try to knock heads together, and there's a possibility of a PM–Von der Leyen–Macron–Merkel call this week as part of the process of finding a way through.

I told Simon that we've prepared a series of concessions if Downing Street needs to throw them some meat.

Ben Wallace, who was on the morning media round, did a first-rate job playing the grown-up. I messaged to thank him.

'I tried to be collaborative with the EU,' he said.

'Yes, you looked the big guy,' I agreed.

'Very kind. They don't let me out much...' he replied.

MONDAY 22 MARCH

As the EU row continues to rage, Jim has poured fuel on the fire by publicly suggesting we might put the whole Schengen area on the red list. This was very definitely not part of the script. The first I knew of it was a furious message from Dan Rosenfield asking what the hell was going on.

'Eh?' I replied.

Dan cut and pasted a quote from Jim to some media outlet in which he expressed his 'enormous sadness' at the sight of our European neighbours rejecting the vaccine policy. 'I don't know how this will play out and it's certainly above my pay grade to speculate, but we are all aware that the possibility lies that we will have to red list all of our European neighbours – but that would be done with huge regret,' he opined.

Downing Street is hopping mad. I promised to talk to him. In fairness to Jim, he covers a lot of ground, and other than taking his top off to get vaccinated, he doesn't normally screw up.

I asked JVT whether we could use human trials to ascertain whether the vaccine works on a new variant from India that's now spreading. He says we can't, because it would take six months to develop a so-called challenge virus to give volunteers. 'The only challenge virus we can use legally is a Wuhan-like one. That took us four to five months to develop,' he explained.

'Why so slow?' I asked.

He replied that any product used in such a way has to be certified free of all other pathogens.

Six months!

'Can't we take our normal "don't let the best be the enemy of the good" view?' I asked.

Apparently not. JVT says that if we try to speed things up, it could end in disaster. 'If we put one foot wrong in this space, we could kill a volunteer,' he told me bluntly. 'Then the whole programme would be put at risk.

Hard to argue with that one.

TUESDAY 23 MARCH

It's a year to the day that Boris gave the British people his 'very simple instruction' to stay at home. We marked the anniversary of the first national lockdown with a minute's silence. Having almost died of Covid himself, Boris understands how emotional a lot of people feel today. The Queen released a statement honouring those who have died, and

Prince Charles asked the nation to 'remember the lives tragically cut short'.

'One year on you should be proud,' Gove messaged.

'Mixed feelings. Wish I'd won the argument sooner in the autumn. Could have saved a lot of lives,' I replied, adding that I am at least proud of the vaccines.

'You should be – you took big risks for the right reasons and were vindicated.'

It's been the longest year of my life.

Meanwhile I think Jim is feeling a bit bruised on borders. He messaged me this evening reassuring me that he's not trying to bounce anyone into going harder. 'I'm absolutely not in any way running pressure in this area. I'm a team player. And by the way, if I did madly take it into my head to do so, it would emphatically be more effective and we would have red-listed the whole world, the solar system and most of the Milky Way by now,' he said.

THURSDAY 25 MARCH

This whole thing about a link between the AZ jab and blood clots isn't going away. I messaged Dan Rosenfield at lunchtime to say that the scientists are trying to work out exactly who is at risk and we'll take it from there.

'Nightmare,' he replied.

By this evening we were in a much better place: having analysed the evidence, the MHRA are not unduly alarmed. We're not out of the woods, but it's not as bad as I initially feared.

Meanwhile MPs have voted to extend the Coronavirus Act for another six months. Labour backed it, so the legislation went through quite easily, with only thirty-five Tory rebels. I hope this is the last time we have to do this. The venom seems to have gone out of the debate, but thirty-five rebels – when we have a majority of eighty – is dangerously close to relying on Labour votes. It all underlines the importance of not opening so fast we have to go back again.

Nadhim's given a slightly wild interview to the *Telegraph* in which he talks about booster jabs this autumn and riffs about obtaining approval for more vaccines to 'future-proof' us against variant changes. I didn't think it sounded too bad until Damon told me he'd also suggested people might need to be jabbed to go to church. Crikey. Damon is trying to hose it down.

Remember Trump's ridiculous intervention almost a year ago about the potential power of ultraviolet light to kill the virus? At the time it sounded laughable, not least because he was also waffling on about people spraying themselves with disinfectant. That bit is still nonsense, but it turns out that the ultraviolet thing might not be so mad after all. Jim, who admits he was also very sniffy at first, messaged to say we backed a research project that is turning out to be promising.

'I am genuinely surprised. Happy, but surprised,' he says.

Perhaps we should send the results to Mar-a-Lago?

SATURDAY 27 MARCH

Boris messaged early afternoon asking for an update on the blood clots. He was clearly very worried and has been speaking to Pascal himself. I didn't have any news.

'Am also waiting with bated breath,' I said.

'Pascal is saying something about the need for labelling,' Boris replied, noting that this 'sounds ominous'.

'This is all about how we handle and I am 99 per cent sure we need to project breezy confidence. But of course will wait,' the PM said.

The thing I worry about most is overreaction. It's a very tiny risk to a very specific group.

We finally got word from the MHRA mid-afternoon. Their conclusion is that any side effect of this kind is very, very rare. The figure they've put on it is between one and five per million.

I messaged Boris right away. 'There's association but they can't determine causality. No indicator by age. So it's a "green light with vigilance",' I told him. It's a huge relief.

While we were waiting for the results, Emma told me that No. 10 is considering announcing social care reform at the Queen's Speech, based on Andrew Dilnot's recommendations. Best of all, HMT has found the money. We've been working on this ever since Boris became Prime Minister and committed to fix it on the steps of Downing Street. Now, out of the blue, this.

'Wow, that's amazing,' I replied. What a breakthrough.

Jeremy Farrar has given a characteristically unhelpful interview to *The Times*, bemoaning the absence of global leadership during the pandemic. That's a statement of the blindingly obvious. Sadly he offers no solution. 'Where are the Mandelas and Kofi Annans of the world?' he laments.

'Have you met Kofi Annan?' Jim texted acerbically. 'Sweet guy. Not the person you'd want running a pandemic though.'

I don't quite agree – I thought Kofi was rather impressive. But that's not the problem: the problem has been Donald Trump in the White House, which means there was no leadership from the United States. And the nature of a health emergency is that each country turns inwards. Then the European Commission has responded to the sorts of pressures we are all under by lashing out.

It is a massive problem and a vital part of learning the lesson that international health diplomacy needs to be in far better shape. We can't just hope for a saviour.

Our G7 calls, when the Americans were completely boxed in by the latest mad position of the White House, were a case in point. Thank God it's got better since Biden arrived, and we've managed to get the G7 agenda into a half-decent shape, but there's a lot more to do. I never quite appreciated how much we have depended on the Americans, and I worry for our future if they are really leaving that role.

MONDAY 29 MARCH

I went on *This Morning* with Phillip Schofield and Holly Willoughby.

Holly's a fantastic presenter, but what I really admire most about her is the way in which she has spoken out about her struggles with dyslexia. She's a great role model for kids, showing that it doesn't have to stop you doing anything. We did the interview outside Television

Centre on Wood Lane and they quizzed me on the chances of having a foreign holiday this summer. Still looking unlikely, unfortunately: there are just too many new variants.

GSK has reached an agreement in principle with Novavax to help them manufacture up to 60 million doses of Novavax's Covid vaccine, still under development, for use in the UK. GSK will provide 'fill and finish' manufacturing capacity at Barnard Castle. When I read the location, I thought I was the one who needed to test my eyesight. Presumably it's a coincidence, but it made me laugh.

TUESDAY 30 MARCH

How did Covid start? A year on, we still don't really know, and there's still an awful lot of pussyfooting around not wanting to upset the Chinese.

Today the WHO released a statement on behalf of fourteen countries, including the UK, US and Japan, which was so lily-livered it's not worth repeating. Jim has been talking to someone important on the WHO's 'origins of Covid' committee, who is a Public Health England official. Unfortunately, in Jim's view, he is also 'a total wet blanket'.

'Lots of stuff about needing to build trust with the Chinese and not being sure that the virus came from China' was his summary of the poor bloke's efforts not to start World War Three.

Jim says he gave the official a 'pep talk' on the necessity of finding out exactly how the virus began so we can make sure that nothing like this can ever happen again, but the meeting sounds as if it was a waste of time. No surprise to learn that the Foreign Office has 'strong views on diplomacy' – in other words, they won't rock the boat with Beijing and just want it all to go away. It all sounds incredibly lame. Unless we ask the awkward questions – and demand answers – we might as well not bother. My own view is that China caused this massive crisis, damaged the whole world, and now refuses to let the world know how it started.

'Suggest you reach out to Dom [Raab] somehow. I gather he's (unsurprisingly) taken a big personal interest. An opportunity to bond.

Also to ensure our own people aren't coming across as ameliorative,' Jim said.

Germany doesn't seem to have got the message that the AZ blood clot risk is minimal and has suspended routine use in the under-sixties. Their medicines regulator has found a total of thirty-one cases of a type of rare blood clot out of almost 2.7 million people who've had the jab. Canada has already suspended use in the under-55s. I am exasperated: these adverse effect figures are so tiny. The benefits hugely outweigh the risk, and the unfounded scaremongering is putting lives in danger.

WEDNESDAY 31 MARCH
Priti has been going through the paperwork on the red list and messaged to ask why India isn't on it. She seems very worried and wanted to know how we go about deciding how to categorise each country and whether it's primarily based on South African variant rates. (It is, but of course that's also determined by the overall prevalence.) She told me rates in India are very concerning. I reassured her that we're keeping a very close eye on it and that only a very small number of people coming in from India are testing positive when they get to the UK.

APRIL 2021

THURSDAY 1 APRIL

Jim has been locked in talks with Rishi's people over funding for Test and Trace. Now that the virus is on the wane, HMT is making worrying noises about pulling the plug. Unless we convince them of the case, Jim fears we might go into winter with nothing. He had a good session with Steve Barclay yesterday, despite the fact that Steve was – in Jim's words – 'a bit grumpy'. He's picked up on the fact some NHS test results aren't being properly registered, therefore we can't collate the data. It's been a problem throughout, but now it's threatening the budget for free tests across the board. For some reason the PM is taking a personal interest in this one and is threatening to speak to Simon Stevens direct.

More enjoyably, Jim's also been liaising with the French junior health minister ahead of the G7 health summit. 'Quite a bracing and constructive meeting with Stephanie and her French G7 sherpa team,' he reported cheerfully, as if they were about to attempt Everest. When the summit was originally planned, we wrongly assumed it would take place 'post-crisis'. Sadly, there's no way we'll be out of the woods by the date of the meeting in June. The EU's appalling antics have complicated the agenda. We were supposed to be talking about how to get the vaccine to developing countries, but that's hardly credible if we are all bickering about our own supplies. Maybe the French could be more helpful reining in the EU's absurd interventions?

As of today, the UKHSA officially exists, terrible name and all. The new boss is Jenny Harries.

SATURDAY 3 APRIL
Pascal Soriot called late this evening worrying about how long the vaccines will stay effective. We know it's not for ever, hence the booster plan, but I found his call unsettling. After I hung up, I messaged the Prof, who has been studying the data himself and is yet to see any sign of the effect waning – and the first vaccinations were almost four months ago. Reassuring.

MONDAY 5 APRIL
A much-loved colleague died of cancer this morning. Professor Paul Cosford was an amazing, inspiring man and I'm so sad. He worked all the way through his treatment as clinical director at PHE, and then stayed on even when he had to give up full-time work to do his bit for his country and steer us through. We have really missed him since he had to stop working. He had been living with cancer throughout the pandemic and working incredibly hard while he was stuck at home. A month or so ago he asked for a call one-on-one and talked to me about what was to come for him. He knew by then that his condition was terminal. He told me that as a doctor he would be able to ease his own pain and would know how to make sure his own end was swift. What he wanted to impress upon me was that others are not so lucky. He asked me to try to change the law. He knew his cancer would lead to a painful death. 'What would *you* want to be able to do in these circumstances?' he asked, encouraging me to reflect hard on how I would feel if I were getting progressively sicker and knew the end would be imminent and inevitably painful. He made such a compelling case.

I then had to turn my attention to the risk of the whole vaccine programme being undermined by more leaks from the JCVI about the blood clot concern. They're meeting to talk about it, but leaks and press speculation are so unhelpful. Take-up rates are already affected, with a higher rate of no-shows at vaccination sites than usual. All this is making me wonder about who's on the committee. They're supposed to be the ultimate authority on these matters, but it turns out that some members aren't even scientists – they have so-called lay members to represent the public. But that's ridiculous – it's meant to be an expert committee, not a social club. Where there are social or political judgements, they should be made by ministers based on expert advice. To my dismay, I've discovered that one of these 'lay' members is a Lib Dem councillor from Lewes. If you've ever met Lib Dems from Lewes, you'll know they are not the sort of people you want on any specialist committee.

TUESDAY 6 APRIL

Jeremy Hunt was on the *Today* programme and knew he'd be asked about the safety of the jab. He messaged me beforehand asking for a steer. 'Planning to say confidence in vaccine programme will not be dented whatever they decide provided there is full transparency about science and any advice is followed,' he said.

'That's a good position to take,' I replied, suggesting he might also highlight the value of having a respected independent regulator.

'Privately are you expecting a change?' he asked.

I demurred, not because I couldn't tell him but because I literally didn't know.

By this evening, the JCVI still hadn't made up its mind. JVT messaged to say that they are worried that the adverse events we've recorded are all after one dose and could double if a similar event rate is seen after the second dose.

'Isn't that why we keep things under review?' I asked.

'Yes,' he replied.

The front page of tomorrow's *Telegraph* has a screeching headline suggesting we should 'pause' jabs for the young until safety is 'certain'.

Sure enough, it's based on an interview with the Lib Dem. It's quite obvious that if you have political figures on a committee like this, they won't be able to resist behaving in a certain way.

The past week has not been a triumph for the vaccine programme, either on substance or on messaging. I hope we present a more united front tomorrow.

WEDNESDAY 7 APRIL

The JCVI has finally made up its mind, recommending that the under-thirties are offered an alternative to the Oxford jab. They've concluded that vaccination with AZ is better than nothing, but we all know this is going to put people off. It's messy.

I spent most of the morning on the phone to newspaper and TV editors, trying to limit the damage. I thought it was going well until Damon sent me a screen grab of a BBC headline declaring that the jab is still safe 'despite halt in under-thirties'.

'There is no HALT!' I exclaimed.

I got straight onto Fran Unsworth, director of BBC News, and told her it's seriously misleading. She immediately accepted my point and had the headline changed. Unfortunately, the message didn't filter through to other parts of the BBC, which made it all sound much more alarming than it is. I listened in dismay as a 5 Live presenter talked about 'stopping' the jab for the under-thirties, and got more and more stressed as other news outlets did much the same. I won't repeat all the expletives in my exchanges with Damon. Suffice to say we need to keep challenging misreporting and hammering home the message that the vaccine is safe. I've asked the team to find some stats to put it all in context.

'As in, "four in a million is as risky as aspirin", or whatever that is,' I suggested.

I have only one positive thing to report from what was a godawful day, which is that the Department of Education has announced they're banning mobile phones in schools. I sent Gavin a clapping hands emoji.

'Long overdue, though I now have two daughters not speaking to me!' he replied.

THURSDAY 8 APRIL

PHE thinks the vaccination programme has prevented as many as 10,400 deaths in the UK. Amid all the fearmongering and negativity about AZ, perhaps that startling statistic will change the narrative. Dr Alison Astles, whose brother Neil died of a rare blood clot on the brain after having the AZ jab, has been reassuring people that these terrible reactions are very rare. It's a very courageous thing to do, and so generous.

I got home to find a letter co-signed by Jim and Ara Darzi. Turns out I've been randomly selected to be part of the REACT survey, which Ara has been running to get more detail on how many people have antibodies. I signed up immediately – it only took a few minutes – and texted Ara to tell him. I'll be REACT's secret shopper...

FRIDAY 9 APRIL

Prince Philip has died. He was ninety-nine. What a remarkable man. The country has gone into mourning. He supported the Queen so magnificently. I met him a few times and he was always as acerbic and witty as his reputation. Because of his great age, most people think of him as a figure of the past, but history shows he was a real moderniser and I've always found him curious and inquisitive – as well as cutting. I diligently donned my black tie. All public events are now cancelled for the period of mourning – but the work inside the department continues.

SATURDAY 10 APRIL

'What do you think of EPI?' Boris asked. After more than a year of listening to scientific jargon, he's gone native. What he meant was the latest infection numbers, which are flat again, at around 3,000 a day. However, the number of over-sixties testing positive is still falling consistently, which is what really matters. The PM seemed pleased with the update.

'Good thanks. We gotta keep testing the school kids,' he replied. Of course.

The Sun asked me to write a tribute to Prince Philip. I'm going to pay homage to his love of sport and modernisation of the monarchy.

MONDAY 12 APRIL

Guto Harri has been talking to Boris about whether the Lions tour to South Africa can go ahead this summer. He messaged Damon to say that it may have to be cancelled if the players haven't been jabbed. Guto says rugby bosses are offering to help in any way they can, e.g. by promoting AstraZeneca or the benefits of the union. They're due to fly out at the end of June. Guto says they don't need vaccinating for a while, but they do need to know whether it's happening so they can book flights and hotels etc.

Damon said he'd see what he could do.

'Top man. They are happy to be jabbed quietly or be engaged in a full-on stunt to promote the vaccine and union,' Guto replied.

Today marks Step 2 of the roadmap out of lockdown, which means I've been able to get my first haircut since Christmas. I sent a photo of the finished product to Jim, who texted to say I've lost weight. I've been working on it and am pleased someone's noticed.

TUESDAY 13 APRIL

Great news that we've hit our vaccine target of offering a first vaccination to the nine highest risk groups two days ahead of schedule. Such brilliant progress by the whole team.

The civil service seems determined to kill off the Covid dogs idea. The animals are amazing – they get it right over 90 per cent of the time – but officials are being very tricky. It's so much more versatile than normal testing that I don't believe it needs to be 100 per cent accurate to be really worthwhile. We should have started training them months ago and then sent them to train stations and other busy places, where they could identify people who probably have Covid so they can then get a conventional test. Unfortunately, even though I've signed off on it, the system just doesn't buy it. So far we've done a successful Phase 1 trial, but Phase 2, which costs £2.5 million, has hit the buffers. Jim messaged to say the civil service are 'pushing back heavily' and have come up with no fewer than eleven reasons to junk it.

Former Tory leader Iain Duncan Smith, who's a big supporter of the scheme, has been like a proverbial dog with a bone and I am dreading telling him I can't get it over the line. Not giving up yet.

WEDNESDAY 14 APRIL

Another blow to AZ today: Denmark has stopped giving the vaccine. This really hurts. They're the first European country to do this and it will fuel the alarm over blood clots. It will also delay their vaccination programme by several weeks. It's so infuriating when this vaccine is already proven to save thousands of lives.

THURSDAY 15 APRIL

'Hey buddy,' Sajid messaged cheerfully. 'Hope well. Hearing really bad stuff coming out of India, and concerns over virulent new variant.'

He's right: they are having a horrendous second wave. He's also right to question why they're not on our red list.

'Lots of Indians I know are heading back to the UK,' he told me. I assured him we're monitoring it very closely.

Meanwhile Moderna has been in touch flagging up a delay with vaccine production. Damon messaged to say that they have a 'headcount issue' at their plant in Switzerland and wanted to alert us before they put out a public statement.

'A "headcount issue"? Can't we find them some more people?' I replied gloomily. Right now it feels like one thing after another – on which note, *The Independent* has run an absurd 'exposé' about my sister's paper shredding company, Topwood, accusing me of cronyism because it has won some NHS contracts. I have just been given a small stake in the firm, but I'm not involved in any way. *The Independent* only know about it because I'm diligent with my declarations. And it's all to do with a contract in the NHS in Wales – over which I have no jurisdiction. The key line in the story is 'Hancock does not have responsibility for NHS Wales and there is no suggestion that he was involved in the awarding of the contract'. It's outrageous that my family should be attacked in this way. I find it very painful that in a desperate attempt to chuck mud at me they throw it at my sister – even when they know their accusations are not true.

FRIDAY 16 APRIL

Angela Rayner's piling into the story about my sister, claiming – ludicrously – that 'Tory sleaze and cronyism' have 'engulfed this government'. Damon sent me a link to a statement in which she accuses me of breaking the Ministerial Code.

'Once Angela Rayner is on the attack, you're safe. This shows Ashworth won't do it,' I replied, more confidently than I felt. I'm so sick of this.

An hour later Damon messaged again to say that Starmer is now going for me. Damon spent most of the day on the phone with journalists, explaining why it's rubbish. Publicly, we can't say much because the ministers' interests adviser Lord Geidt is looking at it. Ever the master of expectation management, Damon has warned me that tomorrow's papers will be messy.

SATURDAY 17 APRIL

Prince Philip's funeral. The Queen sat alone in a pew, in widow's weeds and a black facemask. I cannot think of any more powerful symbol of the sacrifices individuals have been asked to make throughout this pandemic in order to protect others – or a finer example of leadership. Looking at her in her grief, I felt an intense internal conflict, almost an anguish, between the overwhelming sense of duty I have had during all this to save lives and stop the pandemic on the one hand and the painful consequences of my own decisions on the other. I wish she had not felt the need to do what she did, and that I had never had to ask anyone to say goodbye to a loved one without the comfort of friends and family right next to them.

The Queen's extraordinary selflessness fuelled my frustration over the gap between the sensitivity with which I would like the law to apply and the rigidity with which it so often applies in practice. This gap is widest at funerals. I have often been infuriated at the over-interpretation of guidance – yet I am ultimately responsible for it. I wasn't asked my view of these seating arrangements, but they were still my rules. The trouble is that all the advice from public health experts is that funerals are one of the most dangerous spreading events, because they tend to bring together lots of elderly people, and people are very emotional, so have a lot of close contact with each other. Then again, funerals matter more than almost anything. You can postpone a wedding – it's a choice – but you can't postpone a funeral.

Watching the ceremony for Prince Philip, I felt desperately sad. Out of duty, out of an abundance of caution, and to show leadership, the Queen took the most proper and complete approach, as she had throughout the pandemic. It was humbling, and I felt wretched.

Damon's spin operation yesterday clearly worked: there's not much coverage of the (non-) story about my sister's business today, and the Sundays don't seem interested.

India is now in real crisis. Healthcare resources there are limited at the best of times, especially in rural areas, where 600 million Indians live. With Covid on the rampage, hospitals are in a state of collapse and they're running out of everything. According to Priti, who follows it all very closely, Prime Minister Modi is very distracted by elections, which started last week and continue in phases for the rest of this month. She thinks things will improve significantly if, as expected, he wins.

SUNDAY 18 APRIL

There's a major row brewing about putting India on the red list. My clinical advisers are very nervous of perceived pressure on the system on such a major decision because of an upcoming VVIP visit. Ever diplomatic, they've been trying to figure out how to sort the problem. They saw Boris this evening and took him through the numbers. It sounds like we've got movement.

MONDAY 19 APRIL

The situation in India has deteriorated so sharply that we will have to put it on the red list. I told Dan Rosenfield we need to make the decision urgently. He replied that Boris agrees. I spoke to Grant and we put the wheels in motion. By mid-afternoon, the announcement went out. It's amazing how quickly government can move sometimes.

In better news, more than 10 million people in the UK have now received two doses of the Covid-19 vaccine. It's the equivalent of almost one in five adults. An incredible milestone.

In an update to the Commons, I stressed that we need to stay vigilant: we want this to be a one-way street.

I had just returned from this cheerful session when I discovered to my astonishment that No. 10 has got cold feet over the booster programme. What a bizarre volte-face! We've known for ages that people will need third or even fourth jabs, and have had multiple discussions about it at vaccine meetings. Downing Street now sounds very unconvinced and is complaining that the PM 'hasn't seen anything on it', i.e. hasn't been given enough briefing notes. I told the team we will need to swing into action to rescue the situation.

The police rang early this afternoon warning me that anti-vaxxers are planning a march on my London home. They suggested I liaise with Martha so she can tell me if it's happening. Great that they spotted it, but asking my wife to keep an eye out of the window while a baying horde descends on the family home is not exactly British policing at its finest. I asked for more support and messaged Priti saying I was grateful but worried their proposed response is 'lacklustre'. She said she'd personally keep an eye on it. I warned Martha, and thankfully, the Met did end up sending officers to our address.

I went home to make sure I was there if it kicked off, but there was no sign of anyone. I spoke to the policeman, who explained that the anti-vaxxers had posted the wrong details on social media so were busy protesting a few streets away. What complete idiots. I didn't know whether to laugh at their spectacular incompetence or be furious on behalf of the innocent folk who now had a protest on their doorstep. So low.

TUESDAY 20 APRIL

To reassure No. 10, I went through the plans for the booster programme with the PM at lunchtime today in the Cabinet Room. Happily, he loves it.

The EU, on the other hand, continue to screw everything up. They've been trying to do a deal with Valneva but have thrown their toys out of their pram because we have a priority order with the company. One of our officials spoke to Valneva this afternoon and it sounds as if they're so exasperated by their dealings with Brussels that they're going to abandon the whole thing in favour of just striking bilateral deals with member states. EU officials have always known about our contract with Valneva and only recently started complaining about it being a deal breaker. I guess the embarrassment of another UK priority contract, especially with a company that is basically French, is too much for them to swallow.

After work I went for dinner with Gina, Jim and Jim's wonderful wife Melissa. Melissa would not stop talking about inflation. She was incredibly emphatic – almost emotional – that prices are going to soar and can't understand why nobody's talking about it. She's on the board of Tesco, so I guess she has very good insight. I was thinking about it afterwards and it reminded me of the early days of the pandemic, when I kept telling people about the coming storm and people just weren't interested. I also remembered a conversation I had with a historian last year, during which I asked what tends to happen after pandemics.

'Inflation and war,' he replied. Hard to imagine things might get worse than they have been, but it's a dark warning of what could lie ahead.

Jim is extremely worried that the NHS is not going to capitalise on all the progress we've made on modern use of data in the health service. Upgrading NHS technology is so important. The pandemic and – especially – the vaccine rollout have shown just how efficiently things can work when data is used well. Patients have been invited to appointments at the right moment, with next to no queues and a seamless service. The question is how to capture that progress and use what's been learned to make other NHS services as efficient.

Jim came out of a meeting with NHS Digital feeling very depressed. 'This is the "come to Jesus moment". And NHSD are flunking it,' he reported sadly.

He and I both believe the pandemic is a great opportunity for the NHS to become much more patient-centred. 'I would recommend you're really calm and spell it out in really clear language,' he advised. '1. Everything changed last year with the pandemic, on collaboration, privacy, data, tech and all the other hot-button subjects; 2. You did brilliantly with the vaccine rollout; 3. We have a massive crisis in the future; 4. Therefore, expectations of your work are now completely different.'

He thinks I should tell them that everything is going to change and they have got to step up. 'Like Frodo and the ring,' he enthused. I have no idea what this last bit meant, but I'm sure Tolkien would be thrilled to think his trilogy could inspire a revolution in the health service.

WEDNESDAY 21 APRIL

After I finished my box tonight, I found myself in my office, taking my copy of J. S. Mill's *On Liberty*, his great essay about the relationship between individuals and society, off my bookshelf. I want to make the case in my next Commons statement that preventing harm of others is a perfectly liberal action in government. In the back of my mind, I remembered a quote describing this and I wanted to find it. And there it was: 'That the only purpose for which power can be rightfully exercised over any member of a civilised community, against his will, is to prevent harm to others.' From the originator of liberalism himself, just as I remembered it. I took a photo and sent it to my speechwriter, Danny. As well as the practical argument, I should have been making this principled case right from the start.

THURSDAY 22 APRIL

Boris has completely lost his rag over Scotland. He's got it into his head that Nicola Sturgeon is going to use vaccine passports to drive a wedge between Scotland and the rest of the UK and is harrumphing around his bunker firing off WhatsApps like a nervous second lieutenant in a skirmish. There I was, just for one small moment enjoying the satisfaction of knowing that we've hit all our big vaccine targets, when KAPOW! The first round hit my inbox.

'WE MUST NOT LET THE SCOTS HAVE THEIR OWN VACCINE PASSPORTS,' he boomed.

There was a weird gap in his messages, as if he had jabbed the 'return' key a few times, before the all-caps message continued:

'STOP THIS MADNESS NOW.'

For a moment, I imagined him tramping around Parliament Square brandishing a placard with a crossed-out SNP logo. But no: he was not about to march on Downing Street, he was already in it, trying to heave the great government machine in the direction he wanted using one finger and an iPhone.

He's completely right: Sturgeon has tried to use the pandemic to further her separatist agenda at every turn. Because the law says that health matters are devolved, the Scottish government has had considerable latitude, which Sturgeon has consistently used to play politics. But borders are very much a UK responsibility, and the idea of separatists being responsible for borders is dangerous. Now the Scottish government is working on its own system of vaccine certification, which may or may not link up with what's being developed for the rest of the UK. While the Welsh and Northern Irish are being pragmatic, the SNP is trying to harness this crisis to further its agenda. They put everything – everything – subservient to their destructive separatist goal. It's corrosive, and we have to deal with it.

While I was wondering how to manage this latest unwelcome drama and tell him that this is all entirely par for the course for the SNP, he was furiously hitting the phones. Cue another volley of bullets from the bunker.

'Just spoken to NHSX and Cabinet Office re. vaccine passports,' he announced. 'They are proceeding on an England-only basis and relying on the goodwill of the Scottish government. Imbeciles.'

He continued to rant, fretting that the whole thing would 'seriously undermine the UK' and exhorting me to do whatever it takes to solve the problem.

'We must fix this with extreme force,' he urged.

By now I was beginning to feel quite alarmed. What kind of force did he have in mind? Had Ben Wallace been informed?

While he was stomping about, Dan Rosenfield and I tried to work out what to do. 'Needs fixing. PM will go apeshit if not UK-wide,' Dan said, as if I hadn't got the message.

The PM said we need to be 'thinking DVLA style for both international travel and free movement of UK citizens around the UK'.

Well, yes. I obviously agree. The absurdity of different border policies for different parts of the same country has been a problem for months and obviously needs sorting out after the pandemic. But without changing the law now, turning this into a row will only further Sturgeon's destructive agenda.

There's a significant technical problem too: the Scottish government 'owns' Scottish health data, meaning that even if we set up a joint app, whoever controls it won't automatically have access to all the relevant records both north and south of the border. I told the PM that I would instruct our lawyers to find a basis for telling the Scots they can't go it alone. 'We have to find a way to force them to allow their health data to flow into our UK app,' I explained.

Dan wonders if we can play nice with the Scots: make them a UK-wide offer and 'invite' them to use our platform? I very much doubt it and have told him we may need to legislate. We've got twenty-four hours to get back to the PM with solutions, which will start by explaining the realities of the situation.

I'd just finished my box when my phone started pinging again. My heart sank when I saw it was from Simon Case. Surely the PM wasn't still in a lather? Instead it was something lovely.

'I hope you occasionally get the chance to stop and reflect on quite what a remarkable thing the vaccine rollout programme is. Was just looking at the numbers – it is astounding how many jabs are getting into arms.'

Relieved, I replied that it's something the whole country can be really proud of.

FRIDAY 23 APRIL

Liz Truss has been in touch about whether we can help the Indian government with medical equipment, especially oxygen supplies.

'You might already be on this, but Indian Trade Minister Goyal is asking if we can help on oxygen. Is there anything we can do?' she asked.

I told her that we can try but it's very difficult indeed to transport oxygen. What they really need is oxygen production equipment to make pure oxygen from air. I've reached out to my opposite number in India. I told Liz the best thing is to put them in touch with our commercial director, who knows this stuff inside out.

'Goyal, despite being Trade Minister, is also responsible for oxygen supply. He is up for any kit quickly. He helped us out on paracetamol so keen to reciprocate,' Liz replied.

I agree – the government of India went out of its way to help us when we were desperate, and we should do the same for them.

SATURDAY 24 APRIL

The boss wants to get on the front foot donating equipment to India. Cue a completely unnecessary turf war with Dom Raab's people, who seem to think the FCDO should be in the lead. According to Damon, FCDO officials are giving our policy team the third degree, saying it's 'mostly an FCDO thing, which is obviously bollocks'. Medical equipment is clearly a matter for the Department of Health. Unhelpfully, the FCDO has put a very limited spending cap on donations. I told Boris, who didn't know anything about the cap and was suitably dismissive.

'He wants us to drive this and make it happen. We need to stop this FCDO tinpot Chief Secretary thing. They're terrible at it,' I told Damon.

JVT has been to Israel with Michael Gove to see what we can learn from them as they open up. They're one of the first countries in the world to end Covid restrictions. JVT seems to have had a great time, reporting that the trip was 'astonishingly helpful'. Astonishingly fun too, I thought enviously, picturing him in a Tel Aviv nightclub, checking out the vaccine passports. 'We can get there, I'm sure!' he enthused.

Jim has also been talking to the Israeli ambassador, who is going to draft some ideas for us over the weekend. Let's see what we can learn.

Brilliant progress that over half of the UK population have now had the jab.

SUNDAY 25 APRIL

More heartbreaking scenes coming out of India. They announced 349,691 cases today, a record for a single country. There are makeshift beds in the car parks of hospitals, desperate scrambles for oxygen and even mass cremations. I called my counterparts in Scotland, Wales and Northern Ireland to see how they can help. Robin thinks he may be able to source some oxygen manufacturing kits, if we can find a way of getting them from Northern Ireland to New Delhi. I'm seeing if the RAF can help.

The left is complaining about the government's decision not to hold an immediate public inquiry into the handling of the pandemic. I agree we need one, and I am absolutely up for giving evidence, but it's still too soon. The priority has to be delivering vaccines and preparing for a possible third wave. Let's wait till we're through it and then go over what we got wrong and right. Whatever happens, we must learn from this so we're more prepared next time, because sadly there will be a next time.

Liz was on this morning's media round and did a superb job. I messaged to congratulate her. She replied that she was worried that she would have to drop out because she got her jab yesterday 'but no side effects so far'.

'I'm surprised you're old enough to get one!' I teased. My turn soon.

MONDAY 26 APRIL

Big pharma is getting a real battering at the moment, and Jim is worried about the knock-on effect on UK life sciences. Pfizer and Moderna are under fire for charging monopolistic prices and there is a lot of hostile scrutiny of their profits. Much of the developing world still has no vaccines and the industry is being accused of 'pandemic profiteering'.

'After all the wonderful news and good feelings about vaccines, I feel trouble on the horizon,' he said anxiously. 'There's is a chance that pharma may create a massive reputational harm that will make our life sciences ambitions v difficult,' he added, promising to send me a note. I told him that I'm also worried about GSK, a great British company. There's a damning assessment of their performance in today's *FT*.

'Clearly a takeover target. It would be terrible if it either deteriorated or was bought by another pharma,' Jim replied.

The one shining example of course is AstraZeneca, who, by signing up to deliver vaccines at cost to anyone in the world, have undertaken probably the greatest act of corporate generosity in history. It is very upsetting they don't get the credit they deserve for that. Pure jealousy, I suspect, and because it doesn't suit the internationalist left to accept that we Brits have led the charge on this.

Talking of which, I spoke to my Indian opposite number and promised to do everything we can to help them. They are hugely grateful they can manufacture the Oxford vaccine for free. But they need immediate help. I told him we will do everything we can, as fast as we can.

Here, we're now moving further into the under-fifties age group for vaccines. Tomorrow, we open up to 42-year-olds – which includes me! I went to Piccadilly Circus to launch the latest campaign: the vaccine brings you hope. As a politician, I always find launching adverts a weird experience. It's very fake: you're not there to say anything, and the job is to look as comfortable as possible in a situation entirely deserving of parody. I felt odd and awkward as I stood in the middle of Piccadilly Circus under a huge banner brandishing the word 'Hope'.

We had to time the photoshoot very carefully. Amid adverts for JD Sports and Coca-Cola, our own only came up every minute or so and wasn't there for more than a moment. Since nobody was there to see it anyway, I'm not sure how much it mattered. The whole purpose is that we have a sixty-second TV ad that will debut during *Emmerdale* on ITV on Monday and which the BBC will play in between programmes. I'm glad we've finally got the marketing into positive, forward-looking territory. By God, we need it.

TUESDAY 27 APRIL

The boss is still worrying about variants, but so far so good: the vaccine is working. Deaths involving Covid-19 in England and Wales have fallen 97 per cent since the peak of the second wave. I wrote to compliment Pascal and thank him for everything he and his team have done. One in four British adults is now fully vaccinated.

Then, in the car back from our weekly vaccine deployment meeting in Downing Street, I got the magic message myself: 'You are now eligible for your free NHS Covid-19 vaccine.' Hooray! I've been waiting for this moment for so long and felt genuinely overjoyed.

When I got back to the office I went online and booked in for Thursday: no point hanging around. I wanted to test the system myself and was very pleased to find it all worked very well. We've got to make every interaction with the NHS this easy.

I texted JVT to let him know I've booked in for the early morning slot. I hope he can find some way to come and deliver it. After all we've been through together, that would mean a lot.

WEDNESDAY 28 APRIL

Unbelievably, the FCDO is blocking efforts to send some of our spare ventilators to India. We're awash with the things – while they are desperate. In PMQs, the boss reiterated his determination to do whatever we can to help. Yet Dom Raab's officials are throwing up all sorts of obstacles. This afternoon I messaged him direct in the hope of cutting through the red tape. 'I have an instruction from the boss to make this happen, and he talked about it at PMQs. Can you help?' I appealed.

To his credit, once we cleared up the financial arrangements, he said he'd sort it right away.

My Italian counterpart Roberto Speranza has invited me to the G20 in Italy in September. I would absolutely love to go. I've replied saying I very much hope he can come to the G7 in June and then I can make the return trip.

Jamie has asked me to join his box at the Brits. The awards are going ahead as part of a DCMS-led pilot scheme into opening up mass events. Cue an agonised exchange about the optics of the Health Secretary having fun at a celebrity bash while the country is still in semi-lockdown.

'If you were in your old job, what would you advise?' I asked, though I already knew the answer.

He replied that as it's a government pilot programme I would have a very defensible line. Plus, he has some Labour shadow ministers going, so they won't be able to politicise it. 'But in the current climate there would be a small chance that someone would try to make political hay about it, and that small chance isn't worth what would be a really fun night,' he concluded.

I am beyond tempted – who wouldn't be? – but he's right. Sadly, it's a no.

THURSDAY 29 APRIL
Vaccine day! Damon messaged first thing checking everything was still in place. I'd booked the appointment in the same way as everyone else, save that I arranged for JVT to deliver the injection and Damon had invited the press. Of the various venue options, I chose the Science Museum.

'I reckon Union Jack face covering for the jab?' Damon suggested.

I'd had the same thought.

JVT had seemed thrilled to be asked to do the honours and booked a shift at the Science Museum through the vaccinators' online platform, just as simply as I'd booked my appointment. After that, it was brilliantly straightforward. I pitched up like anyone else, waited a minute or two in very short queue, and then went to my booth.

Fortunately for the assembled press pack, there was no question of me subjecting them to a Bethell-style striptease: I had put a T-shirt on under my work shirt. JVT then gave me the same consent briefing that all patients receive, I rolled up my sleeve, and that was it – barely a scratch. I was in and out within eight minutes. Side effect-wise, JVT told me I'll probably wake up around 3.30 a.m. feeling a bit sweaty and that should be that.

Later I received a text from JVT checking up on me. 'How is my patient so far?' he asked.

'Very good. Mild sore arm but nothing serious,' I reported.

'My guess is some symptoms from 3 a.m., but I'll check on you in the morning!' he replied.

I hope I'm in decent shape, because Jim and I are heading north to spend the day campaigning ahead of the local elections. What a novelty that will be!

Jim messaged to say he's spoken to Dido about the sniffer dogs. He told me gloomily that Test and Trace officials are 'still having palpitations about the lack of clinical proof of lab-style sensitivity'.

Infuriating. They are mad to be turning this down.

'I've pushed for a low-cost, low-sensitivity user case that use the existing dogs as a casual screen,' Jim replied with a crossed fingers emoji. Exactly. I told him to add it to tomorrow's agenda.

Simon Stevens has publicly confirmed he's standing down as NHS chief executive at the end of July. He's done seven years and one pandemic: I'm surprised he's still in one piece.

FRIDAY 30 APRIL

Just as JVT predicted, I woke up in the middle of the night feeling strange and sweaty. I looked at the bedside clock and it was… 3.30 a.m.

JVT checked in shortly after 7.30 a.m.

'How's tricks?' he asked.

'I've always thought you're an amazing doctor, but when I woke up feverish at 3.30 this morning I thought that was a pretty impressive prediction… Fine now – bit of a sore arm, moderate sore head, liverish,' I replied cheerfully.

'Sounds pretty standard. Glad you're not flattened,' he said.

After a strong cup of coffee, I linked up with Jim to head up to Teesside for the day. Zooming up north in his Land Rover, stopping off at various campaign points, felt like the good old days before the pandemic, and I loved every minute. For me personally the whole experience was quite surreal. I'm not used to being recognised and everyone seemed to be gawping at me. I lost count of how many people did a double take when they passed me on the street or stopped and stared when I crossed the road. Others came up to me and started talking as if I were an old friend. The first couple of times it happened I was quite taken aback. Like everyone else, since the start of the pandemic my world has contracted: home-office-home; home-office-home. I worked out I'd essentially only been to four places since Christmas: home, Downing Street, Parliament and the department. I hadn't really thought about my face being in people's living rooms almost every night. Hardly anyone used to recognise me; now everyone seems to know who I am. Quite an adjustment.

After the obligatory knocking on doors, we stopped for a photoshoot with Tees Valley Mayor Ben Houchen at a pub. The locals were very positive and supportive. Afterwards I messaged Boris to tell him what a great day we'd had.

'They love vaccines, they love Ben Houchen, they love you,' I told him. Our campaign team shared a surprising statistic: apparently people who have had the vaccine are ten percentage points more likely to vote Conservative. I suppose it's about as physical a manifestation as you can get of your government working for you. Bodes well for the local elections.

MAY 2021

SATURDAY 1 MAY

Boris asked what we're doing to help India ahead of Tuesday's summit with Narendra Modi, which is now being held virtually. I told him that we'd shipped a load of supplies to them yesterday and have more lined up on Sunday (PPE), Monday and Tuesday (more ventilators) and Friday (oxygen machines). We are also working on their request for test kits and cooperation on genomic sequencing. However, as I reminded him, our single biggest gift is the Oxford vaccine.

'Ninety per cent of their vaccination programme is the Oxford vaccine, given to them at cost. We must must must keep stressing this. It's so much more important than anything any other country has done,' I told him.

My parliamentary team received another outright death threat today, finding a message in my inbox that said simply: 'I am going to kill you.' Lovely. These sinister threats from anti-vaxxers are becoming more frequent and alarming. As a result, I am now being assessed for the maximum level of government security.

MONDAY 3 MAY

Dom Raab has written to Boris suggesting we donate half a million vaccine doses to India in time for the G7 in Cornwall next month, which Modi will attend. Nice idea, but not straightforward. We just don't have that many to spare. We've given India the capacity to make the vaccine – and they can manufacture in far greater scale than we can. Instead of proposing a gift of doses that don't even exist, we should be celebrating the far greater gift we've already given. I warned Dan Rosenfield that the proposal might cross his desk, in which case I hope he kills it, though I'll try to sort it out with Dom Raab myself.

Jamie messaged warning me that the other Dom – i.e. Cummings – will try to stitch me up when he gives evidence to the Science and Technology Select Committee later this month. You bet he will!

'We need to watch him like a hawk,' I replied.

'Let me know if there's anything I can do or say. I don't understand why the guy who retrospectively changed his blog to claim he saw Covid coming in 2019 has any sort of credibility in Westminster,' he observed.

'Because he gives good copy,' I replied. The truth is that the public hate him and don't believe a word he says, but journalists like his colourful turns of phrase.

TUESDAY 4 MAY

The Modi summit went well, though Raab is annoyed I killed his 500,000 vaccines donation plan. Emma messaged warning me that I might get a 'grumpy call'.

'He thinks you told the PM to block an announcement on it. I'm calming down his SpAd,' she said.

Meanwhile the new variant from India is a real worry. Jim went to what he described as a 'sombre' meeting about case numbers and says the public health team is 'rattled'.

'Everyone feels that it would be extremely dangerous for domestic hubris to lead to border opening. The big concern is that the domestic situation is SO SO good that it could lead to optimism bias on the borders,' he reported.

India's national cricket team is due to travel to the UK this summer and the England and Wales Cricket Board is in a slight panic. Jim says he's been trying to sort something out.

'You and a whole heap of very talented cricketers!' I replied, because I'm being lobbied by many of my sporting heroes on this. Mike Atherton has been in touch, and even the legendary Ian Botham has been trying to help. Jim is going to liaise with Oliver Dowden to see if we can find a way to make the series happen.

JVT and the Prof have been working on our response to the JCVI's new position on the use of AZ in younger patients. The Prof is happy for us to agree that under-forties should have an alternative if there is one, but we will say that having the Oxford jab is better than waiting for something else. He thinks we can do this without undermining confidence in the programme or derailing our target of offering all adults a jab by the end of July.

After last week's visit to Teesside, today I was out campaigning again in Derbyshire. Gina drove me up. My relationship with Gina is changing. Having spent so much time talking about how to communicate in an emotionally engaged way, we are getting much closer. I took the chance to visit Eyam, where my ancestors were wiped out in a previous pandemic. In one week alone, Mrs Hancock lost six out of eight of her children, as well as her husband, to the plague. I visited the poignant memorial overlooking the Dales, an idyllic spot and a harrowing reminder of the impact of pandemics through the ages.

WEDNESDAY 5 MAY

Michael Gove has organised a ministerial simulation exercise next week codenamed Exercise Barchester to practise our response to a dangerous variant. He's very excited about it and wanted to chair the event, which is fine by me.

Damon messaged warning me that *The Sun* and *The Times* have got a partial leak of our debate over how to respond to the JCVI advice.

I asked whether he thought it was members of the JCVI leaking again.

'Yes,' he replied immediately.

'We MUST sort this out,' I replied. I am utterly sick of certain JCVI members going rogue.

Damon is trying to persuade the papers that it would be irresponsible to publish anything.

Someone has been bending Helen Whately's ear about GP receptionists being told to ask patients who call surgeries asking for an appointment why they need to see a doctor. It's a relatively new policy, designed to reduce the pressure on doctors by filtering out people who can be directed to other help, but everyone hates it.

'I think triage by receptionists is genuinely dangerous,' she told me this evening.

I entirely agree with her.

'It's awful,' I replied. Not everyone needs to see a GP, but the current system puts the onus on the receptionist to work out whose needs are more urgent. They're put in an impossible position – people have every right to expect clinicians to do that triage. It's vital we sort GP access after the pandemic, and I'm determined to do it.

David Cameron's old friend Andrew Feldman is the latest to be dragged into the 'contract cronyism' saga. He's being accused of urging the Cabinet Office to buy PPE from one of his clients. The truth is, we were buying from anyone who had it – but yet more selfless public service is being disparaged. So frustrating. How will we ever get good people to come into government if this is how they're treated?

THURSDAY 6 MAY

The vaccine row is escalating. Now the White House wants pharma companies to give up intellectual property rights to all Covid vaccines. It will never happen – except of course for AstraZeneca, who have been licensing at cost for a year now. We are miles ahead of the curve. Liz Truss has been tweeting that the UK is 'in discussions with the US' and is 'working at the World Trade Organization to resolve this issue'. As a free marketeer, I hope she makes the point that property rights are important but we've chosen to waive profits – and therefore any charge on intellectual property – for the Oxford vaccine. In my view, we should be making the case globally for the British approach, not adopting this counterproductive hard-left narrative that the profit motive is the problem. On the contrary – it's part of the solution!

Oxford vice-chancellor Louise Richardson fears there's a head of steam building that could culminate in demos at the G7 health summit in Oxford next month. Jim thinks we need to get ahead of it in case government securocrats overreact. 'We should have a strategy, or we'll find it's cancelled on us,' he said.

I don't think it will come to this, but it would definitely make sense to have contingency plans.

Thanks to Damon, there was no hint of the JCVI stuff in today's papers. His lecture about the responsibility they have not to whip up anti-vaxxers clearly worked.

'Gold star,' I told him cheerfully.

The local elections passed off smoothly. I'm feeling optimistic.

FRIDAY 7 MAY

Nice outdoor breakfast with Sajid Javid at his place in Fulham. We chewed over what we know of yesterday's results so far. The Tories had a stonking result in the Hartlepool by-election, where we won the seat for the first time ever on a swing of 16 per cent from Labour. In the various mayoral elections, it's looking OK for Andy Street in the West Midlands and good for Ben Houchen in Teesside.

Jim sent me a strange message first thing this morning saying he couldn't sleep last night for worrying about our response to the Indian variant 'and dreaming of AZ bottles encased in glass like Damien Hirst's "medicine" artwork with the word "hope" engraved along the top'.

Context: an idea for a gift for G7 health summit delegates. I like it.

SATURDAY 8 MAY

Jim managed to enthuse Turner Prize winner Antony Gormley about his present idea, which he describes as 'an AZ vial embedded in a glass block, or some such'. We've left it too late to get Gormley himself on board, but Jim managed to find another Turner Prize winner, Richard Wright, who may be able to design something similar. The idea is to give them all a beautiful paperweight featuring a spent AZ one-shot vial, representing a life saved by the vaccine, beautifully presented in a wooden box.

'But we will need some budget,' Jim warned.

'That's amazing,' I enthused.

The idea is to make it in the National Glass Centre in Sunderland.

'I LOVE the National Glass Museum – I've been twice!' I told him excitedly, adding that budget should be no problem. The present ticks every box. With my encouragement ringing in his ears, Jim scuttled off to get everything costed.

'With a Turner Prize winner, it will be more like £100,000. Without, it'll be more like £20,000,' he reported.

After making a few more enquiries, he came back crestfallen. According to the Cabinet Office our budget is fifty quid a head.

'We could get a donor, but maybe too complicated,' he reported gloomily.

That's the end of that idea then.

MONDAY 10 MAY

The life sciences industry is not at all happy about the US gambit on pharma companies ceding their intellectual property rights, fearing it sets a dangerous precedent. I've told No. 10 it's a very bad idea. 'I think we should say we're up for companies waiving IP charges as AZ have, but not up for changing the law,' I told Dan. According to the Foreign Office, Germany is also staunchly opposed.

Separately, Helen has worked up a plan to change the guidance on care home visits. I am cautious. It's a tortuous balance. We know to our very great cost just how vulnerable people in care homes are. Yet visiting matters too – we know that visitors improve residents' health, and frankly for many are what makes life worth living.

'Our last change to visiting guidance was implemented on 12 April,' she persisted. 'Families with relatives in care homes need hope

– especially given we don't have a clear roadmap for social care.' Helen also knows the heavy weight on each side of the scales – and if she's convinced, I find that very persuasive.

'OK, you win. Let's just do it,' I said. She's right. I shouldn't let my paranoia about Covid in care homes make me excessively risk-averse. I know how unbelievably painful all this has been for vulnerable people and their relatives.

Deaths and hospitalisations are at their lowest levels since July last year, so we're moving to Step 3 of the roadmap a week today. Cinemas and museums can reopen properly and we're withdrawing a whole slew of guidance and rules.

TUESDAY 11 MAY

Who am I most looking forward to hugging? My mum! That's what I told Nick Ferrari on LBC this morning, anyway, which didn't go down too well with Dad. I haven't seen either of them since last summer and I can't wait to hug them both. Frankly it's been far too long. I talk to them on the phone, but it's not the same. I just haven't had the chance, because of the rules and the fact that I've been working such long hours.

Covid cases are still rising in certain parts of the country and people are worried we may go back to local lockdowns. Bolton North East MP Mark Logan has warned me he plans to raise it at PMQs tomorrow. He's going to ask the PM to prioritise jabs for people of all ages in hotspots. I told him I'm happy to go down this route and that the boss will be supportive.

Jim was right about the backlash against AstraZeneca over IP. It's their AGM today and there have been minor protests outside three UK offices and labs. Jim is trying to keep everybody calm. He's optimistic that any demo would not amount to much more than a few 'pacifist hippies'.

WEDNESDAY 12 MAY

Tom Newton Dunn has written some absolute drivel in his *Sun* column suggesting Simon Stevens could be given a peerage and then made Health Secretary.

As I told Damon, chances of that happening are 'zero, obvs'.

There's no great love for his team in No. 10 today. Dan Rosenfield messaged me with an expletive after discovering they've put out a briefing on the vaccine rollout for the under-forties without telling the rest of us.

'I have hit the roof. They say it was a mistake,' I told him.

'Bollocks,' he replied.

Meanwhile the airlines are also going rogue. TUI and easyJet are advertising holidays to amber countries despite government advice that people still shouldn't be going abroad. I messaged Raab immediately saying we have to sort it. The advice on the FCDO website is not as categorical as I'd like.

'Totally agree. Reckless,' he replied.

We're looking into whether we can post a banner message on all gov.uk pages, repeating the message that you can't go on holiday to these places. We must protect the domestic reopening.

Earlier I talked Boris through the latest data on the Indian variant. He's alarmed and muttering about local lockdowns. I'm not keen, but I said I'd get back to him tomorrow with some options. I've also asked for legal advice on stopping easyJet and TUI running holidays in amber countries. Maybe we can outlaw travelling to these destinations without a reasonable excuse. It's another of those terrible balances – ruining holidays and stifling the economy because we mustn't wreck the progress we've made with the vaccine here at home.

THURSDAY 13 MAY

Wonderful visit to the vaccination centre at Brent Central Mosque this morning with Lauren from my parliamentary office. There I was, a Church of England Christian, being taken around by the Jewish administrator to watch a Hindu clinician vaccinate the Muslim imam. Very London and very uplifting.

FRIDAY 14 MAY

DOOM: I've been caught speeding. Jim forwarded me a dismal image of a letter he received from the police linked to our trip up north during the election.

'Noooooo,' I said sympathetically. 'Can I pay it for you?' I had momentarily forgotten that we shared the driving.

'I'm afraid I think it might be you. I think I was having a kip,' he said.

For a split second, I thought of Chris Huhne, the Lib Dem Cabinet minister who persuaded his wife Vicky Pryce to pretend she was at the wheel when he was caught speeding. Both of them ended up going to jail. There could be no room for error here.

Armed with Google Maps, Jim identified the scene of the crime, which confirmed that the culprit was me.

My heart sank: I've only just got rid of three points on my licence.

'Sorry, send it my way,' I said gloomily.

'Maybe they'll let you do a course?' he suggested.

'I've done one I'm afraid,' I replied. I'm not sure it would be the smartest option for me anyway. It's all being done online now, but imagine the amusement from the other petrol heads if my face suddenly popped up on the Zoom.

Jim's put my name on the form and I await my fate.

Ben Wallace messaged worrying that we're about to impose new restrictions. His patch – Wyre & Preston North – is a mixed urban and rural seat that has had a particularly rough time.

'My constituents have been in constant lockdown since early Sept!!! Can we keep it in the bigger boroughs like Blackburn? (The problem there is BAME low take-up),' he said.

'Fear not!' I replied. He seemed relieved.

SUNDAY 16 MAY

The *Sunday Times* are on my back again about Covid contracts. The latest is a very weak story about a deal involving lovely former Tory

MP Brooks Newmark. It boils down to nothing more than me telling Brooks to speak to the officials handling PPE contracts. Given it's the civil service who decide, price and sign off contracts, it's desperate stuff.

MONDAY 17 MAY

Did a Commons statement on taking the third step in the roadmap out of lockdown, and the variants. Stuck to the line that we're surging testing and vaccination in badly affected areas but not yet extending jabs to all over-eighteens. I have laid the ground for possible delays to the roadmap but am optimistic we can avoid it.

WEDNESDAY 19 MAY

JVT, Jenny and I fronted the press conference, focusing on what's going on in Bolton. JVT says a significant number of Covid-related hospitalisations are younger people. 'I think the message that in Bolton one whole third of hospital admissions are in under-45s is a really key one *pour encourager les autres*,' he suggested.

The case rate in the area has doubled in the space of a week. Nationally, cases of the so-called Delta variant, as the Indian one is now known, have shot up by almost a third since Monday.

Then again, as of midnight last night, seven out of ten adults have had their first jab; nearly four in ten are fully vaccinated and we're increasingly confident that the vaccines work against the Indian variant. JVT's data, which pools results for Oxford and Pfizer, shows that two doses are 80 per cent effective at preventing infection by this variant, though one dose is just 22 per cent effective. The key is for people to get those second doses in.

Tom Harrison, chief exec at the England and Wales Cricket Board, called for an urgent chat about the Indian team. We decided to let the tour go ahead, but the players are in mutiny because they're not allowed to bring their families. I get it: cricket tours last months. So how do we save the cricketing summer without pissing off every non-cricket fan in the country? A couple of weeks ago, Rod Brans-grove, the Hampshire County Cricket Club chairman, pitched to me that they could use the hotel inside their ground at Southampton as a quarantine hotel. That way, the team can stay there and train at the same time, rather than being cooped up in a separate hotel. Rod had been thinking about English players, but I'm sure he'd be open to of-fering it to the Indian cricket team. Resisting any temptation to put the star Indian batsmen in small underground basement rooms, as one of my cricket-mad advisers jovially suggested, this would mean they can get in some quality practice and their families will be looked after, all in a Covid-secure bubble. Then once their quarantine is over they can all tour the country together. Tom was confident he could sell the plan to the Indian team. Howzat! Fingers crossed it's problem solved.

THURSDAY 20 MAY
No. 10 is still demanding we donate a load more vaccines to COVAX to make the PM look good in the run-up to the G7.

'No, no, no!' I told my private office. We are not doing this! I am not going to put the domestic vaccination programme at risk for the sake of a Downing Street PR exercise. We do not have that amount of spare vaccine and we cannot jeopardise domestic delivery: simple as that. It's so unimaginative – what we should be doing is explaining that the Oxford vaccine is our gift to the world.

What a shame Michael Gove isn't leading on this one: he and I make a good team. This morning the two of us were on a Zoom about something entirely forgettable, both silently losing the will to live as officials went round and round in circles. Letting it all wash over me, I surreptitiously WhatsApped Michael asking what we were trying to achieve in the meeting.

'Letting people express concerns in a therapeutic environment before you and I decide the policy,' he replied mischievously.

'You are glorious,' I said.

Shame it doesn't always work like this.

Good news on the cricket, though: after three phone calls, it looks like we're on. The Indian team and their partners can use the Southampton ground. A summer of cricket is hopefully now saved.

FRIDAY 21 MAY

For the first time in my life, I've appeared under oath in a witness box. It was for the public inquiry into the infected blood scandal, in which tens of thousands of people were given blood tainted with HIV and hepatitis C in the 1970s and 1980s. It's an incredibly important investigation and a small foretaste of the public inquiry into Covid, when it will be my own decisions under the microscope. I told the team I couldn't turn up without sorting out the decades-long wrangle over the issue of compensation. After weeks of back and forth, late last night I was finally given the go-ahead from Rishi to say that of course victims should be compensated. Sometimes even things that are obviously fair and right involve a battle. I hope it doesn't take much longer to get them what they deserve – it's been horrendous for so many people and I want them to know I'm on their side.

SATURDAY 22 MAY

Cummings is flooding Twitter with an angry stream-of-consciousness ahead of his select committee appearance next week. His slot is not for another four days, but he's already working himself into a lather. This afternoon I made the mistake of looking at his Twitter feed, which temporarily transported me into his mad world. Damon sent me a link which took me to tweet number 36 of God knows how many he's going to post[*] ranting about the cowardice and stupidity of the media, the idiocy of 'pundits', the 'BRILLIANCE' of one or two people nobody has ever heard of and what a 'DISASTER' the pandemic response has been.

Apparently the PM lied, the Cabinet Office was useless, DHSC was hopeless and I deliberately misled everyone about everything, especially so-called herd immunity.

---

[*] Sixty-eight, at the last count. All on the same theme. He's never quite grasped the 280-character limit.

I stared at the crazed messages, mesmerised by the ferocity with which he was attacking his keyboard. What is it like to be consumed by such anger? How does it feel to be so utterly convinced of one's own superiority? How frustrating must it be to think you could do everything better than anyone else yet have no power? The arrogance is breathtaking.

I might almost have felt sorry for him, had it not been obvious that he's out to bring me down. The Sunday papers will be full of it – and he's just warming up.

Off to Cornwall on the sleeper tonight to visit some of the hospital building projects, including on the Isles of Scilly, a place I love. We'll fly over to visit St Mary's Community Hospital and get an update on a proposal to build a nursing home next door. Currently, frail and elderly Scilly Islanders have to move to the mainland if they need a care home, frequently separating them from their lifelong spouses who find it difficult to travel. It's heartbreaking, and so I'm keen to find a solution. Apparently I'm the first Cabinet minister to visit since Ted Heath.

MONDAY 24 MAY

Is it wise for politicians who want to be taken seriously to be photographed in a wetsuit? Damon absolutely doesn't think so, Gina is on the fence, and I think it's all about timing.

After we left the Scilly Isles and arrived at Newquay to visit the Wave Project – a wonderful initiative to use surfing to help children with mental health problems gain confidence – this presentational conundrum was causing some angst in the team. Damon, stuck behind his desk in London, felt emphatically that I shouldn't take the risk. Down in Cornwall we were super-relaxed and enjoying the sunshine. Why not get stuck in? 'No good can come of it,' Damon said. 'Just don't go there. Remember what a plonker David Cameron looked?'

I know, I know – but this isn't just about me; it's about publicity for the charity. Who wants another boring picture of a meeting? Worst comes to the worst, at least I'll give everyone a laugh.

By the time I arrived in Newquay no decision had been taken. Back in London, Damon sweated it out, trying not to let his mounting anxiety spill over into a Cummings-style barrage of messages imploring me not to do it.

Eventually he could no longer contain himself.

'Have you said yes to photos of you surfing?' he asked.

'Yes,' I replied. 'Do you think no?'

Silly question: of course he thought no.

'Can you talk to Gina and decide. I get the risks,' I said, but really I had already made up my mind. It was a fine evening, the surf was up and I fancied I wouldn't embarrass myself. What could possibly go wrong? Quite a lot, obviously. What did go wrong? Absolutely nothing.

I slipped on my black wetsuit, donned the grey Wave Project T-shirt they gave me and moved from 'next slide please' to 'next wave please'. In the end, I had no choice. As we arrived at the beach, a TV crew and several cameramen were already there. So I took the biggest board I could find, paddled out through the waves, turned and momentarily stood up, looking as happy and relaxed as if I did this every day. The kids implored me to have another go, but knowing I'd fluked it with beginner's luck, I paddled back into the beach and was interviewed by the local BBC about the brilliant project. All of the angst was a complete waste of time – it's a lesson in life to just get on with it.

The truth is that I'd have liked to have enjoyed the beach for a little longer. Just for a few moments, it was glorious to forget my day job. The minute I peeled off the wetsuit, I had to metamorphose back from salty sea dog to Health Secretary Hancock: the guy who's ruining everyone's summer holiday plans and is about to get a very public kicking courtesy of Dominic Cummings. Word in the lobby is that he's really gunning for me. Jamie messaged asking if I wanted any help shaping the Westminster narrative. 'I think it's so mad we should duck for now,' I replied. I'd had enough risk for one day.

TUESDAY 25 MAY

My tour of the south-west continued, through Devon and to Bristol, interrupted by an hour-and-a-half call with Boris about Step 4. Should we move onto the next stage of the roadmap and ease restrictions even though cases are rising? I'm torn. Pre-vaccine, certainly not, but the whole point of the jab is to replace restrictions with medical protection, so there's a very strong case for sticking to the plan. We've decided to defer a decision until next week. Cummings is up in front of the committee tomorrow.

WEDNESDAY 26 MAY

'Why does he hate you so much?' Laura Kuenssberg messaged me. I was chairing a meeting about clearing the NHS backlog, trying to ignore a flurry of messages about Dom's select committee appearance. Eventually curiosity got the better of me.

'What has Dom said?' I asked Damon. 'Tell me. I'm getting a load of incoming about what a wanker he is.'

Where to begin? According to Cummings, it was 'crackers' that someone like Boris could be PM: it was a case of 'lions led by donkeys, over and over again'. Boris behaved 'like a shopping trolley, smashing from one side of the aisle to the other'. Instead, there should have been 'a kind of dictator' in charge of the pandemic – that way things would have been much more efficient. I wonder who he had in mind for that role – presumably himself. As for me? I should have been fired 'for at least fifteen to twenty things, including lying to everybody on multiple occasions'. Apparently I lied about PPE, lied about patients getting the treatment they needed, lied about this and lied about that. Oh yes, and back in spring last year, the Cabinet Secretary thought I should be fired.

I stared at the screen, gobsmacked. I knew he'd been a destructive force in government, but this was the ultimate ex-employee with a grievance trying to rewrite history.

There were so many accusations, I was struggling to keep up. Meanwhile Damon was trying to work out where to direct our anti-ballistic missile defence system. Which of the pounding rockets should we try to intercept?

'We should have a fifteen-minute chat to discuss handling,' he said eventually.

Fifteen minutes? I wasn't sure whether I needed fifteen seconds or fifteen hours to dispense with these flights of fancy.

'We should definitely say nothing until Dom is off the screen,' I replied.

'We will need something,' Damon reasoned. 'Keep it tight, reject the accusation, back to work. Then we show strength by coming out of the blocks on substance.' I know I'll be up before the committee next month and be able to reply on all the substance. But how to respond to the vitriol?

I tried very hard to focus on the many more important things I had to do, but it was impossible not to wonder just how much rubbish he was talking.

'Did you really call for me to be sacked?' I asked Simon Case. 'I don't really care if you did as the PM was supportive throughout – but important for calibrating how I respond – if I respond at all.'

It turned out to be a case of mistaken identity: Cummings was talking about Simon's predecessor, Sir Mark Sedwill.

'I was a little surprised, to be honest! This whole shit show is a stark reminder of how much easier governing has got these past six months,' I told Simon.

A couple of hours into what turned out to be a seven-hour odyssey, Dan Rosenfield messaged with his verdict.

'The guy is full of shit. And for the record, you are doing a brilliant job, and a hero,' he said.

'Can you imagine what it was like when this guy was doing this stuff internally? Nuts,' I replied gratefully.

'I genuinely can't imagine it,' Dan said.

While I tried to crack on with work, Jamie kept a watching brief on proceedings, periodically alerting me to the latest outrage. After a while, he sloped off for lunch with a couple of colleagues, returning late afternoon to find Cummings still in full flow.

'Bloody hell, he's still going!!??' he exclaimed.

'He's like a big toddler having a meltdown,' I replied, though toddlers usually blow themselves out in twenty minutes max, whereas Dom looked as if he'd quite happily go on all night.

When it was finally over, and Damon and I were catching our breath, the PM called.

'Don't you worry, Matt. No one believes a word he says. I'm sorry I ever hired him. You're doing a great job – and history will prove you right. Bash on!'

Damon told me that Simon, Carrie, Dan and Simone Finn, Dan's deputy, had all been in touch with him to say they are 100 per cent behind us.

'Don't worry for a minute about all the bullshit. We are solid,' Jack Doyle messaged, while Liz Truss WhatsApped to say she was on '#teamhancock'.

'I want to add to your array of supportive messages!' she said.

'Striking that our polling low point was the same day he was fired,' I observed.

'Quite,' she replied.

'Dom's insight is no better than his eyesight,' I told the many lovely people who messaged with support.

At 8.30 p.m., my phone pinged again: a morale-boosting WhatsApp from Gove. 'I ♥ you,' he said encouragingly.

'Your old friend less so!' I replied. Funny to think that Michael, Liz, Cummings and I were once all in the Department for Education together, shoulder to shoulder, trying to drive up standards.

'He is wrong – you are right,' Michael said firmly.

'Yes. And you have been true throughout,' I replied.

'Few people know how hard you have worked, how right you have been and how lucky this country is you have been here – I do and will tell anyone,' Michael said. It was an incredibly kind message and the support meant a lot.

I went to bed thinking, 'Thank goodness I kept vaccines out of Dom's destructive hands or that would have been a disaster like everything else he touched.' As for me, I'm a bit battered but still in one piece.

THURSDAY 27 MAY

Getting out of the house through a huge press pack required elaborate choreography. We knew it would be a bunfight and Damon got himself there early to manage the mob. Ever the professional, he checked the optics, cheerfully offering to move the wheelie bin out of the way to avoid any 'Hancock talks rubbish', 'Hancock's career in the bin' and other garbage-themed headlines. Inside the house, I was pacing around anxiously, waiting for him to give me the all-clear to emerge. My main concern was the kids, who had to leave before I did.

'Tell them to get the house out of the shot,' I asked Damon – otherwise we'll have more nutters with placards on the doorstep.

Around the corner, my ministerial car was waiting. On Damon's instruction, it rolled up to the doorstep, whereupon I made a dash for it, cheerfully telling everyone that I was off to drive forward the vaccine programme.

When I got into work, I heard that the Prof had called my private office volunteering to support me in public if need be. I really don't want to drag him into it, but this vote of confidence meant the most. Jonathan Ashworth messaged to say he thinks I am now in a stronger position than I was last week, which may be true: the Tory Party hates Dom Cummings even more than the public do.

Of all the many accusations Dom hurled, the media seem most interested in his claims that I lied about the arrangements surrounding hospital discharges into care homes at the beginning of the pandemic. Annoyingly, it was only after this evening's press conference – which I led with Jenny Harries – that I received some very pertinent PHE data. They analysed all the Covid cases in care homes from January to October and found that just 1.2 per cent could be traced back to hospitals. The vast majority of infections were brought in from the wider community, mainly by staff. That was a problem tragically faced by care homes around the world.

Colleagues are still rallying round. Emma messaged to say well done after the press conference.

'Not my best,' I replied gloomily.

'It was a hard one, especially without a massive announcement to hook up to. But you did well,' she said reassuringly.

That didn't stop the BBC running some total bollocks on the 6 p.m. news suggesting I 'didn't address concerns over testing'. ITV was even worse, claiming I was 'summoned' to the PM's office last May to explain possible care home negligence.

'This is the most excruciating contortion of rubbish I've ever read,' I said grumpily.

'Thin,' Damon agreed, trying to cheer me up.

While Dom's accusations are unfounded, care homes are one of the issues that weigh on me most heavily. Overall, England did no worse at protecting care home residents than many countries, and better than some – including Scotland. Regardless, the awfulness of what the virus did to people in these settings around the world will stay with me for the rest of my life.

At the beginning of the pandemic, Helen and I were constantly pushing for infection control guidance to be toughened, and it was. Lots of people were contracting Covid in hospital at that time and there were no easy choices, not least because testing wasn't readily available – despite our best efforts to expand it. The NHS needed to get people out of hospitals as quickly as possible to create space and put us under a lot of pressure to speed things up. With hindsight, knowing what we know now, it would have been better if we'd been quicker to stop staff working in more than one care home. That policy was in place from the summer, alongside more testing, so the impact on care homes was much lower in the second wave.

Shortly before I headed home, Ben Wallace sent a nice message asking if I was OK.

'The Cummings evidence can be summed up as the "ramblings of a twat",' he said supportively. 'Your response today was excellent.'

I thanked him and reiterated what I've been telling everyone else who's sent these kind messages of support: that it's a big reminder of what a nightmare running government was when he was on the inside.

'That is the irony,' Ben replied. 'His presence and bullying actually crippled government. He is a phoney.'

Evidently Ben saw Dom's true colours earlier than most: he says he fired him from Boris's ill-fated 2016 Tory Party leadership campaign. Very wise.

FRIDAY 28 MAY

I woke up to find a TV crew on the doorstep again.

'I'm just going to run past,' I told Damon.

'Unless you feel really strongly about running, I would put a suit on and get in the car,' he advised. 'Want to give them absolutely zero chance to take any of it forward.' Fair point. Did I really want 'Hancock running into trouble' headlines?

I grudgingly changed into my suit and made a mental note to fit in an extra run another day.

The reason the media is still on my back is that Dom is still trying to pin what he calls the 'care homes fiasco' on me.

'That is what we MUST bounce out of,' I told Damon, who has been looking for someone to go on the record about Dom's meddling with testing.

'What's Dido's opinion of Cummings?' he asked.

'Very low,' I replied. 'Totally messed up her delivery of Test and Trace.'

In theory, she would definitely be onside, though I don't want to drag her into this already – she has already given extraordinary service.

'Might sound her out,' Damon said.

'You can do everything you think is wise in defending against Cummings,' I said.

Late this evening a ministerial colleague messaged to say the *Mail on Sunday* is working on a story about Cummings. They said they'd tried to be helpful. Sounds like the article will destroy his credibility, if he had any left.

'The thing I really want to prove is he had nothing to do with vaccine and that's one reason it went well,' I replied gratefully.

SATURDAY 29 MAY

Boris and Carrie got married at Westminster Cathedral. Somehow they managed to keep the whole thing secret until it actually happened. I'm not entirely sure how much the PM's mind was on his future with his beloved, though, because this afternoon he was busy texting me about the latest Covid data.

'Lower cases and deaths today. So definitely ne panique pas,' I told him. Then again, perhaps he's just very good at multi-tasking and can examine infection graphs, pick bits of confetti off his jacket and give his new bride doe-eyed looks all at the same time.

One of the best officials – an individual Cummings rated very highly – called Gina to say how furious he was about the attacks. The official said we'd never have reached the 100,000-a-day figure without my target, which Cummings had trashed. Damon has been keeping in close contact with the Sunday newspapers. Apparently Cummings is desperately trying to keep the story going and has been feeding various outlets more material. I genuinely think that he's doing all this as a massive distraction technique, to take away attention from his initial support for herd immunity, and his personal contribution to pushing it so hard, before he eventually U-turned. Perhaps he can't find any other way to deal with his own anguish over his mistakes.

SUNDAY 30 MAY

'Keep going, we have seen off Cummings's bungled assassination,' Boris messaged cheerfully. It was lunchtime and the PM didn't appear to be having any kind of honeymoon, or even half a day off.

'Yes, more of a blunderbuss than a rifle,' I replied, adding my congratulations on his nuptials.

'Lovely pic and perfect weather for it,' I said.

The Prof told me he'd been stopped by two different strangers in the street in Sussex, both of whom wanted him to tell me I was doing a 'very good job'. I bet they congratulated him more than they congratulated me, but he'd never mention that.

MONDAY 31 MAY

Soon I too will be asked to give evidence to the committee. Damon is worried that Dom might supply them with documents they could use to ambush me.

'If we can, we should insist that Dom presents all his evidence before your committee appearance,' he suggested.

I agree that we should try to flush him out.

I spent the evening working on my speech about the story of the vaccine for the G7 health summit in Oxford later this week. Light relief, relative to dealing with Cummings's mad world.

JUNE 2021

TUESDAY 1 JUNE

G7 health summit tomorrow. Jens texted to say how excited he is to be coming to Oxford. Disappointingly, Patty Hajdu, the charming Canadian Health Secretary, has had to pull out because of a domestic crisis. It turns out that when her government drew up international travel restrictions, they forgot about private jets. Result? The super-rich have been coming and going as they please. Patty has taken the heat and has been all over Canadian media talking about the dangers of overseas travel. There's no way she can be seen hopping on a plane right now. Two emotions. One: I'm gutted, as I've got to know her really well on Zoom and was looking forward to meeting her in person. Two: a strange kind of relief that these screw-ups happen everywhere. It could just as easily have happened to us.

I went to watch my son play cricket, then headed to Oxford, where I felt immensely proud to welcome world health leaders to my old university.

Nadhim's constituency association has specifically requested me as their guest of honour and speaker early next year. Nice!

'So they've forgiven me for locking them down?' I asked.

'They appreciate you,' he said.

For the first time since last summer, there were no Covid deaths reported yesterday. We really are coming out of this.

WEDNESDAY 2 JUNE

After a Zoom with the PM about the latest data (good), I headed to the Oxford Jenner Institute to give my speech telling the story of the vaccine. I talked about how the vaccine showed what we can achieve when the 'holy trinity' of academia, industry and government come together to achieve a common purpose. Then to the summit proper, meeting the global CEOs who had flown in. For almost everyone it was their first foreign trip since the pandemic took hold. It was particularly good to see Pascal after so long in the trenches together. He's been stuck in Australia for almost the entire pandemic. In his position as a global business leader, the time difference has been a killer. All this time, he's been working during the Australian nights, unavailable only for four hours at our lunchtime. It must have been exhausting.

I hadn't seen him in person for over two years and to tell the truth, it was pretty emotional: I doubt any corporate leader has ever done as much good as he did with his single decision that weekend last April to make the Oxford vaccine happen at cost, for everyone.

As I left the conference hotel for dinner, I almost walked smack into one of Dido's mobile testing units, which was parked right outside the venue. I went over and talked to the team, thanking them for their work and commitment. I don't know who was more surprised – they were on a scheduled stop to supply testing to central Oxford and certainly didn't expect me to rock up.

THURSDAY 3 JUNE

The first face-to-face meeting of the G7 Health Ministers in two years. After a morning of one-to-ones we had an informal lunch before formal round-table sessions. The goal was to reach an agreement on how the global response can be faster in future, after the failure of international coordination last time round.

Outside Mansfield College, where one of the main meetings took place, a student spotted the Prof and sidled up to him to ask his advice on a minor health condition. The Prof listened patiently before respectfully giving his best advice. What a lovely man he is: equally in his element addressing world health leaders and diagnosing the smallest ailment during a random encounter on the street.

The event I was most looking forward to was the formal dinner in Exeter College Hall this evening. Due to the Rule of Six we couldn't all sit together at one long table, so we broke it up into tables of six, with guests including Jeremy Hunt and Simon Stevens. As Jeremy speaks Japanese, I sat him with their delegation, while I was seated between Pascal Soriot and Albert Bourla of Pfizer – leaders of the two companies that have done so much – and opposite Roberto Speranza, who I knew so well but had never met.

When it came to my turn to say a few words, I suddenly felt unusually nervous: I hadn't stood in front of a real-life audience since before the pandemic. There were only forty other people in the room, but it was still strangely daunting. At least I had a well-prepared speech – or so I thought.

For the first time since the pandemic, I'd decided it was OK to slip in a few jokes – just a few asides to lighten the mood. Delighted to be liberated from drafting the usual dismal proclamations about case numbers and rule changes, Danny, my speechwriter, had set about the task with alacrity.

As the big moment approached, I reached for the print-out – only to realise, to my horror, that I'd left the precious document in my hotel. What to do?

'Can you run back to the hotel and get it?' I asked Danny, frantically doing time/distance/speed calculations in my head to work out whether he had any chance of retrieving it before I had to take to the podium. At best, the answer was 'maybe'.

While he sprinted across Oxford, I darted out of the dining hall and into the senior common room to make emergency notes, trying to talk to Danny at the same time.

'Give me the punchlines!' I urged him, as the poor man panted down the line. 'I know exactly what I want to say on the substance – but I need the jokes.' He rattled off a couple as he sprinted back through the streets of Oxford.

Back in the dining hall, the sudden disappearance of the host was getting awkward. Social distancing rules meant they couldn't just mingle. They were all hovering at their tables, wondering what was going on.

'What are you doing?' asked an anxious-looking Sir John Bell, having located me in the common room. 'Everyone's standing waiting, and they're starting to socially mix.'

Danny still wasn't back, so there was nothing for it but to wing it. Patrick Vallance opened with an impressive speech about the power of science and collaboration between public and private sectors, and then it was me. I knew what I wanted to say – about the vital importance of keeping the progress that we had fought so hard at such cost to achieve – and the audience was a willing one, so happily I didn't embarrass myself. It was a moment of catharsis in which we could all look forward, thinking about the challenges of the future as well as the lessons we've all learned. I managed to remember the jokes, and the audience laughed at all the right moments.

The evening ended with drinks on the roof terrace of the Marriott. I looked out over the beautiful city, which has played such a distinguished role in the greatest public health crisis of our times, and felt beyond proud of it, and of the part the G7 delegates have played in the fight against the virus.

FRIDAY 4 JUNE

After last night's splendour, a mad scramble this morning to arrange a Covid test for one of the global CEOs, who has a cough. Unfortunately, Dido's mobile testing station – so conveniently located on the doorstep yesterday – had vanished. There was nothing else to hand and I was beginning to panic when we remembered that the chief technical officer of NHS Test and Trace lived nearby. Surely he could rustle up a test? He was happy to oblige, and my private secretary gamely provided a taxi service to his house in her Fiat Punto.

The summit concluded with a tree-planting ceremony at Oxford Botanic Garden: one for each country of the G7, plus one for the global health workers who have given so much. Usually on these occasions the VIPs just do one or two symbolic spadefuls, leaving a gardener to do the rest. I was doing my token shovel when out of the corner of my eye I saw that Stella Kyriakides, the EU health commissioner, was still going. She seemed determined to plant the whole tree. I didn't think it would be right to stop before she did. Seeing us shovelling away, everyone else felt they had to do the same. Cue earth flying everywhere and a bunch of sweating G7 leaders – plus some very fully planted trees.

SATURDAY 5 JUNE

Blair and I are both on *Marr* tomorrow and there could be fireworks. He messaged to warn me that he will be banging the drum for vaccine passports. His think tank has produced a report which – in his words – makes the case for 'distinguishing between the vaccinated and unvaccinated'. I thanked him for offering to ping me a copy of the report ahead of the show and told him that Roberto Speranza had said lots of nice things about him at the G7 dinner.

'Ha! He's generous,' Blair replied cheerfully.

After receiving the report, I wasn't feeling quite so friendly. It gets a few things wrong and seems to go out of its way to invite criticism of the NHS app. Choosing my words carefully, I messaged Blair back saying we are 'pretty surprised, tbh', which, as a seasoned operator, he will know means that we are not at all happy.

'I'm told the briefing has been pretty hostile and there's a load of inaccuracies. It's a bit bizarre as the NHS vaccine app is very successful and popular, and we are planning to do the various things the report is calling for. I'm told, disappointingly, the team didn't talk to us about it, so maybe that's why it's wide of the mark,' I said.

I added – meaning it – that I don't want to get into a tangle with him on *Marr* tomorrow, so we'd better discuss. The more I thought about it, the more annoyed I felt, so I sent him a small selection of the commentators who think the NHS app is actually rather good.

'I would be disappointed if the team got a load of incoming when they've actually nailed this one,' I said.

No reply as yet.

SUNDAY 6 JUNE

Blair got back to me first thing trying to smooth things over. He claimed he hadn't intended to criticise the app and that it was all 'a bit of a misunderstanding'.

In the event, he went out of his way to praise the app on *Marr*. I messaged afterwards to thank him, and he decently volunteered to say something supportive of me and the team any time it would help.

'That's very kind. I do think it would help when it feels appropriate. The incoming from a certain former adviser certainly was quite a thing,' I replied gratefully.

MONDAY 7 JUNE

After Blair's intervention yesterday, I had to go through the whole vaccine passport idea again with Gove. To have any chance of working, so-called 'freedom certificates' – as Boris likes to call them – would need to cover everything: going to the pub, going shopping, eating out etc. To my mind, that's both practically and politically impossible. If they're only used for big events, they will have no clinical benefit. The whole concept is toxic and I really don't see the point. Gove seemed very reluctant to let it go: the only major disagreement he and I have had since the start of the pandemic.

TUESDAY 8 JUNE

The Boundary Commission has published its initial proposals for changing the way parliamentary constituencies are drawn. For some MPs, this is a matter of political life or death, as their existing seats either disappear completely or suddenly incorporate areas full of people who vote for other parties.

Evidently Gove isn't too upset about our differences yesterday, as we've been riffing about winners and losers.

'Newmarket or Haverhill?' he asked, looking at the way my patch will be carved up.

'Like choosing between my children,' I replied.

Nadine did brilliantly in the Commons today, slapping down theatrical attempts by Labour's Rosena Allin-Khan to go viral on social media. 'The Queen of the Tik Tok clip is always looking for the Oscar,' she sniffed later.

Two days to go till I'm in front of the select committee. Cummings still hasn't produced any evidence to back up his accusations.

Today marked six months since we first vaccinated Margaret Keenan in Coventry University Hospital; now we're opening up vaccinations for the over-25s.

WEDNESDAY 9 JUNE

I spent the day prepping for the committee hearing, after which we had a proper rehearsal, with each of the SpAds playing different roles. I was armed with a 'superdoc' with replies to everything we could think of that I might be asked. We even filmed it so we could play it back in the office afterwards. Ahead of the session, the SpAds deliberately locked me out of the room for an extra ten minutes to make me more nervous.

I hate watching myself back on these things, but it was crucial. Looking at the footage later, I winced more at my body language than at my answers: I was slouching in my chair and fiddling with my pen, as well as being combative whenever I was asked anything I found irritating. I was particularly poor when the 'attack-dog' character played by Damon asked provocative questions. Am I really this bad? I've done dozens of select committee appearances and am very dismayed to think that I might have looked so slovenly. The whole exercise was extremely useful: I've got to improve my reactions under pressure and sit up straight.

Later Simon Case messaged worrying about the latest figures in the north-west, where there's been a significant rise in hospital admissions. 'That real world data from NW on cases/admissions is the first thing I have seen that makes me feel pretty gloomy about 21 June,' he said, referring to the proposed reopening date.

'Me too,' I replied.

'I was quite bullish yesterday afternoon!' he said.

'On the principle of cautious and irreversible we should be cautious in the hope we can be irreversible,' I replied.

'I think that logic is strong. It has been a sound logic for getting the country through this year – we abandon it at our peril (probably),' he agreed.

If we do decide to delay reopening, the question is when and how we open up again, given that case numbers will continue to rise for a while and we cannot go on with restrictions indefinitely.

In better news, over a million people booked their vaccine in the past twenty-four hours. Incredible to see young people coming forward to get vaccinated in their droves.

THURSDAY 10 JUNE

A fiery message from Nadine ahead of my select committee appearance.

'Good luck today Matt. You will knock it out of the park.'

'Thank you,' I replied.

'He is a little shit and you are a good man. Karma does its stuff,' she said.

I half-expected Cummings to have planted something awkward in today's papers in an attempt to back up some of his delusions, but there was nothing. Encouraged, I headed over to the Commons at 9 a.m., arriving at the committee a few minutes early. After all that prep, there were no questions we hadn't anticipated and plenty of opportunities to explain the truth. I found no need to mention Cummings at all and simply explained what had happened: that government had run a whole lot better since November, when he left. I didn't look like a sack of potatoes and I didn't fiddle with my pen. Job done.

Later Chris Wormald messaged to say he thought it had gone OK.

'Well done – bits I saw you were doing really well, hitting just the right tone,' he said.

'Yes, seemed to go well. I got a bit of [stick over] PPE, but nothing new,' I replied.

Chris, who'd had his own hearing in front of the Public Accounts Committee, said he was also criticised over PPE, mainly on why we over-ordered.

'V v v happy to be attacked for having too much PPE!' he said.

'Quite,' I replied.

Late tonight I also got a nice message from Boris.

'Apparently you were great. Well done,' he said.

Doubtless Cummings will soon hit back. He doesn't let go.

FRIDAY 11 JUNE

Privately, it looks like the PM has decided to delay unlocking. The case rate is clearly rising and the health advice is clear: waiting just a bit longer will save thousands of lives.

Michael Gove has given a big interview to tomorrow's *Times* in which he's made a number of promises about the future of the NHS.

'Are you happy with this?' Damon asked, running me through various pledges on hospitals and waiting times. Er, no. It's just not the done thing for Cabinet ministers to make promises in areas that aren't their responsibility. He's parked his tanks all over my lawn.

'Not at all happy, no,' I said grumpily.

'He might give you a call,' Damon replied evenly.

Now we have journalists asking what we think of his ideas: not ideal.

Michael clearly knew he'd gone too far and sent a slightly sheep-ish message trying to smoke out how upset I was. He called later with a profuse apology. The truth is I believe him when he says it was cock-up not conspiracy. It usually is when something goes wrong in government and, anyway, you have to believe that or ministerial life would drive you mad.

My team is uneasy about delaying unlocking.

'We said vaccine is the way out. So will likely be accused of moving the goalposts,' Emma warned.

Allan, who spends a lot of time talking to our MPs, worries that pointing to rising rates in the over-sixties will not fly. 'MPs will point to death rates and will have anecdotal evidence of old people in their patches admitted to hospital but having fairly mild symptoms. And others saying, "The hospital in my patch has zero Covid patients,"' he said.

We all agree that we can't just delay reopening without making a specific commitment about how the time will be used, for example delivering more vaccines. It's a fine judgement call.

It was my son's birthday. I was overjoyed that for the first time since before the pandemic I managed to make it back for tea and cake.

SUNDAY 13 JUNE

We had a formal meeting on whether to delay reopening by four weeks. I thought it was a very tricky, balanced decision, but the PM was in no doubt and it all went through fairly quickly. Even Rishi wasn't opposed. We all resolved, though, that this delay will be the last. I told the team that the narrative is 'the race'.

'The [Delta] variant gave the virus more legs. So now we must give the vaccine some extra time. We are doing this by both accelerating jabs and delaying opening.' The truth is that I'm not really very comfortable with the decision: the delay risks jeopardising all the goodwill around the vaccine programme. And we know cases don't translate into hospitalisations and deaths in the way they once did. Yet the modelling is clear that one more month will save thousands of lives. Presented with data like that, it's hard to say no.

MONDAY 14 JUNE

A mark of how far we've come is that I'm now able to spend about half of my time on non-Covid matters. Today I was focused on our women's health strategy – a piece of work I've kept going throughout the pandemic. Medicine has been a man's world for too long. Up until now, men have commissioned and carried out the vast majority of research. The result? Some very common female conditions, like endometriosis, are woefully under-researched. I want to change that. An astonishing 112,198 people have contributed to the consultation, over 100 times the normal figure, which shows just how much this matters.

I announced the delay in unlocking in the Commons this evening amid an almighty row about MPs not being told first. No. 10 has done far too much media briefing and the Speaker is furious. Ahead of my speech I messaged Dan Rosenfield warning him that MPs are also going nuts.

'This evening is going to be a total shit show. There is a way to handle Parliament and today was not it. Don't be defensive about it – but you need to strengthen the [parliamentary] operation,' I said.

Dan blamed the Speaker. Apparently the original plan was for the PM to make a statement tomorrow, but the Speaker suddenly changed his mind. 'I reached a new agreement, which he then reneged on too,' he explained wearily.

For his part, the Speaker clearly blames us. I told Dan he's hopping mad. I hope this isn't some great wheeze to get Boris off the hook of making the statement. I'll have to believe it's cock-up not conspiracy again.

'Now I'm off to receive a massive kicking from the Speaker and all his mates on the Tory benches,' I said gloomily.

In the end, the response to my statement in the Commons was weary acceptance – grumbles rather than fireworks. Everyone is just really tired of the whole saga.

TUESDAY 15 JUNE

Unbelievably, someone on the JCVI is briefing again! This time it's about vaccinating children: tomorrow's *Telegraph* claims we'll be advised against doing so until there's more evidence about possible risks. The story wasn't even on the website before we started getting calls from the JCVI asking how they should manage the furore they knew it would create. I messaged JVT and the Prof demanding a crisis meeting.

'Their briefing to the *Telegraph* is completely unacceptable and I no longer have any confidence in their advice,' I told the Prof.

The chairman of the committee, Wei Shen Lim, certainly isn't behind it. However, he's clearly struggling to manage dissenting voices.

'Their increasingly erratic decisions are born of his attempts to maintain consensus,' I said to JVT. 'They do not take into account all health considerations, let alone all considerations. They have been captured by a hardline group – who are willing to use ultra vires means to prevent government from taking proper decisions.'

The Prof is characteristically calm; JVT less so.

The problem with the JCVI is that they only take a narrow view of the health impact of vaccines. They argue that if an individual can't be proven to benefit from a vaccine, they shouldn't have it. But there are much wider health considerations: the lower likelihood of passing Covid on to others if you're vaccinated, for starters. That can't be measured directly, but it really matters. Again, it comes down to a question of political philosophy: in a pandemic, when you might harm someone inadvertently, the harm principle makes a liberal argument for state action. It's not as if we're forcing people to get the jab: we're just encouraging it. But some on the JCVI are determined to push a much narrower political philosophy based on individual benefit. My beef isn't just that I don't agree with that judgement: it's that judgements of political philosophy aren't for expert committees but for elected politicians operating on the *advice* of expert committees.

The Prof points out – rightly – that we need the JCVI's backing for public acceptance of the vaccination effort, and we put that at risk at our peril. So there's not much point getting cross as there isn't much we can do about it. Oh to be so phlegmatic!

WEDNESDAY 16 JUNE

A furious JVT messaged at 6.25 a.m., having read the *Telegraph* front page. Now he gets why I was so wound up yesterday.

'It's disgusting and it damages the whole committee,' he said.

I told him I'm hauling Wei Shen in.

'I've no doubt of his integrity at all, of course, but we cannot have such an important matter driven by these tactics,' I said.

Wormald agrees that this can't go on.

'We now have to deal with the JCVI. We keep putting it off – but their behaviour is totally outrageous,' I said.

He thinks this leak – of actual advice before we've got it, as opposed to JCVI members giving their personal views – is much more serious than the other problems we've had with them.

That thing I said about Cummings not being done with me? He's already burst back out of his box. He's clearly spent the last few days fulminating about the fact that he's failed to get me sacked and is now upping the ante. Heart sinking at this latest stupid distraction, I read the stuff he's leaked in full. It's a text exchange from last year. It's based on a long, aggressive and inaccurate message he sent Boris, clearly designed to be provocative, to which the PM replies, 'Totally fucking hopeless'. It's obvious he's referring to the situation falsely reported to him, not me personally.

'This isn't "evidence",' I told Damon. 'All this shows is that Dom was just shit-stirring. Thank God he's gone!'

Damon suggests 'no war of words, reject accusations, rebut anything substantive, stay close to No. 10 and crack on'.

Simon Case checked in this afternoon, clearly worried that I might be feeling bruised.

'Totally fine. What a plonker,' I replied firmly.

The vaccines for kids story is running hard. I've read Wei Shen the riot act.

THURSDAY 17 JUNE

Huge press pack on the doorstep again.

'Is it helpful if I trek over?' Damon offered.

I told him there wasn't much point – I didn't plan to say anything beyond 'good morning' and perhaps that I'm off to deliver some more vaccines. The story's going nowhere and I don't want to give it legs.

In the evening Damon messaged to say he'd had an interesting discussion about our budget with some No. 10 policy types. 'They think we will need to offer up some shiny piece of NHS reform (on efficiency) to help get HMT over the line for good funding to deal with post-pandemic recovery,' he said.

Fine – there is so much to do on efficiency, this will be a good prompt to the system.

Tomorrow, we're able to open vaccinations up to all adults. Incredible to think that just over six months ago, no one in the world had been vaccinated with a clinically authorised Covid vaccine, and now all adults can get theirs. The NHS has done such a brilliant job.

FRIDAY 18 JUNE

Businesswoman Baroness Michelle Mone has sent me an extraordinarily aggressive email complaining that a company she's helping isn't getting the multi-million-pound contracts it deserves. She claims the firm, which makes lateral flow test kits, 'has had a dreadful time' trying to cut through red tape and demanded my 'urgent help' before it all comes out in the media.

'I am going to blow this all wide open,' she threatened.

In essence, she's not at all happy that a US company called Innova has secured so many contracts while others 'can't get in the game'. She claims test kits made by the company she's representing, and by several other firms, have all passed Porton Down's rigorous quality control checks but only Innova is getting the business.

'This makes it a monopoly position for Innova, who to date have received £2.85 billion in orders and counting from DHSC, while all the other ten suppliers are not able to participate in the home testing kit market...' she complained.

By the end of the email she seemed to have worked herself into a complete frenzy and was throwing around wild accusations. 'I smell a rat here. It is more than the usual red tape, incompetence and bureaucracy. That's expected! I believe there is corruption here at the highest levels and a cover-up is taking place ... Don't say I didn't [warn] you when Panorama or Horizon run an exposé documentary on all this.'

She concluded by urging me to intervene 'to prevent the next bombshell being dropped on the govt'.

'I say a level playing field for all,' she demanded, accusing us of offering 'golden tickets' to others.

I read the email again, stunned. Was she threatening me? It certainly looked that way to me. I asked Jim if he could deal with her, but he's running a mile from it. 'Her tests have not passed validation,' he says – which would explain why the company hasn't won any contracts. Jim says she has not been pleasant to our staff and that he has had to intervene. 'I am very, very wary of any engagement whatsoever,' he said. He has told her that he can't have any informal contact with her on this.

'I will simply not reply!' I concluded.

'I think that's right,' he replied.

He does acknowledge issues with this particular piece of procurement and says we need to publish more data, especially on why we are turning down tests. Fine – but I won't be pushed around by aggressive peers representing commercial clients.

Later I was glad to get out of London to visit King's Lynn Hospital, which is, I'm afraid to say, in dreadful shape. The ceiling is falling down and the whole place desperately needs renovating. It absolutely *has* to be in the forty new hospitals programme, and it is essential that that programme is more than an endlessly repeated promise.

MONDAY 21 JUNE

Back to Covid, working on the booster plan ahead of a planned launch in September. In an ideal world there would be a vaccine that protects against both flu and the latest Covid variant. That's pretty unlikely. Next best is that people can get a flu and Covid jab at the same time. 'One in each arm,' as JVT put it cheerfully. Helen has been talking to No. 10 about social care reform, over which there's more foot dragging. Not entirely encouragingly, she says they 'seem to agree with the need for it' but aren't ready to commit. On and on it goes.

TUESDAY 22 JUNE

I've been thinking about what a massive boost the vaccine has been for the union. The Scots have had very tangible evidence of the benefits of sticking with us. As a result, support for independence – or separatism, as I think we should call it – has plummeted. I'm glad to have played my part. Let's see how long the vaccine effect lasts. In any future referendum, we can make the case that the union got Scots vaccinated first in the world – and would do the same again.

WEDNESDAY 23 JUNE

To Buckingham Palace for an audience with the Queen. I was thrilled when I got the invitation. It was the first Privy Council in person since the pandemic. Since it was also the first in-person meeting between the Queen and the PM since Covid, a TV crew filmed them greeting each other.

THURSDAY 24 JUNE

What price love? I've always known from the novels that people will risk everything. They are ready to blow up their past, their present and their future. They will jeopardise everything they have worked for and everything that is solid and certain. Accompanying the joy of falling in love – if you are supposed to be happily married – is the turmoil. You know, with terrible black dread, that sooner or later the relationship must be revealed and everything will come crashing down.

To others it may seem mad, but for the person in love, the judgement to do it anyway feels right. You know there will be consequences and are afraid and ashamed but are compelled to carry on. Each day without discovery is another day without inflicting pain on others.

For some time now Gina and I have been getting closer. Both of us being married, we knew the devastating implications of our feelings for each other.

That we were trying to work out the least painful way of being together when the call came is of no consequence now. People I love are in agony, and I am fighting for my political career.

The day began quite well, with news that we'd overtaken Israel to become the most vaccinated country in the world. I then met the Prime Minister and Rishi, and for the first time we managed to thrash out a plan to cap the costs of social care. There followed a meeting with Thérèse Coffey to push forward much-needed reforms to sick pay, and then a discussion with the JCVI about next steps on vaccination. So far, so good. I then went to Parliament for a debate on the use of data in the NHS. It's unusual, but David Davis was leading the charge, and out of respect for him – and the trouble he can cause – I answered it myself, off the cuff. I was feeling good and, if truth be told, at the top of my game.

When I saw a missed call on my phone from the editor of *The Sun*, I thought nothing of it. I know Victoria Newton well and have spoken to her regularly throughout the pandemic, so I had no misgivings as I called her back.

'I'm sorry, but I've got a story about you and Gina. I've got pictures, so there's no point in you denying it, but we're giving you a straight, factual write-up, and won't call on you to resign,' is what she said.

As she talked me through what they planned to write in tomorrow's paper, I knew immediately what I had to do.

I needed to tell Martha right away, because it needed to come from me and nobody else. I also knew I had to tell the children – it was going to be incredibly painful, but I couldn't hide away from them. They deserved to know too. Having the Health Secretary for a husband or father during a global pandemic has been incredibly tough for the family, and I feel wretched.

Knowing the *Sun* story would trigger a chain of events I would be unable to control, I decided to go straight home. Before I set off, I called the PM: no stranger to personal turmoil and, it turned out, the kindest of confidants in these ghastly circumstances.

Whatever anyone may say of him, I'll always be immensely grateful for our conversation. He was thoughtful, considered and as supportive as he could be for everyone involved.

I explained it all: that Gina and I had recently fallen in love, and fallen in love very deeply. I told him how I had known Gina for more than half of my life – we first met working together on student radio at Oxford – and I brought her into the department to help with public communications, in the same way we'd brought in brilliant people in so many areas. I told him that we had spent a huge amount of time together during the pandemic and fell in love. Foolish as it sounds, it felt completely outside my control.

Boris listened carefully.

'First, I'm going to talk to you as a friend, and then we'll talk about the politics,' he said.

He gave me some personal advice, after which he assured me that my private life should not affect my public position.

I thanked him for his support and explained that while I had already decided that I would be with Gina there were two political problems. First, *The Sun* is accusing me of bringing Gina into the department because of our affair. This is categorically untrue. I appointed her for her skills and experience, and our relationship only began very recently, as a result of working so closely together.

The second issue is more difficult: while we never broke the law, social distancing guidelines had been in place at the time our relationship began a few weeks ago. Nothing happened between us until May, after legal restrictions ended. We'd always been acutely conscious of all that. Nonetheless the recommendation remained that everyone should follow the one-metre-plus rule, and we clearly had not.

'Well, you haven't broken the law. The guidelines aren't binding – they're recommendations. So I will stand by you,' Boris replied generously.

With those words ringing in my head, and in utter turmoil, I headed home to talk to Martha. It was – and remains – the very worst conversation of my life.

FRIDAY 25 JUNE

The Sun published the story at 2 a.m. as a 'world exclusive'. The picture was a grainy CCTV image of me and Gina embracing in my departmental office. It was immediately obvious that the story would be huge. I knew I had to get out of London, so my wonderful driver Mark came to pick me up last night and take me to stay discreetly in the countryside.

By 5 a.m., photographers and reporters were swarming outside both of our homes. We told the press we weren't there. They camped out nonetheless. Every distant member of the family they could find was called or doorstepped.

Around 8 a.m., a welcome call from No. 10: Dan Rosenfield, to say they'd got my back. He offered any support we might need, including sending a Conservative Party press officer to my house.

By 9 a.m. I'd had half a dozen sympathetic messages from ministerial colleagues: a terrible sign. They knew I was in deep trouble. Nadhim sent me a piece of advice 'from a brother', which sounded very much like an appeal not to resign.

Damon advised that we say as little as possible. Meanwhile I went back over all our movements and tried to think of any other rules we might be accused of breaking. Other than the one-metre-plus rule, I couldn't think of any.

'Should I do a fast apology for letting everyone down/breaching guidance?' I asked.

Gina thought it was a good idea, so Damon began crafting a short statement. He sent me several variations of: 'The Health Secretary has not broken any rules, but he acknowledges that he breached the social distancing advice in this instance. He deeply regrets this, recognises that he has let people down and apologises for it.'

I tried to focus on the words, but my head was spinning.

The final version of the statement, which went out at lunchtime, accepted that I breached social distancing guidance and said I was still focused on working to get the country out of the pandemic. I hoped it would quiet the furore.

Yet the story continued to rage: on all the news websites, on the BBC, on Twitter and on just about every other conceivable news outlet. By mid-afternoon, there were still suggestions that we'd broken the law. It was categorically untrue, and Damon thought we needed to brief harder or put out another line.

'What's wrong with "no laws were broken"?' I suggested.

Round and round in circles we went, trying to find the right words.

Damon's mobile phone was practically melting, and I was more stressed than I have ever been in my entire life.

All afternoon, the 'what, when, where, who, why, how much?' questions continued. Journalists began suggesting I might have broken the Ministerial Code. I hadn't, but I could see the way this was going.

My local association in Suffolk was wonderfully supportive. Allan worked the phones, trying to get MPs to say something helpful. My spirits lifted a little when former party leader William Hague publicly declared that I shouldn't resign. Not for long though: by late afternoon it was clear tomorrow's papers will hideous.

SATURDAY 26 JUNE

The mood was sour and journalists were becoming more aggressive. Privately, I was still getting positive messages from colleagues. Publicly, few were willing to defend me. Politically, I was increasingly isolated.

I feel desperate for my family, my children and Gina's family and her children, and powerless to protect them. Worse is the knowledge that Gina and I have brought all this on them. Gina's feelings of shame and guilt are nearly overpowering her. The jokes and cartoons on social media are excruciating. We are being publicly humiliated, again and again.

While close friends and family were amazing, I also had messages from friends and colleagues who had terrible lockdown experiences and were very upset. Their disappointment in me – and their sense of betrayal – was agonising. It is all my fault of course. I knew I had to take responsibility. I knew in my heart that I had to resign.

I went to Chequers to see the PM. I explained that I had been thinking about what had happened and how it had made people feel – and that my mind was made up. The damage to my family and to the government was too great. I told Boris I had to resign. He was regretful but didn't argue. We sat on the patio and talked about what this would mean for the management of the rest of the pandemic. An exchange of letters was prepared, offering and accepting my resignation, and we each edited our letters. We had to decide how to make the announcement, what to say and how. I must have shot a thousand videos over the course of the pandemic, levelling with the public and thanking the NHS for their dedication. This would be the last. In the end the great machinery of the state was nowhere. It was just me and the PM, fumbling around with an iPhone.

He stood on the grass, holding the phone while I said my piece. It took a few goes to get right. He nodded sympathetic encouragement so much throughout the first take that the camera waved up and down. In the end it wasn't perfect, but I was beyond caring: I had to get it out.

Now messages of sympathy and support flooded in: from my team, the Prof, JVT, Pascal – and just about everyone else who worked so hard alongside us to save lives. I'm incredibly grateful to all my team, especially my SpAds and private office, for going above and beyond in supporting me over in what is such a difficult time for them, too.

'I'm so sorry,' I told them all. 'I mean, the honest truth is I made a mistake due to love and it doesn't matter that it was only guidance. I should not have broken advice that I myself signed off.'

This evening Jamie, whose endless advice – offered long after he stopped working for me – has been so valuable throughout the pandemic, messaged to say I'd done the right thing.

'There is so much you have done that you should be incredibly proud of. There are people alive today who wouldn't be if you hadn't made the decisions you did,' he said.

'I love her. That's what screwed my judgement,' I replied wretchedly.

'Love does that to us all. I hope you can both be happy,' he said.

'Of that I have no doubt,' I replied.

As for Boris? If anyone knows how to survive a catastrophic political and personal mistake, it's him.

'Time to dive beneath the ice cap' was his advice.

EPILOGUE

The aftermath of the pandemic is all around us. As so often through history, pandemic has been followed by inflation and war.

A year on from the events of this book, reviewing my papers, notes and messages has given me the chance to reflect on those extraordinary times. The overriding sense of the huge quantity of communications is of a team of people working incredibly hard to do their best to get the country through an unprecedented challenge, in a world where information was scarce, judgements huge and roadmap non-existent. Of course there were mistakes. Who has ever done anything meaningful where there were not? The task was to learn along the way. As I often told the team: to make a mistake once is understandable; to make the same mistake twice, inexcusable.

Now that learning must be captured, with the full benefit of hindsight.

There will rightly be a full public inquiry to consider every aspect of the response, and to ensure the country is as well prepared as possible for next time – as we were not for this. How can we best use the knowledge, experience and resources we built at such speed? It's vital we learn the right lessons from what went wrong. Importantly too, we must learn from the things that went right. And we must think about the things that didn't happen and so were often absent from the debate – the dogs that didn't bark.

We were lucky, for example, that this virus hardly affected children. Yet we must imagine and prepare for a pandemic that does. We learned painful lessons about how to protect people in care homes: next time we must apply them from the start. We were lucky that both of the first two vaccines approved were able to be manufactured at speed and scale: we must ensure that capacity is retained.

Generally, where we had institutions and experience, we performed well. The scientific response, building on the might of our universities. The NHS response, building on its enormous capability. Clinical trials and genomics, building on our global leadership. The vaccine rollout, building on how we deliver millions of flu jabs every year.

Where we had no such background, we found it much harder, because starting from scratch is much more difficult. Building a testing system. Distributing PPE when the supply chain company collapsed. Implementing lockdowns when nothing like it had been done within living memory.

What's critical is that we learn from all this. And, especially, that we peel back and find the failures in the projects that really worked and the successes in the projects that struggled. It's an easy response, too often made, to idolise every success as successful throughout and to criticise every challenging project as a catastrophe. This would be a failure of learning.

WHAT WE KNOW NOW

The passage of time also means we now know more about what actually happened. In particular, some of the facts are clearer with hindsight.

During the pandemic, it was acknowledged that the worst impact – the extra deaths – could only accurately be measured afterwards. This so-called 'excess deaths' measure is important because it measures all those who died because of the pandemic – whether directly from Covid, from treatments that couldn't be done or from the many negative side effects of lockdown.

While at the time the UK was thought to have one of the worst impacts, measurement errors elsewhere mean we now know this was wrong. Taking everything into account, fewer people died here, over and above a normal year, than in most European countries, and our excess death rate was well below that of the United States. Far-eastern and Australasian countries fared better.

We know more too about the nature of the disease. We know about the long-term impact on the NHS, and the extent of the backlog. We know far more about how the virus spread, including the importance of ventilation, and infection in both health and social care through staff, which were not properly understood until well into the pandemic. And we know about the economic consequences: both the impact of the pandemic on supply chains leading to inflation and the surprising and very welcome lack of mass unemployment.

Taken all together, the UK's response looks better than it did at the time. This doesn't take away from the need for lessons. But it is a vital factual basis from which to learn them.

Now is the time for hindsight. I offer ten thoughts here to begin.

1. PHILOSOPHY OF PANDEMICS

First, on philosophy. Pandemics are communitarian. They affect us all because we are all human. This presents a particular challenge to countries which, like the UK, are governed in the liberal philosophical tradition.

Some say we abandoned liberal principles in the response. That is wrong. For sure we had to restrict personal freedoms. But the liberal political tradition is not one of unfettered libertarianism but rather one constrained by the harm principle: people should be free to do as they choose so long as they do not harm others. So in a pandemic, when anyone can harm another person without even knowing, the liberal state has not merely a justification but a duty to prevent harm.

In practice, the public understood this. Support for lockdown was incredibly strong. The vast majority of people were prepared to make enormous sacrifices to prevent harm to others. In fact, the public pressure was for more formality to the rules, not less.

This principle was strained at points other than lockdown too.

There was great resistance to human challenge trials: but if people fully consent to participating, where is the problem? The expert bodies like the JCVI struggled with the question of vaccinating those for whom a vaccination did not bring clear individual benefit but did benefit society. But in handling a communitarian problem like a pandemic, sometimes difficult actions are necessary for the greater good. It's different from normal medical ethics: but that's because in a pandemic, liberal individualism doesn't work.

The public understood this too. We put huge thought into how to communicate with them effectively. Like so many at the time, I was surprised, and impressed, at how much people came together and did their bit – whether actively, like the explosion of voluntary activity, or simply by staying at home.

Some now say that guidance, not law, was necessary, but we found the public sought clarity and certainty, not ambiguity and advice. Some argue that national lockdown was not necessary altogether. But the evidence does not back this up. Huge efforts to run less onerous regional lockdowns were largely ineffective – we could not even protect the Isle of Wight. Excess deaths in Sweden – the most liberal European country – were ten times that in its nearest comparators of Norway and Finland. Other countries that took less action, like the United States and Brazil, fared far worse.

Judgement will always be required in deciding when and what drastic action is needed in response to a new pathogen. But to argue that the tool of social distancing shouldn't be used is reckless and wrong. Just imagine a disease that kills the young more than the old, with greater transmission and deadly ferocity than Covid-19. Would we seek to use all the tools at our disposal to save lives, with the greater confidence we can now have that a vaccine would be developed and deployed at speed? Of course we would. This could happen at any time. For any leader to rule out a lockdown is foolish.

Pandemics affect us all because we are a community. We must face them as a community.

2. BE GUIDED BY THE SCIENCE

In a democracy, elected ministers should make decisions of significance, guided by the best available evidence. I always tried to say that we should be guided by the science, not that we followed the science.

After all, 'science' is not a fixed set of facts, but a framework to form an opinion based on the best available understanding and information. The scientific method rests on a sceptical challenge to current thinking, and so, as the facts change, conclusions and recommendations change – sometimes rapidly. This is not to criticise scientists – far from it. The brilliant scientists who played such a leading role – including Chris Whitty, Patrick Vallance, JVT, Jenny Harries, Susan Hopkins and their teams – all understood that their role was to give the best information so that ministers could make decisions that took into account both the science and everything else. The role of SAGE is much scrutinised and criticised. When SAGE worked well, it brought scientific advice to Patrick and Chris as the government's chief scientific and clinical advisers, who took that advice – including the weight of the evidence and contrary views – to ministers.

It was a matter of fact that during the early lockdown decisions, we as ministers followed the advice of our scientific advisers. So in that specific case, it is correct to say we 'followed' the science. But in a much broader sense, we were *guided* by the science. Advisers advise, ministers decide.

In many cases, we chose not to follow recommendations. I overruled scientific advice not to quarantine those returning from Wuhan. I disagreed with advice that PHE was expanding testing as fast as it could. I rejected advice to contract the Oxford vaccine to Merck. There were myriad small examples where the scientific advice was balanced or ambiguous and a decision was required one way or the other. These ended up sometimes being the most difficult calls, like on handshaking or the use of masks, where the science was ambiguous but the public wanted clarity.

What is not ambiguous is the vital importance of the very best scientific advice. Those who reject the use of forecasting – even though no forecast is absolute – are wrong. Listening to challenging and dissenting voices is valuable – even if you ultimately choose to reject what they say. We constantly discussed the scientific trade-offs and the balance of judgements – and actively tried to communicate that the decisions we took were what we felt to be the best judgements in very difficult circumstances.

The pandemic demonstrated to me the power of science. We need more science in public life, not less.

3. DATA UNDERPINS EVERYTHING

Scientific advice is of course based on the best available data. We worked incredibly hard to improve the availability and use of data throughout. This covered many forms.

First, we needed to build data about the extent of the pandemic itself. We started with anecdotes from the front line and gradually, over more than a year, built a monitoring system that was about as accurate as you can get. In this science of measurement, it is vital not to muddle the measured from the true fact. For example, while testing was sparse at first, we knew that the actual number of cases were much higher in number than positive tests – but not by how much. It was only when the ONS finally, and brilliantly, put together their representative sample survey that we really had a decent handle on it. Likewise, it was only when we had a representative sample serology survey that we knew approximately how many people had had the disease. You can't manage what you can't measure, and over time we got better measurement and so better management of the virus. By the end, we had incredibly sophisticated data tools and first-rate data visualisation techniques to help inform decision making.

Then the public communication of the uncertainties around the data was a huge challenge. The example of how to measure, and explain, the number of people who tragically died shows that even for the most important of measures the methodology is not straightforward. We put huge thought into how best to communicate the fact that statistics are often estimates, when people understandably clamour for certainty and language can give more credence to hard numbers than they deserve.

We needed to radically improve data about the wider response and the capabilities we had to deal with the consequences. At the start, data on NHS capacity was limited. Social care data was almost non-existent. Over time, with the support of amazing companies, we built data dashboards better than I have known in any organisation. This high-quality management data must be retained and improved.

Data is then a vital tool for the operation of services – not just their management. We used the urgency of the pandemic to break decades-long taboos about the modern use of data in the NHS and to link data that ought to have been linked years before. When effecting any organisational change, changing attitudes is the majority of the task, and the pandemic afforded us the chance to do that. Horrifically reactionary attitudes to data from vested interests had cost lives in the NHS for years, and it's vital that this progress to vanquish those attitudes is not just maintained but taken further.

The shining example of this is the vaccine programme. Modern data techniques underpinned: the analysis of the virus as a target; the acceleration of the clinical approval; the prioritisation of patients; the efficiency of the rollout; the customer experience (how long did you wait for your vaccine?); the measurement of the impact of vaccination; and the observation and response to side effects. We started with the data architecture and built the rollout from there. This is how modern healthcare can and should be done. We used modern data techniques to deliver the largest civilian operation in the country's history, before anyone else and faster than any comparable nation. There are no longer any excuses.

It wasn't just the vaccine rollout. We had to build many new systems at great speed: testing; furlough; PPE delivery; the app; genomic analysis – to name just a few. The digital build was the rate-limiting factor in each case. We couldn't have built them as quickly without modern data capabilities – but getting the tech right was often the hardest part.

But it was worth it to then be able to reach scale. We must learn how we did that and how we can do even better in future.

I have always been a champion of science and innovation, but the pandemic brought home their critical value, not just as nice-to-haves, but as mission-critical requirements for a national response to the challenges of modern times. There is real jeopardy here. I fear that, for all our strengths in science and research, our failure to grapple with the sharing of data is a disaster. We are missing out on the industrial revolution of our times, and we will be held back for a generation if we fail to capitalise on it.

4. BACK MANY HORSES

It is typical, especially in the public sector, to pursue projects only when there is a very high likelihood of success. The nature of public debate is that successes are briefly cheered or go unnoticed, while failures are attacked and picked over. Heads must roll!

This dynamic incentivises caution, stymies innovation and undermines the uptake of better ideas. I think this last point – that great ideas lie unused for years because there is not enough incentive in the system to make them widespread – is one of the major reasons bureaucracies are so unbelievably slow. It's more often the failure to implement than a failure to innovate that holds back progress.

In the pandemic, we didn't have the luxury of only backing projects we knew would work. We had to back many horses. Again, the best example is the vaccine programme. We bought six vaccines initially. Some of them didn't work, and some that did work couldn't be manufactured at scale. I insisted we began manufacturing before we knew if the Oxford vaccine was safe and effective, but because we had backed so many horses it wasn't just luck that the two that were fastest to pass the clinical trials could also be manufactured at scale so fast.

Less well known is that we took the same approach to testing. Over the spring and summer of 2020, we backed many different testing technologies – from 'Covid dogs' to 'cough-in-the-box' AI technology – to achieve mass testing on a population-wide scale. We didn't know which would work. In the end, the decades-old technology of lateral flow devices came off, in massive scale, in autumn 2020, and we in the UK built the one of the best testing infrastructures in the world. It might have been a different technology, like Oxford Nanopore's cutting-edge genomic test – used by President Xi in the early weeks of the pandemic – but we simply couldn't get it to scale at pace. Frankly, I was astonished at where we ended up. But I'm glad we kept the trusty LFT project on the table amid the excitement of the new solutions, and, like you, I've used hundreds of them.

Ministers should have a higher risk tolerance and drive their departments to stretch further. Take a portfolio approach. Back projects even before they know if they will work. Explain that they don't expect every one of them to succeed. Compete different solutions and keep an open mind. Back many horses.

5. TRUST THE PUBLIC

Public health attitudes can too often be very patronising about the public. Too often the assumed attitude is that people's behaviour is wrong in some way. Yet the pandemic showed that when you trust the public, and explain clearly the reasons for any action you're taking, they get it.

We explained to people why they had to take extraordinary measures in lockdown, and by and large they obliged. We put huge effort into objectively and clearly explaining the truth about vaccines – including publishing reams of information about side effects and their consequences – and the public grew increasingly warm to them. We trusted people to test at home, and they did in vast numbers.

Huge thought and research were put into how best to communicate these messages. Not all of them worked. But the overriding philosophy to publish and be transparent was an undoubted success.

I hope we don't backslide. There's a natural instinct against transparency in government, but it's usually better to publish and explain. That way you can change attitudes too. For example, people are now used to taking a test at home when they don't feel well. I think we should have a consumer diagnostics revolution, so that when you feel ill, the first thing you do is take a test at home to find out what's wrong with you – what bug have you got, and what should you do about it? Is it essentially harmless, or do you need to act?

But there's a wider lesson for government that could help accelerate changes in fields like education and transport, and for the media in how it interacts with government. Trust the public. Communicate, communicate, communicate. Complicated concepts can be effectively explained, and changes of approach in response to new information are not embarrassing but sensible. The public are smarter than you think.

6. LEADERSHIP

In something as big as a pandemic – and in many smaller things – leadership by central diktat and interference rarely works. As the Russian Army repeatedly discovered in its invasion of Ukraine, top-down command and control is an incredibly poor form of leadership.

Instead I tried to deliver system leadership: set out a clear mission or objective, find the resources to make it possible, set the guide rails, trust people to deliver and hold them to account.

The formal, statutory independence of some of the health bodies generally got in the way of this approach, because it implied bodies could set different strategic goals, whereas their effective ability to get on with the job without operational interference was what was really valuable. A good example of this was in sharing data. I took the strategic decision that sharing data was valuable and important. The statutory independence of NHS Digital legally required its leadership to make a separate judgement as to whether such data sharing was a good idea. This was extremely obstructive and caused huge practical difficulties. Instead they should have accepted the strategic decision and got on with the part they were brilliant at: their operational ability to execute and deliver the data sharing. The leadership I tried to provide was to give clarity about the objective and resources but delegate flexibility on how to make it happen.

In the pandemic response there are endless examples of both failure and success. The starkest failure was No. 10's constant interference in the delivery of testing from May to November 2020, which held back the project and caused huge difficulties in its operation. By its nature, anyone, at any level of seniority, in No. 10 can cause waves in a department with even the smallest interference. But by frightening people into thinking their jobs were on the line and tinkering with small details over the heads of appointed leaders, they too often got in the way of what they were trying to help deliver. If there's a difference in goal, then it needs to be thrashed out and resolved. But trying to run a department from No. 10 is a mistake.

I put effort into protecting the team from this sort of aggressive top-down interference so they could get on with achieving agreed objectives rather than constantly responding to instructions, commissions, questions and requests from all levels at No. 10 that distracted from the urgent and important work they were doing. Refraining from issuing such instructions is an important lesson for any Downing Street operation – especially in a crisis. We got it right on the vaccine effort when we developed plans with no interference whatsoever and had a weekly meeting with the Prime Minister during the delivery phase for him to set objectives and hold us to account.

Ultimately, the pandemic demonstrated the importance of collaborative leadership. We live in an era of great teams, not great men. The job of leadership is to set the goal and motivate people to play their part in delivering it.

7. GOVERNANCE AND ACCOUNTABILITY

To get the best out of people requires accountability. Where we had clean lines of accountability, things tended to work better. This is always difficult in government, but the basic approach of Cabinet government, with government bodies accountable to departments, and departments accountable to the Prime Minister, has never been bettered. For long periods, No. 10 insisted on confused lines of accountability, with people at different levels formally or informally reporting directly to parts of No. 10 or the Prime Minister. This confused matters. Likewise, a big, interventionist Cabinet Office, often setting out with the best of intentions to drive improvement, causes messy accountability and allows people to play off each other.

One huge success that must be retained was our Beaverbrooks: Kate Bingham, General Sir Gordon Messenger, Dido Harding, Camilla Cavendish, Paul Deighton, Gina Coladangelo, Mike Coupe and many others. We brought more people into government during the pandemic than at any other time I know of. The result was to strengthen and enrich its operational capacity by broadening the capability and experience of the teams delivering the huge range of things that needed to be done. They deserve our huge thanks.

Bringing people in from outside government brought challenges too. Lines of accountability needed to be clear. Different attitudes, pay, terms and cultures often clashed. These need to be resolved better in future. Government should ensure there is a more porous border with the private sector, academia and the clinical world in normal times too.

Likewise, the role of expert bodies needs to be right. Experts should report to ministers, who then make decisions grounded in the expertise. Experts should not try to second-guess wider social or political considerations. For example, it is wrong for the JCVI to have lay members. Their scientific experts should advise ministers, who should make decisions based on expertise alone. It is also a mistake for SAGE members to comment in public on their views. They are either government advisers, who are accountable for their advice and abide by collective responsibility, or they are academics, in which case neither need apply. Public health officials should make recommendations based on their professional judgement, not considering what might or might not be politically acceptable. The clarity of this approach brought better decision making, because it allowed ministers to make judgements based on all considerations and unfettered advice.

8. PROCURE AT PACE
During the pandemic we had to buy many things in huge quantities at

enormous pace. Yet government procurement rules are slow and laborious. In normal times, some of this is defensible to ensure value for money and to protect against corruption – though it can and should be improved. The emergency procurement rules set aside many of those restrictions. It was necessary, for example, to set aside the rule that government should buy PPE in the bottom quartile of prices, because that meant buying nothing at all.

The problem was that the emergency procurement rules have allowed the wholly inaccurate accusation that those involved were somehow wrong to act as they did. Officials were right to spend their limited time buying life-saving equipment and fill in the paperwork later. Yet they were quite wrongly criticised afterwards for acting to save lives in this way. Officials and ministers alike were entirely falsely accused of corruption for moving fast and taking forward proposals that were brought to their attention.

None of these accusations have any substance whatsoever, yet the accusations were painful to many people who worked incredibly hard to buy what was needed – including me. A new system is needed to allow the emergency buying of equipment that protects those procuring it from such baseless and frankly offensive suggestions. My fear is that unless this is put in place, undue caution will prevail from those who have seen the unfair public criticism of those who worked so hard during Covid, and lives will be lost as a result.

9. LOOK TO THE LONG TERM

Even in the depths of a crisis, it's important to look to the long term. I mean this in terms of both the positives, like using the pandemic to change the culture around the use of data, and the negatives, like taking into account the long-term impact of lockdown.

It is inevitably hard to do this during a crisis. We knew, for example, the very serious negative impacts of lockdown. We tried our hardest to limit damage with regional lockdowns, which failed despite our best efforts. We discussed and debated the trade-offs in public and in private. We set out what we knew, for example, of the negative impact on education of closing schools. The impact was impossible to quantify, yet we knew – and know now – that the impact of failing to lock down would have been much worse.

We know, too, that until the vaccine, there was no trade-off between protective health measures and economic factors. As we painfully saw in the autumn and winter of 2020, failure to act early or hard enough on local lockdowns led to a much bigger, full-blown national lockdown instead. It is a sad irony that those who argued during that autumn that we needed to balance economic factors against health impacts simply caused a bigger, longer, tougher lockdown in the end. I found it baffling that Treasury economists, of all people, couldn't see the dynamic impact of a failure to get R below 1 in the autumn of 2020: that failure to act early led to worse long-term effects.

By contrast, once the vaccine was rolled out, there was a trade-off between economic and health considerations, because we had done all we could to protect people. At the start of 2021, when asked what we should do after all the vulnerable had been vaccinated, I said, 'Cry freedom.' Come summer 2021 when that vaccination effort was well under way, we delayed the final step of removing lockdown as cases rose. There was a good argument presented for doing so at the time, based on estimates of the lives it would save. Yet we now know that the vaccine was already working its magic, and the subsequent judgements not to lockdown in response to rising case numbers were correct.

10. RESILIENCE

The pandemic has been just one of several big shocks we will have in my lifetime, including war, inflation, energy crises, climate change, further pandemics and the impact of technology. We live in an era when global forces, rather than the affairs of states, are coming at us hard. As a country, we need to be resilient to these forces. For many years, optimistic assumptions about the continuity of global systems stripped us of the resilience we need. The pandemic opened my eyes to how fragile our economy and our society have become. I want to see Britain stop being a low-cost, fragile economy and society and become the confident, buccaneering nation we can be, with the resilience to thrive in these turbulent times.

For that, we need institutions that are ready and prepared. This is a huge task and I offer just a few specific examples. First, I formed the UK Health Security Agency so we always have a health body whose job it is to prepare for pandemics, even when there isn't one on the horizon, just like in the financial system, which must retain its prudential, systemic defences, separately from the day-to-day regulation of conduct that otherwise draws attention away.

Within public services we must allow for redundancy so we are better prepared when pressure mounts. We should have the confidence to back domestic manufacturing and research, not watch it move offshore. Our testing, vaccine and clinical trial systems must be kept ready to go, just as we maintain miliary defences in peacetime. To disband such systems would be to fail to learn the lessons.

But this is just the first step. A huge plan of work is necessary before we can say we are well-prepared for the next pandemic. We must update the law and the regulatory powers so they work better, especially where a single approach is called for across the UK. We must take forward the consumer diagnostic revolution so it becomes the norm to test when you're ill. New ministers and officials need regular war games to train in how to respond. And we absolutely must ensure vaccines can be available in an even shorter time – within 100 days at an absolute maximum. This can be done.

PERSONAL

For me, the pandemic is likely to be the most consequential time of my life. When I reflect, it is with deep, mixed feelings. I am proud of the things I did well and know what I'd do differently.

As in any large organisation, many decisions are essentially collective ones, in which any one person plays a small part. Our decision to buy vaccines early, for example, was a collective one in which many people deserve credit. I played my part and urged the team from the start to go as fast as possible, but it was a true collective effort.

Other decisions were personal. For example, I acted against advice to stop the Oxford vaccine going to the US company Merck. I was advised to sign off the deal, but without my putting a spanner in the works we couldn't have got exclusive supply for the UK, and there was a significant risk the global at-cost production wouldn't have happened. Likewise, without my intransigent insistence – much resisted by the system – that we must vaccinate the whole population, only 30 million vaccines would have been bought first time round, and so only the vulnerable vaccinated. Away from the vaccine, I know that without my reputationally risky 100,000 testing target, our testing capacity would not have grown as fast as it did, and many more would have died.

In the same way, I take responsibility for areas where I failed. For example, I failed to drive home the importance of asymptomatic transmission. I had my suspicions from the start, and voiced my concerns, but I failed to insist that all policy be based on the worst-case assumption that the disease could pass on without symptoms. It doesn't matter that I was battling a global scientific consensus: there was enough evidence that this consensus was wrong, and I should have insisted it be challenged. That failure had very significant consequences.

The burden will always be with me. The best way for me to discharge that burden is to ensure the right lessons are learned for the future.

A crucial consequence was around how we went about protecting care homes. The consequences of the wrong assumption on asymptomatic transmission were significant.

The most important lesson to draw is that there should not be staff movement between care homes: that is how the virus mostly got in – asymptomatic transmission from staff. Instead, most of the debate focuses on the wrong lesson: the movement of patients out of hospital into care homes. I understand how this is intuitive, but the evidence shows it was a very small part of the problem. The timing of the big peak in care homes was later than this explanation would allow for, and nor does the distribution of cases across care homes bear it out. What's more, there were no easy answers to what to do with people in hospital who were medically fit to discharge and had no symptoms, at a time when we were being told the tests didn't work on people with no symptoms and there weren't enough tests anyway. Leaving these people in hospital also carried significant risks for them and others.

This is just one example, important as it is. What matters is that we learn the right lessons, with humility and evidence. That is why I wrote this book. I want to explain the essence of what happened, warts and all, as seen from where I sat as Health Secretary.

Overall, I believe history will show that those at the centre of the response worked with enormous dedication and public service, and despite the huge challenges, the British response was far better than portrayed at the time.

I have a sense of duty to write down what happened to inform the lessons we learned as we battled our way through – and more we must learn now as we look back.

In order to respond to a new and unknown virus, we made unprecedented decisions in the face of overwhelming uncertainty. We often struggled. I felt very deeply the lack of a guide: there was no plan, nor lessons from those who had gone before. I read what history I could find and turned to fiction to seek insights. I have written this book to help those in the hot seat next time.

On a personal level, I learned other lessons too.

My approach to life has always been to make the most of it. I am an optimist: I have a positive view of human nature and believe in the great, generous, kind spirit of people as individuals. I work hard, at full tilt, and see public service as a great privilege. I deeply regret where I fell short, but I learned that all of these values are stronger, deeper and more important to me than before.

I also learned many lessons about myself and my character – strengths and flaws – and the sometimes significant and often unavoidable personal cost of huge responsibility. The pandemic took a toll on me, my family and my marriage. I have more grey hairs and more perspective. I learned lessons, too, about what really matters. I learned that in the darkest of hours, you can find light.

CAST LIST

Ed Argar: MP for Charnwood from 2015, Health Minister from September 2019. Passionate One Nation Tory and quiet, loyal and completely reliable Minister of State, responsible for the NHS budget. Rock-solid parliamentary and media handler in the depths of a crisis.

Sir John Bell: Blunt-speaking, Canadian-born regius professor of medicine at Oxford University. Played a huge part in Oxford's scientific triumphs and liaised with the government on testing, vaccines and treatments. Was instrumental in the agreement between the government, university and AstraZeneca to enable mass production of the Oxford jab at cost for the world.

James Bethell (Jim): Health Minister in the House of Lords from March 2020. Constant friend, adviser and fixer through the pandemic. Could spot problems coming down the track and take on all manner of almost impossible challenges. Acerbic wit, particularly about political colleagues.

Kate Bingham: Venture capitalist who chaired the Vaccine Taskforce from May to December 2020. Despite occasional disagreements, her success at spotting potential vaccines and negotiating contracts was vital to Britain's vaccine triumph.

Lee Cain: The Prime Minister's director of communications throughout the pandemic. At Boris's side for almost a decade, he was an ally in many of the substantive discussions, despite his proximity to Dominic Cummings. Has come a long way since he spent the 2010 election campaign dressed as a chicken for the *Daily Mirror*.

Simon Case: Permanent Secretary for Covid at No. 10 from May 2020, then, from September 2020, youngest Cabinet Secretary in history. Previously private secretary to Prince William. A vital, sometimes indiscreet, line into No. 10 and an ally in good government and competent management of the crisis.

Jo Churchill: Public Health and Primary Care Minister from September 2019. Worked as finance director of a scaffolding firm in Lincolnshire before becoming MP for Bury St Edmunds in 2015. Practical, personable and good at sorting things out on the ground.

Gina Coladangelo: University friend and high-flying communications and corporate leader. Brought into the department to improve public health comms. DHSC board member from September 2020. Tasks included helping Matt communicate in a more emotionally intelligent way. Their relationship started in May 2021.

Dominic Cummings: Ran the Brexit campaign in 2016. Chief adviser to Boris Johnson from 2019 to November 2020. Wanted to shake up the British state but failed and caused chaos. Broke Covid rules with trip to Barnard Castle at the height of lockdown. Flawed character who alienated many through arrogance, even when they agreed with him.

Emma Dean: Senior special adviser and leading political thinker in the department throughout the pandemic. Newcastle-born and full of northern grit, never shy of telling her boss when he was wrong. The brains behind Britain's first women's health strategy, which she kept on the road through all the turbulence of Covid.

Nadine Dorries: Not your classic Tory. Working-class Liverpudlian of Irish Catholic extraction, novelist and former nurse. As backbencher was famous for riling David Cameron. Minister for Mental Health from 2019 and became an unlikely personal counsellor to Matt in the pandemic. Fiercely loyal, never afraid to speak her mind, and not to be underestimated.

Asher Glynn: Recruited to parliamentary team at age eighteen to run social media, later became Matt's researcher. A-levels cancelled because of the pandemic, then went to study at the London School of Economics, juggling it with the day job.

Dido Harding: Tory peer. Former jockey and boss of TalkTalk, headed NHS Test and Trace May 2020–April 2021. One of the toughest and most important jobs in fighting the pandemic. Took over testing when it was already expanding quickly after being removed from PHE responsibility. Under constant attack, she turned a cottage industry into the biggest testing programme in the country's history.

Dr Jenny Harries: Deputy chief medical officer from June 2019 to March 2021, then head of UK Health Security Agency. Data genius who designed shielding programme for vulnerable people. Hard as nails behind softly spoken exterior.

Elizabeth Hitchcock: Parliamentary office manager with expert grasp of every nook and cranny of the constituency, in effect she was the MP for West Suffolk when Matt was handling the pandemic. Fierce opponent of lockdown on libertarian grounds; never gave up trying to change her boss's mind, much to her colleagues' amusement.

Allan Nixon: Japanese-speaking Glaswegian and special adviser responsible for parliamentary liaison. Phenomenally hard-working and fiercely intelligent, he was pivotal to handling the many parliamentary challenges.

Jamie Njoku-Goodwin: Media special adviser who joined Matt when he was Culture Secretary and served until October 2020. International-standard chess player and concert pianist with uncanny knack for seeing political trouble round corners. Continued to look out for Matt after leaving to run UK Music. Musical passion awakened as a teenager when a charity took him to hear a string quartet.

Steve Oldfield: Probably knows more about medical supply chains than anyone else in British history. Brought into DHSC from industry to improve value for money in buying drugs, he then spent a year preparing for no-deal Brexit. This planning became invaluable during the pandemic, helping to keep supplies of critical medicines flowing. Without Steve we almost certainly would have had medicine shortages in the worst of the peak.

Damon Poole: Replaced Jamie Njoku-Goodwin as media special adviser in October 2020. Previously head of broadcast for No. 10. Trusted by all, soon established himself as sage adviser on all communications and media relations.

Natasha Price: Head of private office at the DHSC. Profoundly dedicated to good government, efficient organiser and popular leader of the hard-working private office team. Knew which Whitehall levers to pull to get things done. Prevented countless dramas from turning into crises. Kept the show on the road.

Pascal Soriot: French-Australian head of British–Swedish pharmaceutical giant AstraZeneca from 2012. Architect of one of the greatest acts of corporate responsibility in history – non-profit global production and licensing of the Oxford vaccine. Never wavered in the face of baseless, vindictive and irresponsible attacks on him and the vaccine. Saved countless lives. A hero.

Jens Spahn: Fresh-faced German Health Minister and key pandemic ally. He and Matt struck up a friendship over beers at a particularly boring summit. Always ready to lend each other's country a hand behind the scenes when Brussels was obstructing.

Sir Simon Stevens: NHS chief executive from 2014 to 2021. Oxford contemporary of Boris. Former Labour councillor, then adviser to Tony Blair in No. 10. Led the NHS through the pandemic. Consummate political operator who saw off repeated attempts by Dominic Cummings to knife him.

Sir Patrick Vallance: Chief scientific adviser to the government, former professor of medicine at UCL and head of research at GSK who brought his huge academic experience to the task of providing scientific advice to the Prime Minister and others. Chaired SAGE jointly with Chris Whitty and became one of the public faces of the pandemic. Ambition was to be a chef.

Professor Jonathan Van-Tam (JVT): Deputy chief medical officer since 2017, and grandson of former Prime Minister of Vietnam. Wears his deep expertise lightly with cheerful, modest manner and deployed a lively turn of phrase at press conferences. Specialist in vaccines. A trusted adviser with sage wisdom and direct honesty.

Helen Whately: MP for Faversham and Mid Kent from 2015, thrown into the pandemic at the deep end when appointed Minister for Social Care in February 2020. Brought laser-like focus and efficiency from a career as a healthcare management specialist. Passionate supporter of social care.

Professor Chris Whitty (the Prof): Chief medical officer from 2019. Unflappable epidemiologist with unsurpassed public service ethos. Trusted by the public, highly respected by everyone, able to advise Boris Johnson with aplomb. The right man in the right job.

Sir Chris Wormald: Permanent Secretary at DHSC from 2016, previously served as Permanent Secretary at Education. Led the official response and reorganised the department to respond to the crisis in double-quick time. Rock-solid adviser and phlegmatic sounding board.

Nadhim Zahawi: Came to Britain as child refugee from Baghdad. Co-founder of pollsters YouGov, MP for Stratford-on-Avon since 2010 and co-author with Matt of *Masters of Nothing* in 2011. BEIS Minister from 2019, with responsibility for vaccines, then promoted on Matt's recommendation to Minister for Vaccine Deployment in November 2020. Bulldozer ability to break down barriers to help ensure millions were jabbed.

GLOSSARY

1922 Committee: The grouping for all backbench Conservative MPs. Discusses how well (or not) government is doing and gives feedback to ministers. Runs contests for the party leadership. Chaired by Sir Graham Brady.

AZ: AstraZeneca. The British–Swedish pharmaceutical giant led by Pascal Soriot that took on responsibility for manufacturing, worldwide licensing and non-profit provision of the vaccine developed by Oxford University.

BEIS: Department for Business, Energy and Industrial Strategy. Alok Sharma was Secretary of State until January 2021, when he was replaced by Kwasi Kwarteng.

BHAG: Big Hairy Audacious Goal. A US business-school catchphrase much favoured by Rishi Sunak to describe ambitious targets such as mass testing.

BioNTech: German biotechnology company that developed the vaccine Pfizer went on to manufacture. BioNTech developed the first vaccine approved in the UK.

BMA: British Medical Association. The main doctors' trade union.

Cabinet Office: Cross-government coordinating department, led by Michael Gove from February 2020 to September 2021.

CCGs: Clinical commissioning groups. The local bodies responsible for planning and commissioning healthcare services.

CDC: Centers for Disease Control and Prevention. US government organisation responsible for fighting infectious disease as well as injury and disability.

CDL: Chancellor of the Duchy of Lancaster. Cabinet-level post, held by Michael Gove throughout the pandemic, responsible, as much as anyone is, for the operation of the Cabinet Office.

CIS: Covid-19 Infection Survey. A vital UK-wide study run by the ONS and Oxford University to estimate how many people have Covid antibodies. Uses repeat home visits to test 150,000 people.

CMO: Chief medical officer. The government's most senior clinical adviser on health. Co-chairs SAGE with CSA. Post held by Chris Whitty throughout the pandemic.

COBRA: Colloquial name for the Civil Contingencies Committee, which coordinates cross-government response to emergencies. The acronym comes from Cabinet Office Briefing Room A, where it usually meets.

Coronavirus Act: Passed March 2020 to give government emergency powers during the pandemic. It was a temporary, draconian piece of legislation that had to be renewed every six months.

COVAX: Covid-19 Vaccines Global Access. The worldwide body set up to support access to vaccines for poorer countries. UK was its biggest early funder.

Covid-O: Cabinet committee responsible for operational management of Covid, reporting to Covid-S. Established September 2020, chaired by Michael Gove.

Covid-S: Cabinet committee responsible for Covid strategy, established September 2020, chaired by the Prime Minister.

CRG: Covid Recovery Group. Backbench group of Conservative MPs sceptical of lockdown measures, set up November 2020. Chaired by Mark Harper, former Chief Whip.

CSA: Chief scientific adviser. Provides scientific advice to Prime Minister and Cabinet, co-chairs SAGE with CMO. Post held by Sir Patrick Vallance throughout the pandemic.

CSF: Covid Support Force: 20,000-strong military organisation mobilised March 2020 to support civilian response, including air evacuations, logistics, testing and building Nightingale hospitals.

CST: Chief Secretary to the Treasury. Number two minister to Chancellor of the Exchequer. Rishi Sunak was CST up to February 2020, before being replaced by Steve Barclay.

CQC: Care Quality Commission. The inspectorate for hospitals, care homes and other health and care organisations.

Cygnus: The three-day cross-government pandemic preparedness exercise held in 2016. Tested resilience to a major flu outbreak.

DCMS: Department for Digital, Culture, Media and Sport, led by Oliver Dowden throughout the pandemic.

DEFRA: Department for Environment, Food and Rural Affairs. Secretary of State during the pandemic: George Eustice.

DfE: Department for Education. Secretary of State during the pandemic: Gavin Williamson.

DfT: Department for Transport. Secretary of State during the pandemic: Grant Shapps.

DHSC: Department of Health and Social Care. Matt's department throughout the pandemic.

DWP: Department for Work and Pensions. Secretary of State during the pandemic: Thérèse Coffey.

FCO: Foreign and Commonwealth Office, renamed Foreign, Commonwealth and Development Office (FCDO) from September 2020. Secretary of State during the pandemic: Dominic Raab.

FDA: Food and Drug Administration. US federal medical regulator responsible for authorising medicines, including Covid vaccines and treatments.

G7: Group of seven leading developed economies plus the European Union. Holds ministerial meetings and summits of national leaders. Health Ministers met weekly during the pandemic and provided huge amounts of mutual support.

GMC: General Medical Council. Manages register of and sets standards for doctors in the UK.

HMT: Her Majesty's Treasury. Chancellor of the Exchequer: Sajid Javid from July 2019 to February 2020, then Rishi Sunak.

Human challenge study: Clinical trial in which people are intentionally infected with a disease to test the effectiveness of a vaccine or treatment. Also known as controlled human infection trial.

JBC: Joint Biosecurity Centre. Established May 2020 to provide analysis and advice on Covid policy to government. Merged with UKHSA in April 2021.

JCVI: Joint Committee on Vaccination and Immunisation. Advises DHSC and devolved equivalents on vaccine policy, including order of priority for who gets vaccinated when.

LAC: Local Action Committee. Network of regional representatives to assess Covid hotspots around the country, helping government to decide on local lockdowns. LAC had three levels, with the Gold meetings chaired by Matt.

LFT: Lateral flow test. The technology used in antigen tests for Covid-19. Often said to be less sensitive than the PCR, but quicker and easy to self-administer, so more suitable for mass self-testing at home.

Liaison Committee: The powerful House of Commons committee comprising all select committee chairs. Questions the Prime Minister twice a year.

Lighthouse Laboratories: Network of mega-labs launched by Matt in April 2020 for rapid mass expansion of Covid testing capacity. Run by universities, hospitals, private companies. Name taken from fluorescent light used in PCR tests to detect virus.

Lobby: Collective name for political journalists authorised to work inside Parliament and attend No. 10 briefings.

MACA: Military Aid to the Civil Authorities. Procedure for armed forces to support government in emergencies.

MHCLG: Ministry of Housing, Communities and Local Government. Secretary of State during the pandemic: Robert Jenrick.

MHRA: Medicines and Healthcare products Regulatory Agency. Responsible for safety, efficacy and licensing of medical products, including vaccines.

MoD: Ministry of Defence. Secretary of State during the pandemic: Ben Wallace.

MoJ: Ministry of Justice. Secretary of State and Lord Chancellor during the pandemic: Robert Buckland.

Moonshot: Informal name for the work on population-wide mass testing, developed during summer and autumn of 2020.

National Institute of Allergy and Infectious Diseases: US government disease-research agency. Director: Anthony Fauci.

NERVTAG: New and Emerging Respiratory Virus Threats Advisory Group. Committee of specialist scientists reporting to SAGE.

NHS Confederation: Representative body for trusts, CCGs and other groups that provide NHS services in England, Wales and Northern Ireland.

NHS Digital: Provides IT to the NHS in England, collects and manages data, runs NHS website.

NHSE: NHS England. Runs the NHS in England.

NHS Providers: Mainly represents England's NHS foundation trusts, which are more independent of the DHSC than other hospital trusts.

NHS Test and Trace: Launched in May 2020 under the leadership of Dido Harding. NHS Test and Trace oversaw mass expansion of testing and tracing of contacts of those who tested positive for Covid. Merged with UKHSA in April 2021.

NHSX: Set up by Matt in 2019 to push through digital transformation of NHS and social care. The X stands for the X in 'user experience'.

Nightingale hospitals: Seven temporary NHS facilities built at high speed to provide extra beds on standby in case existing capacity proved insufficient for the number of Covid patients. First one opened at the ExCel Centre, London, April 2020.

NIHR: National Institute for Health and Care Research. Biggest UK government funding body for health and care research. Funded the Recovery Trial.

NMC: Nursing and Midwifery Council. UK regulator for nurses and midwives.

OLS: Office for Life Sciences. Joint DHSC/BEIS body that provides government funding for biotech research and other technological innovation in health and care.

ONS: Office for National Statistics. Remit includes gathering all UK Covid-19 statistics. Runs Covid-19 Infection Survey jointly with Oxford University.

Perm Sec: Permanent Secretary. The civil servant in charge of each government department. Sir Chris Wormald held the post at DHSC throughout the pandemic, later supported by David Williams as Second Permanent Secretary.

PHE: Public Health England. Agency of the DHSC responsible for infectious disease response, promoting healthy living messages and health and safety at work. Broken up in April 2021.

PHEIC: Public Health Emergency of International Concern. A cross-border health crisis declared by WHO, requiring member states to coordinate their response.

PMQs: Prime Minister's Questions. Weekly half-hour slot at midday on Wednesdays, when the Prime Minister is questioned by the Leader of the Opposition and backbench MPs.

PPE: Personal protective equipment. Masks, gloves, gowns and other equipment used to safeguard healthcare workers and others from infection.

PPS: Either parliamentary private secretary – an MP who acts as a minister's eyes and ears in the Commons – or principal private secretary, the civil servant in charge of a minister's private office in their department.

Private office: The civil service team working directly for a minister or senior official. At the peak of the pandemic, Matt's numbered twenty officials, working in shifts, compared with usual four or five.

Public Health Act 1984: The legal basis for many of the emergency government powers in the pandemic, complemented by the emergency Coronavirus Act.

Public Health Scotland: The equivalent of Public Health England. Answers to the Scottish health ministry. Started work April 2020 in succession to Health Protection Scotland.

Quad: Informal core decision-making group of ministers that met regularly during pandemic, consisting of Boris Johnson, Matt, Rishi Sunak and Michael Gove.

RCN: Royal College of Nursing. UK-wide trade union for nurses.

REACT: Real-time Assessment of Community Transmission. Ongoing study set up in April 2020, led by Imperial College London and Ipsos MORI, to discover how many people are infected or have been infected by Covid in England. Analyses PCR tests on 100,000 volunteers a month.

Recovery Trial: Randomised Evaluation of Covid-19 Therapy. Large-scale trials run by Oxford University to test Covid treatments on hospital patients. Established at remarkable pace in March 2020. Concentrated on repurposing existing drugs rather than newly developed treatments. Evaluated medicines including dexamethasone and hydroxychloroquine. Arguably the most successful clinical trial in history, Recovery has saved millions of lives.

SAGE: Scientific Advisory Group for Emergencies. Expert body that sifts the evidence to provide formal advice to government decision makers. Jointly chaired by CMO and CSA.

SII: Serum Institute of India. World's largest vaccine maker and major supplier of Oxford AZ vaccine.

SpAd: Special adviser. Close confidant advising the Secretary of State in areas such as policy, media and parliamentary relations. Unlike impartial civil servants, they can provide party political advice. Matt usually had three, rising to five at the peak of the pandemic.

SPI-M: Scientific Pandemic Influenza Group on Modelling. Sub-committee of SAGE that produced models and forecasts for how the pandemic might grow.

UKHSA: UK Health Security Agency. Government body launched by Matt in April 2021 to focus on response to infectious disease, absorbing PHE's role in that area.

VTF: Vaccine Taskforce. Created April 2020 to manage Covid vaccine development and purchasing. Chaired by Kate Bingham to December 2020.

WHO: World Health Organization. United Nations body that coordinates international health policy and crisis response. Director general: Tedros Adhanom Ghebreyesus.

GLOSSARY OF SCIENTIFIC TERMS

Antibody test: Detects presence of antibodies in the blood, which can mean either that the person has previously been infected or that the vaccine is doing its job. Also known as serology test. Antibodies are blood proteins that attack antigens.

Antigen test: Detects if someone is currently infected by swabbing for virus in the mouth, nose and throat. Can be done at home using LFT kits, which give results in a few minutes. An antigen is any foreign substance in the body that produces an immune response such as production of antibodies.

Coronavirus: A family of viruses that cause infection in respiratory tracts and a variety of illnesses ranging from the common cold to Covid-19. There were six known coronaviruses that affected humans before the pandemic.

Covid-19: Coronavirus disease 2019. The illness caused by the SARS-Cov-2 virus. Despite the scientific distinction, in practice the term is often used interchangeably with coronavirus.

Efficacy and **effectiveness:** Efficacy measures how well a drug works in controlled trial conditions; effectiveness is how well it works in practice on the general population.

Incidence rate: Estimated number of new PCR-positive cases per day of Covid-19 per 10,000 people.

MERS: Middle East Respiratory Syndrome. Coronavirus infection that emerged in 2012 in Saudi Arabia, killing about 900 people, 35 per cent of infected patients.

mRNA: Messenger ribonucleic acid. Vaccine technology that uses lab-created genetic material rather than adapted virus. The mRNA enters cells and stimulates them to produce the Covid-19 spike protein, which is then recognised and broken down by the immune system. Used in Pfizer/BioNTech and Moderna vaccines.

PCR: Polymerase chain reaction. Lab test that works by making billions of copies of genetic material in a sample, enabling it to detect tiny amounts of virus. More sensitive than an LFT, especially in early stages of infection.

R number: The reproduction number is the number of people infected by one person with a communicable disease such as Covid-19. A vital metric in pandemic management.

SARS: Severe Acute Respiratory Syndrome. Viral disease that broke out in 2002 and killed more than 800 people by 2004, mostly in China. Caused by a strain of coronavirus.

SARS-CoV-2: Severe Acute Respiratory Syndrome Coronavirus 2. The coronavirus that causes Covid-19. Named in February 2020. Genetically related to virus that caused SARS in 2002.